Starting *Your* Practice

A Survival Guide for Nurse Practitioners

Starting *Your* Practice

A Survival Guide for Nurse Practitioners

JEAN NAGELKERK, PhD, APRN, BC

Assistant Vice President for Academic Affairs
and Professor of Nursing
Grand Valley State University
Allendale, Michigan

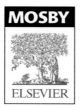

MOSBY

ELSEVIER

MOSBY
ELSEVIER

11830 Westline Industrial Drive
St. Louis, Missouri 63146

STARTING YOUR PRACTICE: A SURVIVAL GUIDE FOR   ISBN-13: 978-0-323-02488-4
NURSE PRACTITIONERS   ISBN-10: 0-323-02488-2

Notice

Neither the Publisher nor the Editor assumes any responsibility for any loss or injury and/or
damage to persons or property arising out of or related to any use of the material contained
in this book. It is the responsibility of the treating practitioner, relying on independent
expertise and knowledge of the patient, to determine the best treatment and method of
application for the patient.

This publication is designed to provide accurate and authoritative information in regard to
the subject matter covered. In publishing this book neither the Editor nor the Publisher is
engaged in rendering legal, accounting, or other professional service. If legal advice or other
expert assistance is required, the services of a competent professional should be sought.

The Publisher

ISBN-13: 978-0-323-02488-4
ISBN-10: 0-323-02488-2

Acquisitions Editor: Sandra Clark Brown
Senior Developmental Editor: Cindi Anderson
Publishing Services Manager: John Rogers
Senior Project Manager: Cheryl A. Abbott
Senior Designer: Kathi Gosche

Printed in the United States of America

Last digit is the print number: 9   8   7   6   5   4   3   2   1

Working together to grow
libraries in developing countries

www.elsevier.com | www.bookaid.org | www.sabre.org

ELSEVIER   BOOK AID International   Sabre Foundation

Contributors

Ramona Benkert, PhD, APRN, BC
Assistant Professor
College of Nursing
Wayne State University
Detroit, Michigan
8. *Coding and Billing for Nurse Practitioners*
9. *Documentation for the Nurse Practitioner*

Ruth Ann Brintnall, MSN, APRN, BC
Assistant Professor, Adult Nurse Practitioner
Kirkhof College of Nursing
Grand Valley State University
Grand Rapids, Michigan
16. *Professional Collaboration*

Katherine J. Dontje, MSN, APRN, BC
Assistant Professor
College of Nursing
Michigan State University
East Lansing, Michigan
6. *Third Party Reimbursement*

Kathy M. Forrest, RN, BSN, MA
Acting Director of Faculty Clinical Practice & Faculty Practice Manager
College of Nursing, Faculty Practice
Michigan State University
East Lansing, Michigan
6. *Third Party Reimbursement*

Lori Houghton-Rahrig, MSN, APRN, BC
Affiliate Faculty
Kirkhof College of Nursing
Grand Valley State University
Grand Rapids, Michigan

11. Risk Management: Tracking Systems

Kim Litwack, PhD, RN, FAAN, CFNP
Associate Professor of Nursing
University of Wisconsin Milwaukee
Milwaukee, Wisconsin

10. Patient Education

Leona B. Meengs, MSN, APRN, BC
Family Nurse Practitioner
Professional Practice Group
Pine Rest Christian Mental Health Services;
Adjunct Faculty
Grand Valley State University
Grand Rapids, Michigan

13. Using Technology to Enhance Practice
17. Professional Responsibilities

Jean Nagelkerk, PhD, APRN, BC
Assistant Vice President for Academic Affairs
and Professor of Nursing
Grand Valley State University
Allendale, Michigan

1. Starting Out: Deciding What Job You Want
2. Nurse Practitioner Socialization and Marketing
3. Corresponding and Interviewing with Potential Employers
7. Starting Your Nurse Practitioner Business
12. Health Care Quality: Evaluating Clinical Practice

Maureen Ryan, MSN, APRN, BC
Assistant Professor of Nursing
Grand Valley State University
Grand Rapids, Michigan

4. Preparing for NP Practice: Certification and NP State Recognition

Thomas H. Ryan, JD
Grand Rapids, Michigan

5. Negotiating an Employment Contract

Patricia W. Underwood, PhD, RN, FAAN
Associate Dean for Academic Programs
Frances Payne Bolton School of Nursing
Case Western Reserve University
Cleveland, Ohio

14. Community Involvement
15. Professional Involvement

Audrey Westdorp
Healthcare Consultant
Grand Management Group
Grand Rapids, Michigan

8. Coding and Billing for Nurse Practitioners

Mary P. White, MSN, APRN, BC
Clinical Instructor, Adult Nurse Practitioner
College of Nursing, Adult Primary Care
Wayne State University
Detroit, Michigan

8. Coding and Billing for Nurse Practitioners
9. Documentation for the Nurse Practitioner

Reviewers

Sharon G. Childs, MS, APRN-BC, NP/CS, CEN, ONC
Concentra Medical Center
Baltimore, Maryland

Yvette Glenn, MSN, FNP, APRN, BC
VA Illiana Medical Center
Danville, Illinois

Carol Green-Hernandez, PhD, FNS, ANP/FNP-BC
Associate Professor
Primary Care Nurse Practitioner Program
The University of Vermont
Burlington, Vermont

Rhonda Johnston, RN, PhD, C-FNP, C-ANP, CNS
Colorado State University—Pueblo
Pueblo, Colorado

Priscilla A. Lee, MN, FNP-C
Family Practice/Geriatrics Nurse Practitioner
President, FNP Nursing, Inc.
Westlake Village, California

Constance Lepper, RN, MSN, FNP-C
Family Health West
Fruita, Colorado

Maureen A. Madden, RNC, MSN, PCCNP, CCRN
University of Medicine and Dentistry of New Jersey
Robert Wood Johnson Medical School
New Brunswick, New Jersey

Denise G. Max, MSN, ACNP
Mercer Bucks Cardiology
Lawrenceville, New Jersey

Anthony W. McGuire, RN, MSN, CCRN, ACNP
St. Mary Medical Center
Long Beach, California

Karen Koozer Olsen, RN, PhD, FNP-C
Texas A&M University—Corpus Christi
Corpus Christi, Texas

Terry Savan, RN, BSN, MA, BA, CRNP
Lehigh University
St. Luke's Hospital
Bethlehem, Pennsylvania

Barbara Schaefer, MS, RN, ACNP, BC, CCRN
Kaiser Permanente Medical Center
Department of Neurosurgery
Anaheim, California

Elizabeth A. O'Rourke Sweet, MS, CPNP
A.I. DuPont Hospital for Children
Wilmington, Delaware

Theresa Pluth Yeo, MSN, MPH, CRNP
Assistant Professor
School of Nursing
Johns Hopkins University
Baltimore, Maryland

Preface

Nurse practitioners, by virtue of their advanced practice nursing roles, are leaders in health care organizations. In their roles, NPs serve as change agents, expert clinicians, policy advocates, health care educators, and consultants to provide leadership in health care services and policy and access to quality cost-effective care. The complexity of their roles coupled with the rapid changes in health care makes this text an invaluable resource for NP practice. The impetus for this text comes from teaching NP students and from numerous telephone calls from practicing NPs searching for a central resource on career development, contract negotiation, NP state recognition, billing and coding information, professional development opportunities, quality improvement systems for clinical practice, and resources for starting an independent clinical practice. Each of these topics and many more are covered in detail in this text to provide a rich resource using a question and answer format to assist with mastery of chapter content. There are existing texts that provide written descriptions of some of these topic areas, but this text not only provides a detailed coverage of the topics but also examples of tools and resources that can be useful in practice. The tables, figures, and appendixes are full of rich resources and tools that provide a step-by-step approach—the "how to" of accomplishing, developing, or designing specific protocols, processes, or skills. This text is designed to assist individuals in exploring career trajectories, engaging in professional nursing practice, and developing community partnerships and linkages.

Starting Your Practice: A Survival Guide for Nurse Practitioners is a reference book for students, as well as novice and experienced nurse practitioners. The organizational framework of this book groups the 17 chapters into four units. Unit I, "Finding the Job You Want," sets the foundation for exploring career opportunities, marketing oneself, and interviewing with potential employers. Unit II, "The Tools You'll Need to Get Started," examines important elements in establishing a clinical practice. The process and implications of certification, NP recognition, and regulation for professional practice are explored in depth. A key section of this text, which is integral to clinical practice, is understanding information about revenue generation and expenses, as well as the "nuts and bolts" of billing and coding. Unit III, "The Tools You'll Need to Practice," includes essential components of documentation, the key elements and a framework for client education, and the importance of tracking systems and minimizing risk. Essential content on establishing productivity measures and clinical outcomes, as well as the use of technology to enhance clinical practice, is presented with tools to more easily understand and integrate complex material into practice. Unit IV, "Your Place in the Community," includes information on community and professional partnerships and influencing the policy making process. Emphasis is placed on professional development and responsibilities in terms of clinical practice.

With its question and answer format, this text is an easy-to-use reference tool for NPs faced with questions about professional practice. A key feature of this text is the extensive appendixes that provide a rich resource for additional materials, Internet resources, tools, and summaries of useful information. Some NPs will read this text from cover to cover and use it as an NP role text or "survival guide" to practice, whereas others will use chapters or units to explore those areas of clinical practice that they are interested in pursuing at a particular point in time. Regardless of the approach you take, enjoy the tools and resources and have fun applying them to your clinical practice.

Acknowledgments

This book would not have been possible without the invaluable assistance from Cindi Anderson, Senior Developmental Editor, and Cheryl Abbott, Senior Project Manager, at Elsevier; a sincere thank you for all of their help.

Jean Nagelkerk

This book is dedicated to my husband, **Tom,** and my children, **Jonathon** and **Jennifer Nagelkerk,** for their love and caring, and to my parents, **Pat** and **Stanley Sagorski,** for supporting and encouraging my career in professional nursing practice.

To my professional colleagues in nursing and other disciplines who inspire me and serve as examples of excellence in teaching and scholarship, I am grateful. To my former mentor, the late **Beverly Henry,** for her guidance, inspiration, and professionalism, and to my undergraduate and graduate students, who are creative, innovative, and a source of intellectual stimulation, I am thankful.

Contents

U N I T II
Tools You Will Need to Get Started

U N I T **III**

The Tools You Will Need to Practice

Finding the Job You Want

1

Starting Out: Deciding What Job You Want

Jean Nagelkerk

Establishing Your Career and Practice

To establish your career goals, you will need to understand the nurse practitioner's scope of practice, the challenges you may face in providing care to clients, the types of job opportunities available, the four advanced practice nursing roles and how they complement each other, and certification requirements. This chapter provides an overview of information and resources to help you in establishing your career path and professional practice.

What is the role of the nurse practitioner?

Nurse practitioners (NPs) make a significant contribution toward increasing access to community, county, state, and national health care services in primary, secondary, and tertiary care settings. The focus of the NP role has been the provision of direct care using a holistic, family-centered approach often to the unserved, underserved, and indigent clients. The care that NPs provide has achieved equal or better outcomes compared with outcomes of physician providers with concomitant high client satisfaction scores (Brown & Grimes, 1993). NPs practice in a variety of settings with a diverse clientele to deliver high-quality, cost-effective care with positive health outcomes

(Horrocks, Anderson, & Salisbury, 2002; Mundinger et al., 2000; Salkever, 1992; U.S. Congress, Office of Technology Assessment, 1986). Not only do NPs provide health promotion education and management of acute problems, they establish mutual goals to assist clients with adherence to the complex, multi-faceted lifestyle changes required by chronic illness and disease management. Nurse practitioners have played a critical role in redirecting the focus of health care delivery toward primary care.

A vital goal that emerged from the *Healthy People 2010* report was to ensure universal access to health care for all citizens (U.S. Department of Health & Human Services, 2000). To deliver cost-effective quality care to communities, a mix of primary, blended, and acute care health care providers is needed. Nurse practitioners are well positioned to meet the needs of citizens in this country.

Nurse practitioners work independently in many primary care settings and collaboratively in hospital inpatient and outpatient settings, and they develop collegial relationships with physicians, physical therapists, pharmacists, occupational therapists, dietitians, and other health care professionals. Nurse practitioners are developing businesses and becoming savvy in owning and administering companies. They are advocating for access to care and becoming politically astute in influencing public policy that is client focused, enhances NP prescriptive authority, and eases credentialing barriers in practice.

What challenges do nurse practitioners face in providing care?

Restrictive regulatory and reimbursement practices and systems are challenges to NP practice. In many states, prescriptive authority limitations have been imposed (Kaplan & Brown, 2004) that require delegation of prescriptive privileges from a supervising physician or a collaborative agreement arrangement (Buppert, 2004). Depending on the terms of an agreement or collaboration, the delegated prescriptive function can be cumbersome or restrictive to NP clinical practice.

Reimbursement is an essential component of practice and allows an NP to maintain viability in an employed position or business venture. To be reimbursed for services rendered, NPs must be credentialed through insurance companies, a process that often involves lengthy application procedures that require documentation of a physician collaborative agreement. These requirements may either limit or prevent practice. In addition, lengthy processes and multiple levels of authorization are often required for NPs to be credentialed in health care systems or agencies for admitting privileges or special procedure certification.

Despite the bureaucratic challenges that NPs encounter, they have joined together to streamline regulatory and prescriptive processes and develop nurse-managed health centers. As clients have become dissatisfied with the traditional medical health care model, they have become supportive of the NP movement toward promotion of healthy lifestyles and mutual goal setting for illness management. Historically, the medical model has been "cure" oriented. Today, with an aging population, chronic illnesses require new strategies for optimizing the client's quality of life while stabilizing chronic illnesses and comorbid conditions. Clients are looking for alternative health care models that incorporate information, prevention, caring, and case management of wellness and illness care over their life span. NPs are strategically positioned to emerge as leaders in community primary health care (Towers, Dempster, & Counts, 2003).

Advanced Practice Nursing

What is an advanced practice nurse?

The term *advanced practice nurse* (APN) is a designation conferred on registered nurses who have advanced educational preparation at the graduate level. According to the American Nurses Association (2004):

Advanced practice registered nurses are RNs who have acquired advanced specialized clinical knowledge and skills to provide health care. These nurses are expected to hold a master's or doctorate degree. They build on the practice of registered nurses by demonstrating a greater depth and breadth of knowledge, a greater synthesis of data, increased complexity of skills and interventions, and significant role autonomy. (p. 14)

Similarly, the National Council of State Boards of Nursing (NCSBN), in 2002, defined advanced practice nurse as follows:

Advanced practice registered nursing by nurse practitioners, registered nurse anesthetists, nurse midwives or clinical nurse specialist is based on knowledge and skills acquired in basic nursing education; licensure as a registered nurse; graduation from or completion of a graduate level APRN program accredited by a national accrediting body and current certification by a national certifying body in the appropriate APRN specialty. (Section 4. Advanced Practice Registered Nurse, para. 1)

Advanced practice nurses work in a holistic framework advocating for client needs. They involve the client and family in mutual goal setting and help develop the therapeutic treatment plan while working in a collaborative health team approach. The APN focuses on health promotion and risk reduction, aiming to prevent illnesses and manage complex multiple chronic diseases through self-management of care. They tailor interventions to individual needs that reflect the sociocultural care components of clients and family dynamics.

The term *advanced practice nurse* is an umbrella term that encompasses four primary roles: nurse anesthetist, nurse practitioner, clinical nurse specialist, and nurse midwife (Beitz, 2000; Dunphy, Youngkin, & Smith, 2004; Hamric, Spross, & Hanson, 2005). Each of the advanced practice roles has specific educational requirements, but they share similar characteristics in advancing the practice of nursing. Often, these practitioners refer clients to each other through referral networks based on individual specialized expertise. They also collaborate on political issues, work synergistically to enhance positive client outcomes, and improve care delivery systems.

All advanced practice nurses engage in direct care to clients. The differences in APN practice often occur in the emphasis of the role components and the specialty focus. Role components include expert clinician, consultant, client and staff educator, researcher, and administrator. Table 1-1 depicts the four primary APN roles, provides a brief description of the history of each role, lists some of the associated professional associations, and describes the recertification period of each.

How is each advanced practice nurse role defined?

Certified Registered Nurse Anesthetist

Certified registered nurse anesthetists (CRNAs) are graduates of nurse anesthesia educational programs accredited by the Council on Accreditation of Nurse Anesthesia Educational Programs or its predecessor, and have passed the certification examination administered by the Council on Certification of Nurse Anesthetists or its predecessor. CRNAs provide anesthesia and anesthesia-related care in the following domains: (1) the performance of pre-anesthetic preparation and evaluation; (2) anesthesia induction, maintenance, and emergence, including administration of appropriate drugs and techniques and local, regional, and general anesthesia, and the establishment of invasive monitoring; (3) post-anesthesia care; (4) acute and chronic pain management; and (5) associated clinical support functions, such as respiratory care and emergency resuscitation. (American Nurses Association [ANA], 2004, pp. 14-15)

Certified Nurse Midwives

Certified nurse-midwives (CNMs) are registered nurses, educated in the two disciplines of nursing and midwifery, who possess evidence of certification according to the requirements of the American College of Nurse-Midwives. Midwifery practice conducted by CNMs is the independent management of women's health care, including prescriptive authority. This practice focuses particularly on pregnancy, childbirth, the postpartum period, care of the newborn, and the family planning and gynecological needs of women. CNMs practice within a health care system that provides for consultation, collaborative management, or referral as indicated by the health status of the client. (ANA, 2004, p. 15)

Certified Nurse Practitioners

Nurse practitioners (NP) are registered nurses who have a graduate level nursing preparation at the master's or doctoral level as a nurse practitioner. NPs perform comprehensive assessments and promote health and the prevention of illness

Table 1-1 Advanced Practice Nursing Roles

	Nurse Anesthetist (NA)	Nurse Midwife (CNM)	Nurse Practitioner (NP)	Clinical Nurse Specialist (CNS)
History of Role	• 1877: First NA was Sister Mary Bernard. • Promoted as a clinical nursing specialty within the military.	• 1925: first CNM was Myra Breckinridge. • 1932: First CNM program offered by Maternity Center Association in New York.	• 1965: First NP program offered by University of Colorado. • 1977: First graduating class of pediatric nurse practitioners.	• 1943: Frances Reiter proposed the concept of CNS. • 1954: First CNS program offered by Rutgers University
National Associations	• 1931: National Association of Nurse Anesthetists (NANA) founded. • 1939: NANA renamed American Association of Nurse Anesthetists (AANA).	• 1955: American Academy of Nurse Midwifery founded as the first professional organization. • 1956: Merged with the American College of Nurse Midwifery (ACNM).	• 1973: National Association of Pediatric Nurse Associates and Practitioners (NAPNAP) founded. • 1992: National NP Coalition created and later formalized into the American College of Nurse Practitioners. • 1993: Association of Women's Health, Obstetric, & Neonatal Nurses.	• 1965: ANA recognized the role of CNSs. • 1995: First National Association of CNS (NACNS) founded.

Continued

Table 1-1 Advanced Practice Nursing Roles—cont'd

	Nurse Anesthetist (NA)	Nurse Midwife (CNM)	Nurse Practitioner (NP)	Clinical Nurse Specialist (CNS)
Certification Examination	• 1945: First certification exam offered for NA by AANA.	• 1971: ACNM certification.	• 1977: First NP certification pediatric nurse/NP certification exam offered by NCBPNP/N. • 1983: National Certification Corporation offers NP certification exam. • 1990s: American Nurses Credentialing Center offers many advance practice certifications for excellence in practice.	• 1976: American Nurses Credentialing Center.
Recertification	• Recertify every 2 years.	• Recertify every 8 years.	• ANCC recertifies every 5 years. • NCBPNP/N recertifies every 7 years. • NCC recertifies every 3 years.	• Recertify every 5 years.

and injury. These advance practice registered nurses diagnose; develop differential diagnoses; order, conduct, supervise, and interpret diagnostic and laboratory tests; and prescribe pharmacologic and non-pharmacologic treatments in the direct management of acute and chronic illness and disease. Nurse practitioners provide health and medical care in primary, acute, and long-term care settings. NPs may specialize in areas such as family, geriatric, pediatric, primary, or acute care. Nurse practitioners practice autonomously and in collaboration with other health care professionals to treat and manage clients' health problems, and serve in various settings as researchers, consultants, and client advocates for individuals, families, groups, and communities. (ANA, 2004, p. 16)

Certified Clinical Nurse Specialists

Clinical nurse specialist (CNSs) are registered nurses, who have a graduate level nursing preparation at the master's or doctoral level as a CNS. They are clinical experts in evidence-based nursing practice within a speciality area, treating and managing the health concerns of clients and populations. The CNS speciality may be focused on individuals, populations, settings, type of care, type of problem, or diagnostic systems subspecialty. CNSs practice autonomously and integrate knowledge of disease and medical treatments into the assessment, diagnosis, and treatment of client illnesses. The nurses design, implement and evaluate both client-specific and population based programs of care. CNSs provide leadership in advancing the practice of nursing to achieve quality and cost-effective client outcomes as well as provide leadership of multidisciplinary groups in designing and implementing innovative alternative solutions that address system problems and/or client care issues. In many jurisdictions, CNSs, as direct care providers, perform comprehensive health assessments, develop differential diagnoses, and may have prescriptive authority.

Prescriptive authority allows them to provide pharmacologic and nonpharmacologic treatments and order diagnostic and laboratory tests in addressing and managing specialty health problems of clients and populations. CNSs serve as client advocates, consultants, and researchers in various settings. (ANA, 2004, p. 15)

What is the difference between a physician assistant and advanced practice nurse?

A physician assistant (PA) is a health care provider who is licensed to practice medicine under the direct supervision of a physician. The physician assistant movement and program development began in the 1960s during the acute shortage of family practice physicians in the United States. The first program to be developed was at Duke University Medical Center in North Carolina. Many army medical personnel and individuals with health backgrounds were eager to earn the PA credential. A physician assistant may diagnose and treat acute and chronic illnesses, order laboratory and diagnostic tests, conduct physical examinations and provide wellness care, order medications, and assist in surgery. Program admission requirements vary considerably. Some programs require prior medical or health care experience and college credits, whereas others do not. Some PA programs lead to a certificate, others to a baccalaureate or master's degree.

The roles of the PA and APN have many similarities in terms of the direct care component, but the frame of practice is different between these two professional groups. The PA programs have a medical model focus, whereas the APN program has a nursing holistic framework. PA students are bound to the practicing of medicine under a physician's license and supervision, whereas APNs practice under their own license. APNs can establish independent practices, whereas PAs cannot. In many practice settings, APNs are responsible for their own clinical judgment and therapeutic plan of care, whereas the physician is responsible for supervising PAs in their implementation of the medical treatment plan.

History of the Nurse Practitioner Role

How did the nurse practitioner movement begin?

In 1965, Loretta Ford, a nurse, and Henry Silver, a physician, developed the first NP program to improve access to primary health care services. The new pediatric NP program emphasized health promotion and wellness care as well as management of acute illnesses. During the next three decades NP certificate and graduate programs proliferated in the United States with an expansion into multiple specializations. The NP programs were developed in response to a primary care physician shortage coupled with a need for increased access to primary care to meet the national health care needs of urban and rural communities. In the late 1970s, the first documented acute care role, the neonatal NP, was implemented (Greier, 2000). Today there are 326 institutions with graduate NP programs in this country that graduate approximately 7000 NPs annually. These programs prepare women's health, pediatric, adult, family, school health, occupational health, emergency, acute care, gerontological, and mental health NPs. In 2003, 6388 NPs graduated (Berlin, Stennet, & Bednash, 2004). This is a slight decline from 2002 with 6942 graduates (Berlin, Stennet, & Bednash, 2003) and from 2001 with 7172 graduates (Berlin, Stennet, & Bednash, 2002).

How were the nurse practitioner program requirements developed?

The emergence of NPs in the 1960s paralleled a shortage of primary care physicians. Many physicians were choosing to specialize and fewer were electing primary care practice. This provided an opportunity for nurses to expand their practice into primary care with public support and resources. However, nursing leaders disagreed about the appropriateness of the NP role and were concerned that it was too medically focused. Early in the NP movement, this provided a fragmented approach to the development of standards and educational requirements for NPs, resulting in variation of content among graduate programs and the development of multiple certification agencies. This fragmentation decreased the collective strength of NPs and precluded a centralized coordination for credentialing and political power.

The proliferation of NP programs from 1965 to 1980 from 1 to 200 (Pulcini & Wagner, 2002) created significant concerns among medical and nursing associations and among state and federal regulators about increased numbers of NPs and the quality of the programs. In the mid-1970s, a national task force was formed with funding from the Robert Wood Johnson Foundation to develop the first NP curriculum guidelines for educational programs. This task force was the impetus for the founding, in 1980, of the National Organization of Nurse Practitioner Faculties (NONPF). NONPF was created to ensure the quality of NP programs and establish educational standards. NONPF developed the first NP educational program standards in 1990, which were incorporated into the 1995 document titled, *Advanced Nurse Practice: Curriculum Guidelines and Program Standards for Nurse Practitioner Education.* To further promote the development and maintenance of quality educational NP programs, NONPF convened the multi-organizational National Task Force (NTF) on Quality NP Education. The NTF released the first edition of the criteria in 1997 for evaluation of NP education that established a standard framework for the review of NP programs by faculty, students, administrators, accreditors, and others. The criteria for evaluation of NP education were revised in 2002. By 2004, nursing accrediting organizations implemented the evaluation criteria for NP programs through endorsement or adoption.

Nurse Practitioner Education

What is the educational preparation of an advanced practice nurse today?

Preparation for each of the advanced practice nursing roles includes foundational or core courses that all graduate nursing students must take with additional requirements for each specialty. In 1996, the American Association of Colleges of Nursing (AACN) published a document titled *Essentials of Master's Education for Advanced Practice Nursing* that describes the (1) core for all graduate programs, (2) advanced practice core, and (3) specialty curriculum components. The graduate core, which all graduate students must complete, is composed of research, policy, organization, and financing of health care, ethics, professional role development, theoretical foundations of practice, human diversity and social issues, and health promotion and disease prevention, which serve as the program foundation. The advanced practice nursing core includes advanced health/physical assessment and pharmacology. The specialty curriculum content includes the clinical learning experiences germane to the elected specialty focus.

Most NP educators base their curriculum on the AACN *Essentials of Master's Education for Advanced Practice Nursing,* the *Domains and Core Competencies for Nurse Practitioner Practice* (NONPF, 2002), *Advanced Nursing Practice: Curriculum Guidelines and Program Standards for Nurse Practitioner Education* (NONPF, 1995), the NTF's *Criteria for Evaluation of Nurse Practitioner Programs* (2002), and specialty standards of practice and competency statements from these organizations: National Panel for Acute Care Nurse Practitioner Competencies (2004), National Panel for Psychiatric-Mental Health Nurse Practitioner Competencies (2003), and NONPF and AACN's *Nurse Practitioner Primary Care Competencies in Specialty Areas: Adult, Family, Gerontological, Pediatric, & Women's Health* (2002).

The NONPF curriculum guidelines are based on domains and competencies of practice derived from research conducted by experienced practitioners in clinical practice. The domains were formed by grouping similar competencies together. The core competencies are essential behaviors for NP students to master prior to graduation regardless of specialty. The broad domains and competencies provide a holistic nursing foundation and framework for practice and specialty competencies. The client is defined as the individual, family, group, or community. All role components of an APN—provision of direct care, educator, researcher, administrator, and consultant—are used in fulfilling the competencies in NP practice. Refer to Table 1-2 for a listing of the seven domains of practice published by NONPF.

What tools do nurse practitioner programs use to track student clinical experiences?

NP programs use many different tools to track student clinical experiences and facilitate learning experiences to assist graduate students to become novice practitioners. Many graduate programs have developed clinical experience checklists or electronic tracking programs for assessing major areas of nursing

Table 1-2 Domains of Practice

Domain 1	Management of Patient Health/Illness Status
Domain 2	The Nurse Practitioner-Patient Relationship
Domain 3	The Teaching-Coaching Function
Domain 4	Professional Role
Domain 5	Managing and Negotiating Health Care Delivery Systems
Domain 6	Monitoring and Ensuring the Quality of Health Care Practice
Domain 7	Cultural Competence

activities or experiences, life-span issues, procedures, prevention counseling, diagnostic testing, and illness care that students should encounter prior to graduation.

By tracking the age group (using a spreadsheet or an electronic medium), the type of care provided (health promotion, risk reduction, disease prevention, acute or chronic illness management), and procedures completed, students are able to manage and optimize their clinical experiences, develop confidence in their practice skills, and develop a strong clinical portfolio. An example of a Clinical Experience Checklist, titled "Culminating Clinical Behaviors," is given in Appendix 1-1. A tool to track visits across the life span is given in Appendix 1-2.

Nurse Practitioner Practice

What is nurse practitioner practice?

Nurse practitioners provide the public with a distinct choice for the provision of health care services (Turkeltaub, 2004). Nurse practitioners engage in health promotion, risk reduction, disease prevention, and the treatment of minor acute problems and stable chronic illnesses. In a client encounter, they often not only manage and treat the chief complaint, but provide education about health issues (Lin, Gebbie, Fullilove, & Arons, 2004) or diseases and manage complex chronic illnesses by establishing mutual goals in relation to resource availability and client understanding. The emphasis of the client provider role is to encourage support and facilitate the self-care management of wellness, illness, and chronic problems. Nurse practitioners in most states have prescriptive authority and are able to order medications, diagnostic laboratory tests, and medical imaging tests to diagnose and manage client care. They are able to manage a caseload of clients independently or in collaboration with other health care members in diverse settings.

In addition to the direct provision of client care, NPs engage in other role components such as administrative duties, policy development, research, and consultation. Cultivating these skills is critical in advancing your career and the specialty of nursing. Politicking (that is, using strategies to influence key stakeholders) to make significant changes in public policy is important for reimbursement for health care services provided by NPs, as well as for taking leadership roles to improve community health care. Being skillful in leading teams, building coalitions, and delegating is an important aspect of the NP role. In addition to direct client care, NPs lead interdisciplinary teams, provide staff and client education, and analyze strategies to improve the health of communities. They often share on-call responsibilities with their team and triage or manage client care as appropriate. Some NPs have elected to become credentialed in health care facilities and make hospital rounds to manage care across settings and over the life span. Studies show that NPs cost 40% less than physician providers and are effective in managing a caseload (Appleby, 1995). NPs also provide cost-effective care while managing preventive and chronic illness care and often have a reduction in inpatient visits for their population (Spitzer, 1997).

Nurse practitioners are joining existing health care organizations, but some are building their own practices, and owning businesses is becoming more common. The National Nursing Summit on Nurse Managed Health Centers held in Dearborn, Michigan, in fall of 2002 met to build consensus on a strategic vision and direction for nurse-managed health centers. They identified the following directions at the summit for a national network of nurse-managed centers: to become a strong political advocate for nurse-managed centers, to assist nurse-managed centers with operational issues, and to develop a nurse-managed center data repository (Michigan Academic Consortium, 2002).

What is the scope of practice for a nurse practitioner?

The scope of practice for a profession comes from many sources including the profession's practice standards, code of ethics, and state and federal laws, regulations, and rules (Hamric et al., 2005). The scope of practice of a profession provides the structure of practice and is reflected in the state statutes. The state statutes set the practice parameters for professionals. The ability to bill for services emerges from the scope of practice established in the state statutes. Each state has a nurse practice act that governs an NP's scope of practice. There is significant variability among the states for NP practice authority, prescriptive authority, and physician collaboration or supervision for practice. To determine the scope of practice in your state, write your state board of nursing or access its website to request a copy of the nurse practice act with the rules and regulations that govern NP practice. By reviewing this document you will be knowledgeable about the legal parameters that regulate nurse practitioner practice. See Appendix 1-3 for a list of state boards of nursing contact information.

The development and implementation of an adequate scope of practice for NPs has been a historic struggle with many opportunities, as well as barriers and trials. Continued collaboration by NP organizations and groups has provided a unified effort to seek appropriate changes in the breadth of autonomous practice. The professional role statement developed by the American Academy of Nurse Practitioners (AANP, 2002) in their *Scope of Practice* is as follows:

> Nurse practitioners are primary care providers who practice in ambulatory, acute, and long-term care settings. According to their practice specialty these providers provide nursing and medical services to individuals, families, and groups. In addition to diagnosing and managing acute episodic and chronic illnesses, nurse practitioners emphasize health promotion and disease prevention. Services include, but are not limited to ordering, conducting, supervising, and interpreting diagnostic and laboratory tests, and prescription of

pharmacologic agents and nonpharmacologic therapies. Teaching and counseling individuals, families, and groups are a major part of nurse practitioner practice.

Nurse practitioners practice autonomously and in collaboration with health care professionals and other individuals to diagnose, treat and manage the patient's health problems. They serve as health care researchers, interdisciplinary consultants and patient advocates. (Professional role, para. 1)

Members of professional organizations develop standards of practice to regulate and control practice. They provide a self-regulatory process of accountability for professionals to the public (Beitz, 2000). These standards provide a method of professional accountability to protect the public from unsafe practice or unethical behavior. The standards of practice generally provide an overview of qualifications of the professional and include a general job description or functions, care priorities, and role description. Box 1-1 identifies some professional organizations that publish standards of practice for nurse practitioners.

Box 1-1 Professional Associations that Publish APN Standards of Practice

American Academy of Nurse Practitioners (ACNP)

www.aanp.org/Practice+Policy + and + Legislation/Practice/Position + Statements + and + Papers/Position + Statements + and + Papers.asp

American Association of Nurse Anesthetists (AANA)

www.aana.com/crna/prof/scope.asp

American College of Nurse-Midwives (ACNM)

www.midwife.org/prof/display.cfm?id=138

American Nurses Association (ANA)

http://nursingworld.org/books/pdescr.cfm?cnum=15.#03SSNP

Association of Women's Health, Obstetrics & Neonatal Nurses (AWHONN)

www.awhonn.org

National Association of Pediatric Nurse Practitioners (NAPNAP)

www.napnap.org/practice/pnpstandards/

Oncology Nursing Society (ONS)

www.ons.org/xp6/ONS/Library.xml/ONS_Publications.xml/Book_Excerpts.xml/ AdvancedPracticeStandards/II.xml

Nurse Practitioner State Recognition and Certification

What nurse practitioner state recognition is required to practice as a nurse practitioner?

Each state's government establishes minimum standards to protect public safety, often through the licensing of professionals. Licensure is one method used to establish minimal competence for professionals to practice. Each state has a process to license, certify, or recognize NPs. In all states, you must maintain registered nurse licensure. In addition, you will need to apply to the state for recognition as a nurse practitioner. Box 1-2 provides a state-by-state listing of regulatory approaches for nurse practitioners (National Council of State Boards of Nursing, 2003).

What is certification?

Certification is a process used by individuals and certifying bodies to validate competence in a specific area or specialty. The certification body develops specific competencies or criteria that are assessed through an examination or recertification process. Individuals who take the certification examination are then "certified" by the professional organization indicating that they have met the standards developed by the certifying body. In many states, certification is required for NPs to be licensed or "certified" to practice in the state. The first NP certification examination was offered through the Pediatric Nursing Certification Board (PNCB) formally known as the NCBPNP/N (National Association of Pediatric Nurse Practitioners, 2000). Professional organizations that certify NPs include the American Academy of Nurse Practitioners Certification Program, the American Nurses Credentialing Center (ANCC), the National Certification Board of Pediatric Nurse Practitioners (PNCB), and the National Certification Corporation (NCC). Table 1-3 lists professional organization contact information and type of certification offered.

Where to Begin

How do I develop a job description?

A job description is designed for a specific role and is based on educational experiences, specialty practice, and the scope and standards of practice. Job descriptions are designed by private or corporate organizations for specific roles to inform individuals about job responsibilities and expectations and to set performance criteria. Individuals often develop job descriptions to market their unique skills and specialties. Many small clinic practice settings do not have the resources or the knowledge of the full scope of practice of an NP to

Box 1-2 Regulation of Advanced Nursing Practice: Regulatory Approach for Nurse Practitioners

Board-Issued Advanced Practice License = 12 Boards

Alaska, Arkansas, Delaware, Illinois, Louisiana, Maryland, Nebraska, New Hampshire, New Mexico, North Dakota, Utah, Washington

Board-Issued Certificate to Practice = 11 Boards

Arizona, California, District of Columbia, Guam, Kansas, Mississippi, Nevada, New Jersey, Ohio, Pennsylvania, Texas

Board-Issued Letter of Recognition or Authorization to Practice = 20 Boards

Alabama, Florida, Georgia, Hawaii, Idaho, Illinois, Iowa, Kentucky, Maine, Massachusetts, Michigan, Montana, Oklahoma, Oregon, South Carolina, South Dakota, Virgin Islands, Virginia, West Virginia, Wyoming

Other = 10 Boards

Colorado	Listing on registry; title protection, no scope of practice
Connecticut	Department of Public Health issues advanced practice license
Indiana	Will be issued additional credential if apply for prescriptive authority only
Minnesota	National certification required
Missouri	Advanced practice nurse rule; board-issued "document of recognition" specifying clinical nursing specialty area and role
New York	Department-issued certificate to practice
North Carolina	Authorization to practice issued by Medical Board and Board of Nursing
Rhode Island	Board-issued advanced practice license and certification by national organization
Tennessee	Certificates of fitness to prescribe and/or issue legend drugs
Vermont	Endorsement to practice as an advanced practice registered nurse

Other

Alabama	Designation appears on RN wallet card
Connecticut	Advanced practice registered nurse license is for prescriptive authority only; RN is basis for advanced practice
Maryland	CNS: psychiatric/mental health-advanced practice license; Maryland designated CS-P (certified specialist-psychotherapist)
Mississippi	"Certification" is the term used in R/R, but nurse practitioner status appears printed on the registered nurse license card
Nevada	Nurse psychotherapist: certificate to practice
Ohio	APN: board-issued letter of authorization to practice
Puerto Rico	Community health nurses; medical and surgical nurses; perinatal nurses
Vermont	Also signified on RN license by specialty area and prescriptive authority
West Virginia	RN: legislative rule does not restrict practice or regulate practice of nurse practitioner or certified nurse specialist

Data from Crawford, L., & White, E. (2003). *Profiles of Member Boards 2002.* Chicago: National Council of State Boards of Nursing.

Table 1-3 Nurse Practitioner Credentialing Organizations

Credentialing Agency	NP Certification	Credential	Website
The American Academy of Nurse Practitioners Certification Program	Adult, family	NP-C	*www.aanp.org/certification/certification.asp*
American Nurses Credentialing Center	Acute care, adult, family, pediatric, gerontological, adult psychiatric & mental health, family psychiatric & mental health	APRN, BC	*www.nursingworld.org/ancc/*
National Certification Board of Pediatric Nurse Practitioners	Pediatric	CPNP or CPN	*www.pncb.org/ptistore/control/index*
National Certification Corporation	Women's health, neonatal care	RNC	*www.nccnet.org*

design a job description. By having a written document detailing the job description of an NP, applicants can demonstrate their practice capabilities to a potential employer.

The job descriptions that you read or develop are based on the role components of the NP. The major components of the NP role include autonomous practice, comprehensive assessment, differential diagnosis, management of complex therapeutic treatment regimens, and skilled clinical decision making. Depending on your specialty and practice site, you will design a job description to meet the needs of the clients and the practice. Specific components of most job descriptions include a general overview of the NP role, education and experience requirements, and principal duties or responsibilities. A sample job description is depicted in Appendix 1-4. A job description is important because it identifies and describes the scope of practice, role components, and performance expectations in the practice setting in which you are employed.

What is career planning?

Opportunities abound for new NPs in local communities across the country and around the world. So, how do you determine which direction you will select after graduation or with a job change? It is useful to determine a career plan or direction you would like to go as you begin searching for a job. Mapping out your career goals and plans provides a systematic, focused strategy for professional development and assists you to move forward in your specialty area and role. By engaging in a deliberate, careful, and planned approach to researching career options and potential job opportunities, you will begin to establish your career trajectory. By taking the time to map out your career, you will be able to move forward as you gain valuable clinical experience and develop professionally in your specialty and clinical tract.

Whether you are experienced, beginning your career, or enrolled in an NP program, it is never too early to begin developing your career path. Teasdale (2002) describes a flexible approach to career planning to understand your priorities and the available work choices. By exploring varying job opportunities, you can determine the job activities that you enjoy and eliminate jobs that you do not. One activity to help you learn about varying roles is to interview individuals in blended roles, administrative positions, owners of businesses, and various practitioners to determine the types of activities that appeal to you (Teasdale, 2002). Develop a list of activities, skills, and role components that you are interested in pursuing as you explore career choices.

Another strategy to explore job opportunities and requirements is to cut out advertisements for jobs in newspapers or magazines. These advertisements often identify required criteria for successful applicants. Criteria usually include experience, education, and certifications or licensure. Make a table and list the jobs and requirements. Then review the table and note similarities among job criteria. Based on the similarities, you can begin to develop a portfolio of your experiences and education to show potential employers. A portfolio provides highlights of your accomplishments and is an organized way to demonstrate your accomplishments and skills.

Other strategies to explore your career direction include discussing professional goals with a trusted colleague, preceptor, or mentor. They can help guide you in gaining essential clinical experiences and making critical contacts to enhance your professional career.

What factors are important in career planning?

Besides the types of activities and skills you will incorporate into your practice, there are many other areas to consider when you determine the type of job you will accept:
- Salary
- Profit sharing or bonus potential

- Hourly or salaried positions
- Benefits
- Positional power
- Hours of employment
- Temporary or permanent assignment
- Experience required
- Educational preparation
- Geographic location.

Another equally important consideration in career planning is your personal goals. How do your professional goals fit with your personal ones? Without a match between personal and professional goals, a selected job can become burdensome and demanding, creating conflict between home and work life and becoming unrewarding. Personal habits, hobbies, and travel plans should be factored into work style choices. For some, family responsibilities need to be evaluated and will strongly influence work selection; for others, professional goals will be the major focus. To assist in determining your personal preferences, answer the following questions:

- Is time off a central consideration in job choice?
- Is independence or autonomy a major goal?
- Do you enjoy change?
- Do you prefer structuring the environment, making assignments, and allocating resources?
- Are salary and benefits the driving factor in your work choice?
- Do you enjoy direct care or a combination of direct care and other activities?
- Do you prefer a schedule that works around your family's needs?

Once you have identified your priorities you can develop a long-term strategic plan for your career.

Each position you accept will strategically move you toward your career goals.

Personal and Professional Assessment

A long-term personal and professional self-assessment provides goals, objectives, and plans to help you achieve your desired goals. Table 1-4 features a worksheet that can assist in career planning (Nagelkerk, 2005). This worksheet incorporates 1- and 5-year and lifetime personal and professional goals. By writing these goals down, you can note the congruence between personal and professional goals and work toward their accomplishment. Goals should be revisited annually, revised, and updated. Then successes and progression should be celebrated.

Table 1-4 ▪ Career Planning Worksheet

Directions: Complete the following task: In the blank lines below, identify and prioritize by ranking five personal and professional goals for three time periods.

1-Year Personal Goals	5-Year Personal Goals	Lifetime Personal Goals
1.	1.	1.
2.	2.	2.
3.	3.	3.
4.	4.	4.
5.	5.	5.

1-Year Professional Goals	5-Year Professional Goals	Lifetime Professional Goals
1.	1.	1.
2.	2.	2.
3.	3.	3.
4.	4.	4.
5.	5.	5.

Source: Modified from Nagelkerk, J. (2006). *Study guide for Huber leadership and nursing care management* (3rd ed.). Philadelphia: W. B. Saunders Company. All rights reserved. Annually review, revise, and update your career plan. Take time to celebrate accomplishments.

Thinking out of the box

What Types of Job Opportunities Are Available? There are many different ways of gathering information about job opportunities. Written announcements of job openings are listed in professional journals, nursing association websites, newspaper advertisements, health care agency and employment consultant websites, and schools or colleges of nursing bulletin board or web postings. Other successful avenues for locating job opportunities include listening to individuals in practice; contacting primary care clinics (owned by hospitals, health systems, physicians and nurses), hospitals, or health maintenance organizations for openings; and working with an employment agency. There are many opportunities for signing contracts for traveling nurse corporations either in the United States or abroad as well as armed service NP positions. The National Health Service Corporation has many job opportunities available for nurse practitioners in underserved rural and urban areas.

Nontraditional roles are emerging as viable options for individuals seeking creative work opportunities. Blending acute care and primary care roles, carving out tertiary roles, and working in community settings offering specialized services are examples of blended roles. You may choose to open a business such as a nurse-managed center consulting service or specialized clinic. Other approaches to role blending include working in a community college or university teaching theory or clinical courses and contracting for part of your job with the academic health center precepting students or with a local health care center. By blending the role you have a variety of job components to enrich your career trajectory.

How Do I Create a Job? Based on your NP specialty, do a self-assessment and determine the types of activities that you have learned and enjoy. To identify your ideal or preferred job, ask yourself the following questions:
- What types of activities do I prefer?
- Do I prefer a variety of different activities or a normal routine?
- What types of hours do I prefer to work?
- In what type of health care setting or geographical area am I interested in working?
- Is there a specific client population from whom I want to develop an expertise?
- Do I enjoy direct client care more than teaching?
- Do I enjoy administrative tasks such as budgeting, establishing schedules, writing policies and procedures, and engaging in quality assurance activities?
- Do I enjoy completing physical examinations, performing procedures, and diagnosing and treating acute problems or chronic stable illnesses?
- Do I prefer to provide health teaching?
- Do I enjoy public speaking, political action work, or developing client materials?

By answering the questions posed, you will begin to get an idea for the type of job, the environment, the working requirements, and the activities that suit your educational and experiential preferences.

Once you are clear on your preferences and specialty, you can begin to create the "ideal" job. You can blend your NP expertise with a specific specialty to become, for instance, an oncology acute or primary care NP or an end-of-life NP. You can use your skills to develop a wound or ostomy clinic. If you enjoy chronic illness management, you can design self-care management programs and engage in chronic illness management for clients with diabetes, congestive heart failure, or chronic obstructive pulmonary disease. The options are unlimited for blending roles, developing specialty expertise, focusing on pediatric, women's health, or male health care, or being a generalist in family practice. Complementary health programs, skin care, cosmetic augmentation, exercise health, or nutritional care are all potential opportunities. A benefit of NP practice is the multitude of interesting job opportunities available to you.

Entrepreneurship and Intrapreneurship

Developing your career as an NP is an exciting, dynamic, and engaging activity. Planning for the future and exploring job options that fit your practice preferences and specialty focus require considerable analysis and evaluation of existing and potential job opportunities. Many NP positions are available in the more traditional physician or health care system-owned acute, primary, or tertiary care settings, but opportunities also exist in nontraditional settings. Exploring a variety of practice options and potential employment settings enhances the process of obtaining the ideal position for your career trajectory and provides an opportunity to review not only traditional NP jobs, but also emerging role opportunities.

What is an intrapreneur?

Many new and experienced NPs decide to practice within existing organizations, either in health care systems, community health settings, private physician practices, or nurse-managed centers. In these practice settings, NPs often become *intrapreneurs* within their organizations, carving out and negotiating their niche, developing blended roles whereby they successfully integrate primary care visits in a clinic setting with admitting and managing acute care visits for their clients. They may create other blended roles as well. Intrapreneurs are skilled in creating, discovering, promoting, and implementing new programs, product lines, or systems into existing organizations (Huber, 2006). Qualities that intrapreneurs have include these:
- Assertiveness in intense situations
- Ability to take risks
- Strong leadership skills
- Negotiation expertise
- Self-motivation
- Innovation
- Expertise in their specialty area (Antoncic & Hisrich, 2003; Dayhoff, 2003)

What is an entrepreneur?

Other NPs will take a different type of personal risk and become entrepreneurs. An *entrepreneur* is an individual who is innovative and assumes the risk of owning and managing a business (Vollman, 2004). Entrepreneurs possess qualities similar to those of intrapreneurs, but prefer to work outside of existing organizations and enjoy the challenges of managing and leading an independent business operation. More and more NPs are making the choice to own their own practice or business and take the necessary personal and professional challenges, risks, and opportunities to manage their patient care via a new, nurse-centered, holistic, community-centered model of care or via an independent business operation.

What types of businesses are owned and managed by nurse practitioners?

NPs are opting to own and manage many different types of businesses. Examples of different types of business opportunities that NPs initiate are listed in Box 1-3. Refer to Chapter 7 for descriptions of the planning process and implementation steps of owning your own business.

How do I develop a specialized practice?

The health care environment is fluid and constantly changing. Consumer demands for special services create niches for NPs to develop specialized practices. Examples of innovative roles NPs have crafted include congestive heart failure NP, gastrointestinal NP, neurological nurse specialist, acute care NP, oncology NP, and musculoskeletal NP. Many of these new roles not only

---

Box 1-3 Examples of Businesses Owned and Operated by Nurse Practitioners

Day care for the elderly
Group home for people who are elderly or who have disabilities
Women's care specialty store
Billing and coding business
Incontinence clinic
Wound care clinic
Primary care practice
Health care consultant
Weight enhancement program clinic
Genetic counseling center
Exercising spa
Diabetic education center
Quality management and system design
Case management agencies
End-of-life care program
Continuing education business
Psychiatric counseling
Pain management consultant
Risk management consultant
Sexual assault response team
Forensic nursing consultant

include the direct client care component, but use the other APN roles of administration, education, research, and consultation. A *role* encompasses the behaviors and/or characteristics of a person that helps define his or her work. A role is broad and dynamic to include activities, skills, and functions that may change over time as historic events unfold and as health care discoveries emerge. Innovative NPs often craft specialty positions based on societal and specific institutional needs. They are intrapreneurs or entrepreneurs and leaders in their organizations and communities.

Often, NPs who are intrapreneurs begin to carve their specialty roles based on observation of a need within an organization or community. They obtain the facts and figures of volume of clients, procedures, and services that are needed and attach cost and expenses to these data. This begins to set the stage for the development of a presentation, often in the form of a brief business plan. The mission of the new service is identified along with the goals and objectives. A clear description of what service(s) will be offered along with the benefits to the organization are articulated. A job description is crafted for the new specialty position that clearly describes the role components and activities.

During the data collection and job description development phase, the NP begins to make the necessary contacts both internal and external to the organization to plant the seeds and set the stage for the need for this new service. Many NP students have wisely used assignments to sketch out a plan, gain feedback from their professors, and then develop a specialty practice. Others have sought out the organization with which they are interested in pursuing employment and have completed vital clinical experiences in the agency. These strategies often provide important contacts and knowledge of organizational processes that can be used to secure a new position.

Presentation of the information to key administrators and clinicians is an important aspect of specialty role development. A professionally designed presentation using well-developed handouts and a carefully prepared script is an important aspect of securing the new specialty role. Demonstrating your professional appearance and presentation are important marketing aspects that the organizational personnel will use to judge the overall viability and desirability of the newly proposed specialty role.

SUMMARY

As an NP you have many career opportunities, from working in a primary care office, to a specialty practice, to a blended primary and acute care role or owning your own business. Whatever you choose, you will be a leader in your work environment and in the community. Your skills as a leader, educator, consultant, and expert clinician will enable you to impact public policy and the health of citizens in your community. Think out of the box and create that innovative emerging role that fills a need in your community.

Internet Resources

National Council of State Boards of Nursing
www.ncsbn.org
111 E. Wacker Drive, Suite 2900
Chicago, IL 60691-4277
(312)525-3600
Fax: (312)279-1032

National Health Service Corps
http://nhsc.bhpr.hrsa.gov/
5600 Fishers Lane, Room 81-55
Rockville, MD 20857
(800)221-9393

References

American Academy of Nurse Practitioners. (2002). *Scope of practice for nurse practitioners.* Retrieved March 15, 2004, from *www.aanp.org*

American Association of Colleges of Nursing. (1996). *The essentials of master's education for advanced practice nursing.* Washington, DC: Author.

American Nurses Association. (2004). *Nursing: Scope and standards of practice.* Washington, CD: Author.

Antoncic, B., & Hisrich, R.D. (2003). Clarifying the intrapreneurship concept. *Journal of Small Business and Enterprise Development, 10*(1), 7-24.

Appleby, C. (1995, September 20). Boxed in? *Hospitals and Health Networks*, pp. 28-34.

Beitz, J. M. (2000). Specialty practice, advanced practice, and WOC nursing: Current professional issues and future opportunities. *Journal of Wound, Ostomy, and Nursing Continence, 27*(1), 55-64.

Berlin, L.E., Stennet, J., & Bednash, G.D. (2002). *2001-2002 Enrollment and graduations in baccalaureate and graduate programs in nursing.* Washington, DC: American Association of Colleges of Nursing and National Organization of Nurse Practitioner Faculties.

Berlin, L.E., Stennet, J., & Bednash, G.D. (2003). *2002-2003 Enrollment and graduations in baccalaureate and graduate programs in nursing.* Washington, DC: American Association of Colleges of Nursing and National Organization of Nurse Practitioner Faculties.

Berlin, L.E., Stennet, J., & Bednash, G.D. (2004). *2003-2004 Enrollment and graduations in baccalaureate and graduate programs in nursing.* Washington, DC: American Association of Colleges of Nursing and National Organization of Nurse Practitioner Faculties.

Brown, S.A., & Grimes, D.E. (1993). *Nurse practitioners and certified nurse midwives: A meta-analysis of studies in primary care roles.* Washington, DC: American Nursing Publishing.

Buppert, C. (2004). *Nurse practitioner's business practice and legal guide* (2nd ed.). Boston: Jones and Bartlett.

Crawford, L., & White, E. (2003). *Profiles of member boards 2003.* Chicago: National Council of State Boards of Nursing.

Dayhoff, N.E. (2003). You don't have to leave your hospital system to be an entrepreneur. *Clinical Nurse Specialist, 17*(1), 22-24.

Dunphy, L., Youngkin, E., & Smith, N. (2004). Advanced practice nursing: Doing what had to be done radicals, renegades, and rebels. In L.A. Joel (Ed.), *Advanced practice nursing: Essentials for role development* (pp. 3-25). Philadelphia: F.A. Davis.

Greier, W. (2000). The evolving role of the acute care nurse practitioner. *Nurse Practitioner, 25,* 126-129.

Hamric, A., Spross, J.A., & Hanson, C.M. (2005). *Advanced nursing practice: An integrative approach.* St. Louis: W.B. Saunders.

Horrocks, S., Anderson, E., & Salisbury, C. (2002). Systemic review of whether nurse practitioners working in primary care can provide equivalent care to doctors. *British Medical Journal, 324,* 819-823.

Huber, D. (2006). *Leadership and nursing care management.* Philadelphia: W.B. Saunders.

Kaplan, L., & Brown, M.A. (2004). Prescriptive authority and barriers to NP practice. *Nurse Practitioner, 29*(3), 28-35.

Lin, S.X., Gebbie, K.M., Fullilove, R.E., & Arons, R. (2004). Do nurse practitioners make a difference in provision of health counseling in hospital outpatient departments? *Journal of the American Academy of Nurse Practitioners, 16*(10), 462-466.

Michigan Academic Consortium. (2002, December). *Report of the National Nursing Summit Addressing Nurse-Managed Health Centers,* Dearborn, MI.

Mundinger, M.O., Kane, R., Lenz, E.R., Totten, A.M., Tsai, W., et al. (2000). Primary care outcomes in patient treatment by nurse practitioners or physicians: A randomized trial. *Journal of American Medical Association, 283,* 59-68.

Nagelkerk, J. (2006). *Study guide for Huber: Leadership and nursing care management* (3rd ed.). Philadelphia: W.B. Saunders.

National Association of Pediatric Nurse Practitioners. (2002). *NAPNAP position statement on certification.* Retrieved December 22, 2004, from *www.napnap.org/practice/positions/pos_certification.html*

National Council of State Boards of Nursing. (2002). *National Council of State Boards of Nursing model nursing practice act.* Retrieved December 22, 2004, from *www.ncsbn.org/regulation/nursingpractice_nursing_practice_model_practice_act.asp*

National Organization of Nurse Practitioner Faculties. (2002). *Domains and competencies of nurse practitioner practice.* Washington, DC: National Organization of Nurse Practitioner Faculties.

National Organization of Nurse Practitioner Faculties and American Associations of Colleges of Nursing. (2002). *Nurse practitioner primary care competencies in specialty areas: Adult, family, gerontological, pediatric, & women's health* [Health Contract No. HRSA 00-0532(P)]. Rockville, MD: Department of Health and Human Services, Health Resources and Services Administration, Bureau of Health Professions, Division of Nursing.

National Organization of Nurse Practitioner Faculties Curriculum Guidelines Task Force. (1995). *Advanced nurse practice: Curriculum guidelines and program standards for nurse practitioner education.* Washington, DC: National Organization of Nurse Practitioner Faculties.

National Panel for Acute Care Nurse Practitioner Competencies. (2004). *Acute care nurse practitioner competencies.* Washington, DC: Author.

National Panel for Psychiatric-Mental Health Nurse Practitioner Competencies. (2003). *Psychiatric-mental health nurse practitioner competencies.* Washington, DC: National Organization of Nurse Practitioner Faculties.

National Task Force on Quality Nurse Practitioner Education. (1997/2002). *Criteria for evaluation of nurse practitioner programs.* Washington, DC: National Organization of Nurse Practitioner Faculties.

Pulcini, J., & Wagner, M. (2002). Nurse practitioner education in the United States: A success story. *Clinical Excellence for Nurse Practitioners, 6*(2), 51-56.

Salkever, D.S. (1992). Episode-based efficiency comparisons for physicians and nurse practitioners. *Medical Care, 20,* 143-153.

Spitzer, R. (1997). The Vanderbilt University experience. *Nursing Management, 28*(3), 37-43.

Teasdale, K. (2002). Professional nurse study: Taking a flexible approach to career planning in nursing. *Professional Nurse, 17*(5) 309-311.

Towers, J., Dempster, J., & Counts, M. (2003). Nurse practitioner practice in 2012: Meeting the health care needs of tomorrow. *Journal of the American Academy of Nurse Practitioners, 15*(4), 146-148.

Turkeltaub, M. (2004). Nurse-managed centers: Increasing access to health care. *Journal of Nursing Education, 43*(2), 53-54.

U.S. Congress, Office of Technology Assessment. (1986). *Nurse practitioners, physician assistants, and certified nurse midwife: A policy analysis* (Health Technology Case Study 37, OTA-HCS-37). Washington, DC: U.S. Government Printing Office.

U.S. Department of Health and Human Services. (2000, November). *Healthy people 2010,* (Vol 1, 2nd ed.). Washington, DC: U.S. Government Printing Office.

Vollman, K. (2004). Nurse entrepreneurship: Taking an invention from birth to the marketplace, *Clinical Nurse Specialist, 18*(2), 68-71.

Nurse Practitioner Socialization and Marketing

Jean Nagelkerk

The Transition from Student to Nurse Practitioner

Graduating from a nurse practitioner (NP) program and entering the NP job market is an exciting time, but it may also be a time fraught with apprehension and worry about securing a permanent position. Apprehension is a common feeling that new NPs experience on graduation and during the first several months of clinical practice. Research has shown that new NPs experience a transition period as they enter into their first NP role (Heitz, Steiner & Burman, 2004; Rich, Jorden & Taylor, 2001). The transition period from student to confident practitioner generally lasts 6 months to 2 years (Heitz et al., 2004).

What occurs during the transitional year from student to nurse practitioner?

The first year of clinical practice as an NP is a critical time for cementing and expanding the knowledge base established during an individual's graduate program. It is an important time for developing confidence in conducting physical assessments, acute illness visits, and chronic disease management and becoming adept at procedures. Research conducted on the actual experience of NPs who were in their first year or transitional year of clinical practice showed that NPs experienced many doubts and feelings of uncertainty about their skills and knowledge base. During this transitional period, participants described feeling like impostors, feelings of not being "real," fear about missing important or life-threatening data, and uncertainty about diagnoses and treatment decision making (Brown & Olshansky, 1997; Thibodeau & Hawkins, 1994). Brown and Olshansky's research further supports the existence of this transitional period and discusses a model for this role transition from novice to confident practitioner.

Brown and Olshansky's (1997) model, titled "From Limbo to Legitimacy," describes the transitional period as encompassing four major categories: laying the foundation, launching, meeting the challenge, and broadening the perspective. Each category has subcategories that help explain the process an NP engages in to become "real" and confident as a seasoned practitioner. Understanding the role transition process that you will experience and learning helpful clinical strategies will assist you in successful NP role implementation. Important tasks for the NP who is making this role transition include becoming aware of one's self, understanding the change process, and implementing new responsibilities while tackling new challenges (Kelley & Mathews, 2001). The transitional period is an important part of professional development; it is a transition from student to practicing, confident NP.

During the transition process, many new NPs feel that they are in limbo, a period in which they do not belong to their initial nursing role nor to the new NP role. As they develop more skills, embrace the challenges of the NP role, and build on their nursing knowledge, they discover that their nursing skills and experiences serve as a foundation for their professional NP practice. The NP is, first, part of the group of all professional registered nurses and, second, a provider who has expanded nursing skills in advanced practice and has developed a specialized clinical role. By being part of the professional nursing community, the NP role strengthens the role of nurses, assists with influencing policy, builds networks for referrals, and enhances nursing's public image. NPs and RNs support each other and work collaboratively (Gooden & Jackson, 2004). The emerging identity of the new graduate becomes one of an expert nurse and developing NP, one who draws on his or her prior education, experiences, and role socialization to enact an autonomous role as clinician in a distinct specialty. Ideally, new NPs apply the art and science of nursing and the newly acquired advanced nursing interventions to their advanced practice nursing role, while valuing and supporting other nurses in practice and including them in the network of nursing as a society.

In the "limbo to legitimacy" model, the first category of role transition is *laying the foundation for practice*. From graduation until acceptance of an NP position, the graduate is laying the foundation for future development and professional practice. In this category, individuals work through four subcategories: recuperating from school, negotiating the bureaucracy, looking for a job, and worrying about securing an NP position. Depending on economic and family responsibilities, graduates usually take time to recuperate, spend time with family, and vacation before engaging in intense job searches. This time provides a much needed renewal and catching-up period for personal, family, and professional activities. The new graduate, during the recuperating period, begins to negotiate through the bureaucracy. The applications and forms required for national certification and state board of nursing certification, licensure, or recognition are often confusing to the new graduate, and waiting for approval to take an examination and to obtain the required credential(s) to practice seems to take an endless amount of time. Applications that new NPs generally apply for during this transition time often include NP certification, state board of nursing credentialing, and DEA, Medicare, and Medicaid numbers. Conquering the bureaucratic paperwork can increase the apprehension and frustration surrounding the amount and length of time it takes to be credentialed. In many geographical areas, employers will not hire an NP until they have received the appropriate required credential (recognition, certificate, and/or licensure). This requirement tends to delay the employment process and increases worry and apprehension about securing an NP position. New NPs must develop a letter of introduction, résumé, and portfolio and consider potential job opportunities in their local communities or assess whether moving to a new geographical area or doing local tenems work may be a viable option. New NPs must negotiate for salary and benefits, develop a collaborative agreement and job description, and establish their practice.

The second role transition category, *launching*, begins with accepting the first NP position. The launching of the NP role is the most turbulent and often the most difficult time for a new NP. The NP graduate expends significant energy and personal resources in traversing the health care system, becoming proficient in practice, and developing an independent clinical role. The launching phase has four subcategories: feeling like an impostor, confronting anxiety, getting through the day, and battling time. NPs who were actively engaged in this phase reported an overwhelming dissonance of feeling like they were "faking" and not "being real." They were often unsure of their skills or knowledge base when engaged in client care visits and described the overwhelming feeling of "being an impostor." New NPs reported high levels of anxiety that interfered with productivity and used inordinate amounts of energy when entering client rooms and completing client encounters. New NPs also felt overwhelmed by time constraints, client complexity, and the process of surviving the day. Strategies that NPs used during the launching phase included voraciously reading textbooks and scanning online resources, consulting with a trusted colleague, and negotiating with employers for increased length of client visits during their orientation period. These strategies assisted NPs in building confidence, improving their knowledge base, and becoming more efficient in terms of improved productivity in client care.

The third role transition category, beginning approximately 6 months after initial employment as an NP, is *meeting the challenge.* During this time period, NPs became more confident and proficient in the management of client care and also expanded their awareness of and utilized their skills in management of simple office or systems issues. The subcategories in the challenge phase include increasing and gaining competence and acknowledging system problems. With repeated experiences in client care, NPs enhanced their knowledge base and became proficient in routine procedures and skills, thereby freeing time for them to assist in staff orientation, trouble-shoot system problems, serve on quality improvement committees, and develop educational materials or resources for client care. Employers recognize the value-added contribution that NPs bring to practices through their leadership skills in system and practice management initiatives.

The final category of NP role transition is *broadening the perspective.* In this phase, NPs broaden their scope of practice and not only manage a wide range of client care, but engage in system management and professional role development. The NP is able to accept positive feedback and engages in quality improvement activities and system-wide enhancements. The NP confidently enters client rooms and manages complex multifaceted health care problems in reasonably short appointment time frames and manages on-call issues adeptly. Strategies that were used to build confidence in practice were to consult with colleagues, to attend journal clubs with peers where they could review complex client cases, and to negotiate additional time for office consultation during orientation.

In the NP role, individuals are accountable for their decisions in the management of client care. They are responsible for follow-up, diagnostic test interpretation, consultation evaluation, and coordination and management of client care. New practitioners experience periods of uncertainty about their clinical decision making coupled with time constraints, productivity expectations, and economic implications of practice patterns. Attributes that contribute to effectiveness and smooth role transition in the NP role include assertiveness, autonomy, and clear decision making about clinical problems. Those NPs who feel confident, independent, and enjoy making independent clinical judgments tend to be more successful in implementing the NP role (Hawkins & Thibodeau, 1994).

The most successful NPs incorporate the role of case manager in their everyday clinical practice. They recognize the value and power of managing their clients through the health care continuum and assisting individuals with attaining high-quality, cost-effective health care. NPs serve as a client's gatekeeper to health care. "Case management is a collaborative process of assessment, planning, facilitation and advocacy for options and services to meet an individual's health needs through communication and available resources to promote cost-effective outcomes" (Case Management Society of America, 2002, p. 5). A centerpiece of NP practice is the provision of holistic, humanistic care to their clients through case management, coordination, facilitation, utilization management, and discharge planning.

Coordination and *facilitation* refer to the review of services provided to avoid redundancy and to ensure that health promotion, risk reduction, and disease prevention strategies are in place. *Utilization management* includes reviews of client services, diagnostic facilities, and insurance resources to acquire the necessary diagnostics and treatments at reasonable costs. *Discharge planning* is the process of engaging family and community resources to provide essential services and respite care to clients with chronic illnesses. NPs establish community-based care management with clients to capitalize on available internal and external resources, thus establishing long-term collaborative relationships with their clients. NPs assist the client to navigate the health care system to obtain the necessary diagnostic tests, consultations, and treatments required for optimal health and outcomes. They encourage their clients to capitalize on their inner strengths and available resources to implement holistic self-care strategies that are culturally sensitive and individualized. They incorporate the available social support system into the plan of care to enhance successful integration of healthy lifestyle changes and implementation of treatment interventions. By focusing on the client's functional health status, individualizing care with integration of social supports, a holistic, mutually agreed-on plan is set forth. The client becomes a partner in care instead of an individual to whom strategies are dictated and from whom compliance is expected. NP students develop a holistic framework of practice through the socialization, guidance, encouragement, and inspiration of experienced faculty, practicing NPs, and mentors.

What type of socialization processes do nurse practitioners experience?

Socialization into the NP role and practice is a two-part process beginning with a formal educational program and continuing into the work environment. The socialization process assists NP students and practitioners in "feeling real" and having confidence in their practice style. By taking courses and practicing, either as a student or practitioner, clinical experience assists with integrating content into practice and improves confidence. Role courses in NP programs provide the knowledge base and the beginning elements of role socialization for practice. The advanced practice nursing role components of educator, clinician, consultant, administrator, and researcher are covered in detail in such programs. Discussions of scope of practice, licensure requirements, physician collaborative agreements, quality improvement, and policy implications are basic content delivered in professional role development courses. Role content is then integrated throughout the NP program, providing the basic elements for role socialization and implementation during precepted clinical experiences.

Clinical conferences and seminars are used for discussions of role components, integration, and enactment to assist NP students in becoming comfortable with the practice requirements and standards. Student clinical work is designed to help the NP acquire the essential experiences that will lay the foundation for practice. The role of faculty is to secure safe, nurturing, supervised practice sites that will enforce confidence and assist the student in implementation of NP role components. The student is exposed to a variety of preceptors and NP faculty from different specialties and backgrounds who share real-life clinical encounters with students to enhance learning. Preceptors and NP faculty are role models for students in clinical practice (Edmunds, 2002). Faculty, preceptors, peers, and mentors provide informal and formal evaluation measures for student learning in both formative and summative formats. *Formative evaluation* strategies include feedback on papers, charting, and impromptu critiques of clinical performance, whereas *summative evaluation* is the culmination of the semester-long work in a clinical evaluation or performance appraisal. NP students and graduates alike also may seek input through a self-assessment process to determine their strengths and work on growth areas.

Self-Assessment and Professional Relationships

What self-assessment measures are useful during the transitional period?

The NP can choose from among many different mechanisms to obtain input into improving clinical practice. Faculty and preceptors often complete measurement or evaluation tools during each clinical rotation to provide information about areas of growth and excellence and areas where growth and improvement are still needed. These documents are important in the learning process and provide an opportunity to establish goals for the next semester. Clients in the clinical setting and staff members often provide valuable verbal information that assist you in working collaboratively and expanding your skills.

There are also evaluation measures for clinical practice that you may use for self-assessment. Two assessment measures have been developed by Thibodeau and Hawkins, nurse researchers, to measure successful NP practice. Thibodeau and Hawkins (1989) developed the Confidence Self-Assessment Scale, which is composed of 65 questions to evaluate nurse practitioners' level of confidence regarding their knowledge, skills, nursing orientation, and enactment of role components. This questionnaire can be used by students or experienced practitioners. This self-assessment provides feedback about areas in which the NP feels comfortable and skilled and identifies areas for growth opportunities. See Appendix 2-1 for the Confidence Self-Assessment Scale.

Another useful assessment tool was also developed by Thibodeau and Hawkins (1989). The Attitudes and Values Scale was designed to assist NPs to better understand their values on NP knowledge, skills, role components, and professional nursing practice. This useful tool for assessing your nursing values is found in Appendix 2-2.

What is network building?

Network building is a simple and fun process. You have built networks of friends, acquaintances, coworkers, colleagues, and family members throughout your life. Individuals in your network can range from the beautician and gas station clerk to members of your church, professional organizations, or work environment. Diverse networks are important for building connections, information sources, and referrals for personal and professional matters (Roth, 2002). Individuals in your network play important roles in your everyday life and work activities. Networking is an important vehicle in building a successful career. *Networking* is the process of utilizing the contacts in your network to advance your professional interests and promote your career (Roth, 2002). Successful networking involves open, confident, engaging conversations with individuals. Alerting individuals in your network that you are looking for employment can give you leads to potential job opportunities. Therefore, the larger, more diverse, and varied your network is, the more your opportunities for gathering information about potential job offers are enhanced.

During your educational program and clinical experiences, it is important to begin building a network of individuals that can provide you with resources, connections, and potential job referrals. Nurse practitioner faculty are often contacted by employers looking for NP job applicants that meet the requirements for their employment setting. Faculty then contact individuals who are looking for a new employment opportunity or who are engaged in a job search to alert them to the potential job. Faculty members may not contact you if they do not know that you are actively seeking employment or what type of job opening you are trying to secure. Another important network connection is the clinical preceptors to whom you are assigned for clinical experiences during your graduate program. Cultivating strong positive relationships with your preceptors enhances and expands your employment network. During your clinical rotations, your preceptors are able to evaluate your strengths and areas for growth. They know firsthand your abilities and have strong credibility with employers. Preceptors may also be seeking to employ an NP. They will be able to assess your clinical, interpersonal, and work style and may choose to offer you an employment opportunity.

A strategy to improve your opportunity to secure a job is to provide names of potential preceptors to your faculty members for your clinical placements. If you know of a practice that is interested in hiring a new NP you may increase your chances of employment by completing your clinical placement in this setting. The individuals who are making the hiring decisions will be able to evaluate your performance, and you can also use part of the clinical experience to increase your familiarity with the practice requirements.

Another important networking source is the individuals you work with in your current employment situation. Peer employees, managers, and physicians may have networks or connections regarding NP jobs or potential new job creation opportunities. If they know you are close to completing your program and seeking NP employment, they may be a useful source of information and potential job opportunities.

An often overlooked networking source is the services that are provided by professional organization membership. Professional organization member services frequently include networking opportunities, continuing educational opportunities, notices of job opportunities, and journals that carry paid advertisements for job openings. These services can provide valuable links and contacts to enhance your job search. Another valuable networking opportunity is the development of a relationship with a mentor. Mentors provide support and guidance to their protégés throughout their careers and offer them important tips, access to established networks, and resources that protégés would not have developed at that point in their careers.

What is a mentor?

Mentoring occurs in nursing programs and can occur in all stages of a nursing career. *Mentors* are individuals who possess expertise in a specific area or specialty who selflessly provide a safe and supportive environment to guide and coach individuals in their education or work environment. In addition to expertise, mentors provide social support, resources, and networks to assist less experienced nurses in their growth process and skill development as their careers progress (Andrews & Wallis, 1999; Bedini & Anderson, 2003). Mentors are often thought of as confidants, individuals who serve as counselors and advisers. They supervise and guide individuals in their academic journey or work (Dutton, 2003). Over time, the relationship may develop into a supportive, trusting, and mutual friendship that is beneficial to both individuals.

An effective mentor is one who is open and approachable, who interacts effectively, and is a positive role model. Characteristics of mentors are generosity, competence, self-confidence, and openness to mutuality, whereas the characteristics of protégés include being able to take the initiative, committing to a career trajectory, having a strong self-identity, and being open to mutuality (Owens & Patton, 2003). A mentor is self-assured, has good problem-solving skills, is client, is a good listener, shares dreams, ideas, and professional opinions, encourages independence, provides opportunities, and sets high, but achievable goals. Mentors enjoy working with protégés who are self-starters, who listen and communicate effectively, take risks, accepts constructive feedback, and share openly.

Many disciplines such as business assign and encourage formal mentoring relationships. In nursing, however, mentoring relationships often develop informally, although in many places employers may try to offer some type of mentorship. Mentoring relationships are valuable and can help students secure successful contacts, career opportunities, and networks. Mentoring relationships can be valuable to both parties because they offer a collaborative sense of teamwork, which can develop into strong friendships and advance the careers of all parties involved. Mentoring assists both parties with developing innovative, creative ideas, challenges each others' abilities, and stretches each person's imagination and thinking (Owens & Patton, 2003). As the relationship progresses, it provides the setting to develop unique, novel research projects, educational materials, and practice innovations. Mentors and protégés work closely together and are often able to be more productive and provide leadership in employment settings, professional organizations, and community settings.

How do I find a mentor?

Many expert practitioners, educators, and administrators are willing to serve as mentors. If you are interested in developing a mentoring relationship with an experienced nurse, you should identify an individual who you feel is a good professional role model. Introduce yourself and engage in a thoughtful conversation. Make contact with the person you have identified as a potential mentor and communicate frequently. Work with this individual on a project or an assignment. By focusing on a common problem or project to be completed, each of you will provide knowledge and support that will assist in establishing trust and openness in the developing relationship. Frequent, meaningful contact that is productive and goal oriented solidifies the mentoring relationship. Just as in any strong relationship, there will be tense times as well as productive moments. It will take work and time to continue your meaningful partnership. Working in this close, nurturing relationship will be energizing and move your career forward as well as assisting your mentor in his or her professional work.

If you cannot locate a mentor in your organization or university, do some detective work. Identify individuals in a specific area or field who you would like to meet. Contact them by e-mail or in written correspondence with a brief, but succinct message and request a meeting. Before you meet the person, prepare a list of questions that you want to cover in the specified time period of the meeting. This provides the framework for future correspondence and work. Make sure that you send a thank-you note as a follow-up.

A mentoring relationship is a professional partnership established to support and nurture each others' professional goals and careers. Remember, mentors will reap many rewards from the people they mentor, but they will also experience increased demands as they guide the protégé's learning

(Billett, 2003). Strategies that foster nursing mentoring relationships include being willing to go beyond routine expectations, offering to take on a new assignment or project, finding time to enjoy the new relationship, communicating creatively and frequently, being courteous and respectful of time commitments, and allowing flexibility in goal setting (Owens & Patton, 2003). Showing interest and willingness to seriously engage in student-faculty collegial relationships as well as working closely with a preceptor or seasoned manager or clinician in a work setting to learn and integrate advance practice nursing content are two opportunities that will improve the likelihood of developing a mentor-protégé relationship. Becoming active in a professional organization and meeting experienced nurses is another avenue to pursue when looking for a mentor.

Marketing Tools

What is a portfolio?

Competition for an NP position may be challenging in some geographical areas in the United States and the world. To maximize the possibility of securing a desirable position in a tight job market, you will need to be prepared and clearly understand your value and worth. Marketing yourself to potential employers is the first step in a successful job search. Many different strategies can be used to aid you in your job search, but they all require preparation and planning. Marketing is finding out who the target audience is seeking and filling that void. Networking is critically important when searching for a job because at least 50% of jobs openings are never formally advertised. It is important to have a well-written letter and résumé to pique the interviewer's or recruiter's interest to secure an interview. A useful tool to use when marketing yourself to potential employers is a professional portfolio.

A *professional portfolio* is a compilation of information that is relevant to the NP role and job opening. It is an organized collection of materials of educational, work, and professional experiences that documents the NP's achievements and serves as a visible display of evidence to document one's career (Bowers & Jinks, 2004; Crist, Wilcox, & McCarron, 1998; Hayes, Chandler, Merriam, & King, 2002; Weinstein, 2002; Wenzel, Briggs, & Puryear, 1998). A carefully designed portfolio will demonstrate the job candidate's ability to plan, organize, select important documents, and build a case for employment (Burgess & Misener, 1997; Jackson, 2004). The portfolio is a resource in securing an NP position, making job and career changes, highlighting achievements for professional memberships, and enhancing current job opportunities. A portfolio can serve as an assessment of professional activities and provide evidence of knowledge and skills gained through continuing educational or college offerings, clinical experiences, and professional and political involvement. This compilation of materials can be used for self-reflection and directed learning to enhance career mobility and self-development. It pulls together your professional accomplishments and provides a showcase for colleagues, potential employers, and potential partnerships and provides background information should you choose to pursue running for office within a professional organization.

A portfolio also serves the functions of documenting competence and showing continued progress, updating, and knowledge in a specialty (Meister, Heath, Andrews, & Tingen, 2002). It helps present you in the best possible manner by providing evidence of knowledge and skills directly related to the desired position.

How do I develop a portfolio?

A professional portfolio can be developed as you progress through your NP program or it can be designed after graduation. A professional portfolio is a powerful marketing tool. This is your opportunity to create a diverse package of excellent work samples to illustrate your knowledge, skills, organizational ability, and clinical experiences. The components of a portfolio vary according to individual preferences and career trajectory, but often include a résumé, listing of clinical rotations, copy of the appropriate state's nurse practice act and professional scope and standards of practice, an NP job description, examples of scholarly work, depiction of the financial value of NP services to the practice, completed student clinical checklist with procedures, and a sample protocol. Other items that can be included are educational documentation of skills assessment, practice privileges for procedures, clinics, HMOs, or hospitals as appropriate, DEA number, and a sample prescriptive collaborative agreement, if appropriate, for your state.

Prior to designing your portfolio it is useful to engage in a self-assessment and personal inventory analysis. Make sure you take credit for important clinical experiences that you have had during your graduate program (Meredith & Tumolo, 2001). Other important components of the portfolio include awards, certifications, professional memberships and any offices that you have held, articles, abstracts, or papers presented, research experience, employment history, and community service.

Be sure to highlight those aspects of your past or present employment that show the connections of leadership aspects, client care management, and project accomplishment to the job for which you are applying. These past experiences can be a critical component of an employer's interest in your talents. Highlight those skills by providing concise, succinct statements regarding your experience not only with direct care, but with the projects and assignments you completed that encompassed teaching staff and clients; negotiating for quality improvement updates, equipment changes, or documentation refinements; effective interpersonal communication and team building; and financial management skills.

Portfolio design

Designing a portfolio is a fun and creative process. There is no one right way to develop the end product, and portfolios vary depending on individual experiences and creativity (Meister et al., 2002). Meister and colleagues recommend including a table of contents with accomplishments that include professional introduction, clinical, scholarship/research, and service accomplishments. Box 2-1 provides a sample table of contents for a professional portfolio that showcases the NPs knowledge and skills.

The documents should be placed in a high-quality binder, notebook, or other repository, approximately 1 to 3 inches deep and large enough to hold $8\frac{1}{2}$-by-11-inch typed pages. Careful attention should be paid to proper spelling, grammar, and legibility of each page. A heavy outer, protective covering is recommended for protection and appearance. First impressions of the professional portfolio cover and binder will influence the reviewer's reaction to

---

Box 2-1 Professional Portfolio Table of Contents

Section 1: Professional Introduction

Narrative introduction (may be letter format)
Résumé
References (two or three written references)

Section 2: Clinical Accomplishments

Clinical rotations or practice
Educational or administrative experience
Clinical checklist
Sample protocol
Certification and/or license
DEA number
Sample prescriptive collaborative agreement
Privileges or credentials for procedures, clinics, HMOs or hospitals
Medicare and Medicaid numbers
Statement of financial value to the practice

Section 3: Professional Accomplishments

Publications and presentations
Awards and honors
Community service
Committee leadership and membership
Scholarly work
State practice act
Professional scope and standards of practice
Job description

the content. An organized portfolio makes the reviewer's job simple and guides the individual through the content, simply by showcasing those portfolio components that are pertinent to the desired job.

Professional cards

Business cards are another potential marketing tool as you graduate and begin networking and looking for an NP position. A business card should include your name, credentials, title, address, telephone and fax numbers, and e-mail address. Providing a business card to colleagues, individuals at professional meetings, recruiters, and potential employers assists with providing a quick reference for your personal contact information.

Strategies for marketing yourself

Many strategies can be used to market yourself to a practice or strengthen your standing in the practice where you already are employed. Listed here are a few strategies that can help you market yourself:

- *Respond flexibly to ambiguity.* When interviewing and negotiating for a new position, be flexible and creative in salary and benefit negotiations. Be willing to take on new assignments and learn new skills.
- *Be a change agent.* When you notice that a system is not working in your practice, offer to work on the project with key stakeholders to solve the problem. Your leadership skills and willingness to contribute to the practice will be noticed and rewarded.
- *Be a positive role model.* In every practice there will be challenges that arise, whether it is a difficult client situation, staff conflict, or difficult working conditions, you can model positive behavior and assist with conflict resolution.
- *Problem solve.* You have the opportunity to demonstrate proficiency in solving minor and major problems in your practice. Common problem areas in practices include lack of consistency in tracking systems, problems with telephone triage systems, inefficiencies in clinical staff, conflicts among staff members, and fairness in distribution of office work. Helping to improve any of these systems will demonstrate your leadership skills.
- *Communicate effectively.* Taking the time to communicate effectively by e-mail, written correspondence, or verbal interaction will pay large dividends. Take care to write e-mails that are clear, courteous, and accurate. E-mails can be copied, forwarded, and distributed widely without your authorization. So it is important that they be well written and professional. You will also be required to write referral letters to specialists to describe the client problem(s) and to request evaluation services. Verbal interactions are equally important because 70% to 90% of the message can be interpreted from your facial expression, body language, and tone of voice. Being client,

taking the time to listen, and responding in a thoughtful manner will foster positive communication and build friendships and partnerships.

- *Be a self-starter.* By careful observation, you will notice many activities that need to be done. You have the option of doing your designated work activities or, during slower periods, working on a project that benefits your practice. In many practices, educational materials need updating or organizing. Other activities may be assisting with medication assistance program form completion, revising an office form, or assisting with orienting a staff member.
- *Nurture interpersonal relationships.* Once you land a job, the work has only just begun. An important aspect of any position is the development of relationships. Fostering supportive relationships with staff, administrators, and the other providers is important for collegial relations. Strong relationships build teamwork and members who are more willing to work together to solve problems. Often colleagues and staff share valuable information about practice patterns, client information, and office functioning that you might not be aware but that can help you practice more effectively. You can share your expertise with others to strengthen linkages as well.
- *Build skills.* Continue to expand your knowledge base and skill level to enhance your clinical practice. By increasing your skill level and ability to perform a variety of procedures, you will be able to expand your client base. By performing suturing, casting, or mole removal, you will be able to provide comprehensive, convenient care for your client. The procedures you perform will also be a source of revenue for the practice.
- *Show enthusiasm.* Successful individuals often smile, acknowledge their colleagues' contributions, and are interested in the work they are doing. They demonstrate enthusiasm when working on new projects and are willing to take on new challenges, complete complex client visits, and work collaboratively with staff and peers alike.
- *Cost-effective measures.* With capitated payment systems, Medicare and Medicaid reimbursement, as well as other forms of negotiated fees, many practices are looking for strategies to hold costs down or eliminate them. Some practices are requiring increased productivity to help the bottom line or sustainability of the practice. By assessing the office environment you can determine areas to potentially eliminate costs and identify ways to streamline systems or bring revenue to the practice.
- *Set personal and professional goals.* First you must determine what your personal goals are in order to establish your professional goals. Once you have completed this task, you can embark on your career trajectory. By determining your long-range goals, you can establish strategies to reach them. Each position you accept and professional activity that you engage in will then build a path to your long-range goal.
- *Maintain a positive appearance.* Dress for success! Depending on the event or occasion, you will want to dress professionally. When presenting a policy, procedure, poster, or paper you will want to have a nice suit or skirt and

blouse or slacks and blouse combination. Casual dress may be appropriate for some activities.

- *Don't whine.* Everyone complains about a job once in a while, but constant complaining becomes annoying. Individuals who are negative often become isolated from the other workers and administrators. If a problem arises, instead of whining, put forth an idea or strategy that could potentially alleviate the situation. Individuals who are problem solvers are respected for their knowledge, skill, and insight.

SUMMARY

There is a transitional period as students graduate from an NP program and begin work in their first NP position. As the new NP progresses through the four stages in the transitional period, they develop confidence and comfort in their new role. Being proactive and finding a mentor, joining a journal club, and reading voraciously assists in the transition to a seasoned NP. The socialization process is important for an NP's growth in professional practice. Developing professional relationships, building a network, and choosing a mentor assists in the clinical, scholarly, and professional advanced practice activities. The documentation of professional practice through a portfolio is effective in marketing yourself and identifying areas for future growth. Marketing is an important tool to showcase your abilities and accomplishments, as well as attracting new clients to your practice and portraying a positive image of nurse practitioners.

References

Andrews, M., & Wallis, M. (1999). Mentorship in nursing: A literature review. *Journal of Advanced Nursing, 29*(1), 201-207.

Bedini, L.A., & Anderson, D.M. (2003). The benefits of formal mentoring for practitioners in therapeutic recreation. *Therapeutic Recreation Journal, 37*(3), 240-255.

Billett, S. (2003). Workplace mentors: Demands and benefits. *Journal of Workplace Learning, 15*(3), 105-113.

Bowers, S.J., & Jinks, A.M. (2004). Issues surrounding professional portfolio development for nurses. *British Journal of Nursing, 13*(3), 155-159.

Brown, M.A., & Olshansky, E.F. (1997). From limbo to legitimacy: A theoretical model of the transition to the primary care nurse practitioner role. *Nursing Research, 46*(1), 46-51.

Burgess, S.E., & Misener, T.R. (1997). The professional portfolio: An advanced practice nurse job search marketing tool. *Clinical Excellence for Nurse Practitioners, 1*(7), 467-471.

Case Management Society of America. (2002). *Standards of practice for case management.* Little Rock:, AR: Author.

Crist, P., Wilcox, B.L., & McCarron, K. (1998). Transitional portfolios: Orchestrating our professional competence. *American Journal of Occupational Therapy 52*(9), 729-736.

Dutton, C. (2003). Mentoring: The contextualization of learning-mentor, protégé and organizational gain in higher education. *Education & Training, 45*(1), 22-29.

Edmunds, M. (2002). Market to the media. *The Nurse Practitioner,* 27(3), 72.

Gooden, J.M., & Jackson, E. (2004). Attitudes of registered nurses toward nurse practitioners. *Journal of the American Academy of Nurse Practitioners, 16*(8), 360-364.

Hawkins, J., & Thibodeau, J. (1994). 25+ and going strong: Nurse practitioners and nursing practice. *Journal of the American Academy of Nurse Practitioners, 6*(11), 525-531.

Hayes, E., Chandler, G., Merriam, D., & King, C. (2002). The master's portfolio: Validating a career in advanced practice nursing. *Journal of the American Academy of Nurse Practitioners, 14*(3), 119-125.

Heitz, L.J., Steiner, S.H. & Burman, M.E. (2004). RN to FNP: A qualitative study of role transition. *Journal of Nursing Education, 43*(9), 416-420.

Jackson, R. (2004). Behold the power of a portfolio. *Nursing Management, 35,* 12-14.

Kelly, N., & Mathews, M. (2001). The transition to first position as nurse practitioner. *Journal of Nursing Education, 40*(4), 156-162.

Meister, L., Heath, J., Andrews, J., & Tingen, M.S. (2002). Professional nursing portfolios: A global perspective. *MEDSURG Nursing, 11*(4), 177-182.

Meredith, P., & Tumolo, J. (2001). Landing your first NP position: Your RN experience does count! *Advance for Nurse Practitioners,* pp. 73-74, 94.

Owens, J.K., & Patton, J.G. (2003). Take a chance on nursing mentorships: Enhance leadership with this win-win strategy. *Nursing Education Perspectives, 24*(4), 198-204.

Rich, E.R., Jorden, M.E., & Taylor, C.J. (2001). Assessing successful entry into nurse practitioner practice: A literature review, *Journal of the New York State Nurses Association, 32*(2), 14-18.

Roth, M. (2002). How networking works. *Career World, 31*(2), 18-19.

Thibodeau, J.A., & Hawkins, J.W. (1989). Nurse practitioners: Factors affecting role performance. *Nurse Practitioner, 14*(12), 47, 50-52.

Thibodeau, J.A., & Hawkins, J.W. (1994). Moving toward a nursing model in advanced practice. *Western Journal of Nursing Research, 16*(2), 205-218.

Weinstein, S.M. (2002). A nursing portfolio: Documenting your professional journey. *Journal of Infusion Nursing, 25*(6), 357-364.

Wenzel, L.S., Briggs, K.L., & Puryear, B.L. (1998). Portfolio: Authentic assessment in the age of the curriculum revolution. *Journal of Nursing Education, 37*(5), 208-212.

3

Corresponding and Interviewing with Potential Employers

Jean Nagelkerk

Preparing for Your Job Search

Effective correspondence with potential employers is critical when marketing and securing an NP position. Today's health care provider job market is competitive and demands skilled preparation for employment searches. Careful attention to the preparation and design of a letter of introduction and professional résumé that convey both nursing and medical knowledge, skills, procedural capability, and specialty expertise is essential to securing a job interview. Developing documents that highlight your professional achievements and promote your career provides a competitive edge over other applicants for available primary, acute, and tertiary employment opportunities. The introductory materials demonstrate your organizational skills and showcase your professional and educational accomplishments in a succinct, but clear and descriptive format (Teasdale, 2002). These materials should be interesting, precise, attractive, and readable.

How do I prepare for a job search?

You have worked hard to earn the credential of nurse practitioner and know that NPs provide value-added services to communities. Nurse practitioners provide quality, cost-effective care to clients and emphasize health promotion, disease prevention, and risk reduction. In addition, NPs practice holistic client care that incorporates nursing theory and clinical experience along with diagnosing, treatment planning, and counseling to improve the health of clients (Meredith, 2001). NPs have knowledge and skills that are unique to their advanced practice nursing role, and part of effective marketing is the ability to articulate this role to potential employers. Besides describing the NP role in a job interview, you must also define your practice and explain financial reimbursement and prescriptive authority as they relate to NP practice in your state.

The first step in the job search is to conduct a self-assessment of your educational and clinical experience and professional achievements. Document your registered nurse (RN) experience. Highlight RN skills that are central to the advanced practice role such as leading family and team conferences; delegating tasks and making assignments; collecting client histories; performing comprehensive and focused physical examinations; administering oral, intramuscular, and parenteral medications; drawing blood; assessing; and providing wound care. All clinical rotations completed during your NP program should be documented as experience (Hauri, 1994). Illustrate the complexity of the clinical rotations by identifying the type of practice (i.e., family practice, internal medicine, gynecology, dermatology) and length of time spent in the clinical placement. For practicing NPs, include volunteer experiences at health clinics; temporary, part-time, and full-time clinical experiences with type of specialty practice or populations; skills; and length of time practicing in the health center or organization. In addition to clinical experiences, include professional activities that demonstrate your professional commitment, writing skills, scholarly work, and committee activity.

What materials do I need for a job search?

To document your clinical experience and professional accomplishments, you will want to develop a portfolio that includes a letter of introduction, curriculum vitae or résumé, and samples of professional works and accomplishments. By using a software program to design your job search materials, you will be able to customize them for each position to which you apply.

Introductory Letter. A cover letter is a formal business document that introduces you to potential employers and piques their interest in your résumé or curriculum vitae. The cover letter is the first contact with potential employers. It should be memorable and create interest in your skills and talents. Begin the cover letter by personalizing it to the individual who will be screening job applicants.

Use the correct name, credentials, and title of the individual. Pay special attention to the correct spelling of names and accuracy of titles because potential employers may feel that lack of attention to detail will be exhibited in work habits as well.

The cover letter should be three or four single-spaced paragraphs with double spacing between each paragraph. The first paragraph should provide an introduction, purpose of inquiry, and brief description of how you learned of and reason you applied for the advertised position. The second and third paragraphs are your opportunity to market and sell yourself to the employer. This is the place where you should expand on significant contributions and experiences identified in your résumé or curriculum vitae and make them relevant to the job for which you are applying. If appropriate, write a brief statement of why you desire to change employment. For many it is a transition from a registered nurse position to a nurse practitioner role, but for others it may be a desire to expand your role or to specialize. These paragraphs should make the employer want to interview you. The final paragraph provides a summary and a statement of what you plan to do. The letter should be no more than one to one and a half pages in 12-point type and it should be printed on the same quality bond paper as your résumé or curriculum vitae.

The use of employer letterhead should be reserved for scholarship or grant applications and should not be used for NP job searches. It is a good idea to ask a faculty member or esteemed colleague to review your cover letter for format, content, and grammar before mailing it to a prospective employer. The cover letter provides the first impression to individuals in an organization and spelling errors or grammar problems may decrease your opportunity for an interview. It, along with the résumé or curriculum vitae, is the tool that will secure an interview and provide the opportunity to market your skills. Box 3-1 provides an example of a cover letter.

Résumé or Curriculum Vitae? There are major differences between a résumé and curriculum vitae; however, the purpose of both is the same: to obtain a job interview. A *résumé* is a brief written statement of your education, job experiences, and professional achievements. It is succinct and comprises one to two pages of information (Harper, 1999). A résumé is often used for application to clinical positions. In contrast, a *curriculum vitae* is a document that is composed of one's career experiences. It is longer, more detailed, and structured to describe credentials, education, and professional experiences, activities, and scholarly work (Hinck, 1997). Curriculum vitae are often requested for academic openings, consulting, research, grants, awards, and corporate positions (O'Conner, 1999).

Résumé. The major categories of information that should be included in a résumé are listed in Box 3-2. A résumé should include your name address, and phone number. This information should be placed at the top of your résumé. The second item should be your professional objective stated in one or two succinct sentences. The objective should be tailored to the prospective job. The third section includes your qualifications for the position you are applying

Box 3-1 Example of a Cover Letter

August 5, 2005

Nurse Alley Bristle, RN, MSN
Human Resource Recruiter
Palm Springs Medical Center
2487 Palm Drive
Palm Springs, California 19877

Dear Ms. Bristle,

I am interested in applying for the family nurse practitioner position that was advertised in the Palm Springs Centennial. I work as a registered nurse in the Emergency Department at St. Izabelle Hospital in Sacramento, California, and I am in my final semester of the Family Nurse Practitioner Program at Grand Lodge University.

In my 10 years of emergency room experience, I have provided direct care that includes completing comprehensive and focused assessments, administering medication, leading teams, and working as the evening charge nurse. In the Family Nurse Practitioner Program, I completed clinical rotations in family practice, dermatology, orthopedics, obstetrics and gynecology, emergency, and psychiatry. The skills that I am proficient in are casting, splinting, suturing, reading electrocardiographs, and conducting basic X-ray interpretations.

Professional activities include membership in the Academy of Nurse Practitioners, the Sacramento Nurse Practitioner Journal Club, and a member of St. Izabelle's Emergency Room Quality Initiatives Committee. Other professional activities include co-authorship of an article on diabetes care published in the *Nurse Practitioner Journal* and recipient of the Award for Excellence in Clinical Practice from St. Izabelle's Hospital.

My enclosed résumé provides further details about my skills, clinical experiences, and educational preparation. I look forward to hearing from you to discuss the family nurse practitioner position and my qualifications. I may be reached at my current address, by telephone at (301)555-8767, or by e-mail at *halspej@oil.com*. I look forward to hearing from you.

Sincerely,

Janice Halspen

Janice Halspen, RN, BSN
9842 Triston Ave.
Sacramento, California 29876

Box 3-2 Major Categories for a Résumé

1. Name, address, and phone number
2. Professional objective
3. Qualifications
4. Educational accomplishments
5. Professional employment
6. Certification and licensure information
7. Professional activities and memberships/award/honors/publications
8. References

for. In this section, include the completion of your NP program, clinical experience, and skills. The fourth section should be your educational accomplishments beginning with the highest level of education. Each entry should include the college or university attended with address, degree awarded, and graduation date.

The fifth section should list your professional employment. The employment section should be structured in reverse chronological order, beginning with your present or most recent position. List all nursing positions and any other employment that contributes to the present job opportunity. Include the employer's name, address, and telephone number, dates of employment, and a brief description of job responsibilities. The sixth section is certification and licensure information. In this section, identify the certifying body, specialty certification, and the certification period dates. Include your registered nurse licensure information as well. The seventh section should identify professional activities and memberships. Include the name of the organizations you belong to with dates of membership and be sure to include any offices that you have been appointed or elected to in the organization. This section is also used for including any awards, honors, or publications.

The final section is for references. You may write "available upon request" or you may list two or three references. If you choose to list references, make sure you have checked with the individuals listed and obtained their support. It is important to have the correct spelling of the name, title, address, phone number, and e-mail address of individuals willing to serve as a reference for you. Employers are busy and do not have time to track down your references if the data you provide is invalid. An example of a résumé is shown in Box 3-3.

Curriculum vitae. A curriculum vitae (CV) is used to showcase your professional activities and accomplishments. Unlike the résumé, a curriculum vitae has no page limitations and no specific rules for format and content. However, general guidelines for development of the CV do exist as well as a guide for the appropriate length of the document. As a general guide, the CV should be no longer than four or five pages for a bachelor's applicant, five or six pages for a master's applicant, six or seven pages for a doctoral applicant, and seven or more pages for an experienced educator, clinician, administrator, or researcher. The length guideline can be modified based on the intended use

Box 3-3 Example of a Résumé

Jennifer Sampski, RN, BSN, MSN, APRN, BC

3462 Meadowbrook Street
Grand Rapids, MI 49503
Phone: (616)555-8246
E-mail: Jennif21@webaddress.com

Professional Objective

To provide quality patient care to patients of all ages, races, and states of health as a family nurse practitioner in a primary care setting.

Qualifications

Successful completion of a family nurse practitioner program. Primary care clinical rotations include Meadows Family Practice, Grand Rapids Health Center, Dermatology Associates, Women's Care Center, Orthopedic Care, and St. Mary's Emergency Room.

Education

University of Michigan Ann, Arbor, Michigan	MSN	2005
Nazareth College Kalamazoo, Michigan	BSN	2000

Professional Experience

Staff RN, Nursing Resource Pool (2003-2005)

- Staff nurse in Adult Critical Care at Barkley Hospital, Ann Arbor, Michigan.
- Member of the nursing resource pool professional practice committee and preceptor for undergraduate nursing students.

Staff RN, Intensive Care Unit at Cedar Hospital (2000-2002)

- Staff nurse at Cedar Hospital, Kalamazoo, Michigan.
- Member of the Resuscitation Team and Ventricular Device Core Team.
- Preceptor for undergraduate nursing students and for new nurses.
- Conducted inservices for staff.
- Co-author of the standard of care for the patient with an aortic aneurysm.

Certification and Licensure

- Certified as a Family Nurse Practitioner, American Nurses Credentialing Center (2005-2009)
- Michigan State Board of Nursing Registered Nurse Licensure (2000-2009)

Professional Activities

- Michigan Nurses Association/American Nurses Association (2000-Present)

References

- Professional references are available upon request.

Box 3-4 Major Categories of a Curriculum Vitae

1. Name, address, and phone number
2. Professional objective
3. Educational experiences
4. Employment history
5. Certification and licensure
6. Professional memberships
7. Professional service
8. Research activities
9. Awards and honors
10. Professional presentations
11. Publications
12. Community service
13. Continuing education
14. References

for the CV, and the information presented should be modified for the specific activity. There are many uses for a CV, but historically they have been used most often for application to academic positions at universities. More recently, CVs have been used as career documentation to apply for career advancements, committee positions, awards, scholarships, or grants. Box 3-4 identifies the major categories of a curriculum vitae.

As with the résumé, the first item on your document should be your name, credentials, address, telephone and fax numbers, and e-mail address. This is the first information that a potential employer will see and hopefully remember. The second item is the professional objective. This statement should be specific and tailored to the position you are seeking. The third section is a listing of your educational experiences including the college or university, inclusive dates of attendance, city and state of the educational institution, degree awarded, and honor designation if applicable. Grade point average is not expected, but and, if it is important, can be conveyed in the interview. The high school attended and year of graduation need not be included in the CV. The fourth section is the employment history. This section is important and demonstrates career advancement, types of experiences, and skills. Beginning with reverse chronological order, list your present employment with dates, address, position title, employment status (part or full time), and a description of job responsibilities. Military experience may be included in this section or be listed in its own section.

Remember to note dates and activities for any employment gap so that employers do not begin to speculate about what might have happened in your career. Indicate specific activities such as attending graduate school or taking personal leave to raise family, care for elderly parents, or travel. *Gap years,* for instance, when taking one or more years off to travel, raise children, or attend school, are becoming more popular and acceptable. The fifth section is a listing of your certificates or licenses. Be specific with the name of the certifying agency and specialty certification. Also include your RN and any other licenses. The sixth section is professional memberships. This section includes membership in local, regional, national or international organizations. The seventh section lists professional service. Examples in this category include offices held in organizations or committee or task force membership.

The eighth section of a CV lists the research activities that you have completed including your master's thesis and if applicable your doctoral dissertation. Provide detailed information on the title of the research, funding sources, and agency that supported your work. The ninth section is for awards and honors. Include local, regional, national, and international awards with dates and specific titles of the awards and their sponsoring organizations. Scholarships, research or teaching assistant positions, or community service awards should all be documented. The tenth category is for professional presentations. Paper and poster presentations should be included with date, title of presentation, sponsoring organization, and city and state of the conference. These should be placed in reverse chronological order. The eleventh section includes all publications. List all publications that have been accepted and are in press and those published. Document the author, year, title, journal, and page numbers in reverse chronological order.

The twelfth section is community service. In this section, include nursing-related community volunteering. Teaching health-related educational programs, raising money for community programs, leading or coordinating health-related work groups, and setting policies or procedures related to health care issues should all be included in this section. Section thirteen is continuing education. This section can become very long and exhaustive, so it is important to list only the major conferences or those that highlight the skills you are trying to illustrate to a potential employer. Typically, only the last 5 years of continuing education events are included. The conference title, dates, sponsoring organization, and location of the conference should be recorded. The final section lists your references. It is appropriate to indicate that references will be made available upon request—this is your preference. You may choose to include them on the CV or wait until the potential employer contacts you to provide them. At times, applicants may not want their employer to know they are seeking alternative employment opportunities and you may choose to wait until you are a finalist candidate before alerting your supervisor to a job opportunity that you are seeking. An example of curriculum vitae is shown in Box 3-5.

What Not to Include on a Résumé or Curriculum Vitae. Personal information such as age, marital status, religion, health status, and number of children should not be included on a résumé. Do not add extraneous information to your résumé; it is the first impression you will make with your employer. Be sure to review, double check, and have a trusted colleague review your résumé for typing errors, incorrect spelling, poor grammar, and improper punctuation. Do not use thin, colored paper or paper other than $8\frac{1}{2}$ by 11 inches in size; do

Box 3-5 Example of a Curriculum Vitae

Samantha Ann Rekus

459 Gambus Street
Madison, Wisconsin 48787
Phone: (813)555-9477
E-mail: Same@itv.com

Professional Objective

To provide superior quality patient care to adult patients in a rural health
care setting.

Education

Educational Setting	Degree	Date
University of Wisconsin Oshkosh, Wisconsin	MSN	2005
University of Arizona Tucson, Arizona	BSN	2000
Bronson Hospital School of Nursing Kalamazoo, Michigan	Diploma	1990

Employment History

Organization	Position	Date
St. Lucy Medical Center Oshkosh, Wisconsin	Charge nurse	2000-2005
University Hospital Tucson, Arizona	Staff nurse	1990-1999
Bronson Hospital Kalamazoo, Michigan	Nurse aide	1987-1989

Certification and Licensure

- Certified as an adult nurse practitioner, American Nurses Association Credentialing Center (2005-2009)
- Licensed as a registered nurse, Wisconsin State Board of Nursing (2005-2009)

Professional Memberships

- American Nurses Association
- Wisconsin Nurses Association
- Association of Critical Care Nurses
- Oshkosh Nurse Practitioner Journal Club

Professional Service

- Delegate for Lakeshore Chapter of the Wisconsin Nurses Association (2003-2005)
- Nomination Committee Member for the Association of Critical Care Nurses (2000-2005)
- Treasurer for the Oshkosh Nurse Practitioner Journal Club (2005-2007)

Continued

Box 3-5　Example of a Curriculum Vitae—cont'd

Research Activities

- Caring for the Care Giver: Supporting Critical Care Nurses. Thesis. 2005.

Awards and Honors

- Excellence in Clinical Practice, April 9, 2003; awarded by St. Lucy Medical Center
- Nursing Scholarship, August 25, 2004; awarded by University of Arizona College of Nursing

Professional Presentations

- Rekus, S. (2005). Caring for the Care Giver: Supporting Full-Time Critical Care Nurses. Paper presentation at the Wisconsin Nurses Association Annual Convention.
- Rekus, S. (2005). Assessing Critically Ill Patients. Paper presentation at the Oshkosh Nurse Practitioner Journal Club.

Publications

- Rekus, S. (2005). Caring for the Care Giver: Supporting Critical Care Nurses. Unpublished master's thesis, University of Arizona, Tucson, Arizona.
- Rekus, S. (in press). Caring for the Care Giver. *Nurse Practitioner Journal*, Springfield, Connecticut.

Community Service

- Member of the Arizona Heart Association (2000-2005)
- Teach "Healthy Heart" to community members biannually (2000-2005)

Continuing Education

- Annual Meeting of the American Critical Care Association, Wixom, California, April 20-22, 2005
- American Nurses Association Annual Convention, Las Vegas, Nevada, April 1-3, 2004

Reference

Available upon request.

---

not use an extremely small or large font size. Professional appearance is important. Be sensitive to highlighting, underlining, and italicizing of words. The judicious use of these techniques can be very effective, but overdoing it can detract from the content and substance of the résumé (Hobins, 2003). Professional appearance is important for initial impressions.

Techniques that Will Make Your Résumé or Curriculum Vitae Stand Out. It is much easier to make changes to your résumé if you use a word processing program. The use of technology also provides ease in individualizing the résumé objectives, references, and other pertinent information with each job application. By using a computer, you can easily keep your résumé up to date and tailor it to the job for which you are applying. Keep the presentation of the résumé clear and concise. Do not use special fonts or characters. Follow the instructions or guidelines of the job advertisement and application form. Be sure to include key experiences and professional activities that are indicated in the advertisement. Only include those experiences that you have completed. Honesty and truthfulness are essential for a strong employer-employee relationship. Should you have employment gaps, list activities or experiences that explain this time period. Examples of activities include attending graduate school, volunteering in community agencies, or raising a family.

Other helpful guidelines for writing a good document includes using double spacing to separate sections and single spacing to write descriptions. Be consistent with headings. If you decide to capitalize the major categories and make them bold, make sure they are all treated consistently. Do not use italics in one section, then boldfaced and capitalized subheadings in another. The use of a manual for style for punctuation and grammar usage such as the latest issue of the publication manual of the American Psychological Association is valuable in designing your job application materials. Use action verbs to describe activities.

Interview Process

What should I expect during the interview process?

An interview is an opportunity for employers to learn more about you and for you to learn more about them and the employment opportunity. Your careful preparation of a letter of introduction and résumé helped you to secure the interview. Preparing for the interview is as important as your written correspondence. An interview is the first face-to-face impression that you will have with the interviewer and is central in the application process. Research shows that an employer's initial impression occurs within 60 seconds of the initial meeting (Restifo, 2002), and that employers form 80% of their opinion in the first 4 minutes of the interview (Lind, 2001). Preparation is extremely important because approximately 80% of job applicants cannot accurately and completely describe their skills or experiences at an interview (Restifo, 2002). A favorable impression will enhance communication, job opportunities, and negotiations.

Employers evaluate each job applicant to determine the match between the applicant's goals and skills and the organizational mission and work. They try to determine the best fit by assessing the applicant's skills, work ethic, leadership characteristics, and communication style during the interview. Just as potential employers are evaluating your skills and characteristics, you should be assessing the organization and environment. Is this an organization where you would like to spend a significant portion of your time? Does the organizational philosophy fit with your nursing practice framework? Is the environment supportive of continued professional growth? Are employees working together as a team and enjoying their work? What is the potential for advancement?

One of the first steps in preparing for an interview is reviewing the literature that is mailed to you when applying for a position, searching the organization's website (also a good place to search for job openings; see Box 3-6), talking with employees regarding their job experiences and satisfaction, and reviewing any rankings or awards the potential health care employer has received. The more knowledge you have of the organization, the better prepared you will be to ask questions and the more relaxed and confident you will feel. By knowing the organization and job qualifications and by rereading the job description, you can highlight, in the interview, the skills that you have which are identified as essential for the position. In your introduction, describe your education and work experience and outline your qualifications to set the stage for the interview. Remember, not everyone will have the time to read your materials prior to the interview, and if they did, they may have reviewed several applicants and, hence, may not remember your particular qualifications. A brief, but clear and informative introduction will set the stage for the interview and provide a strong initial impression.

What should I wear to the job interview?

Initial impressions are often lasting and can make a difference between getting a second interview, landing a job, or being sent a "thank you for applying for the position, but we have found a more qualified applicant" letter. Therefore, dressing appropriately for an interview is important. Make sure that you schedule your interview on a day that you are not working so that you have time to prepare yourself by dressing appropriately, reviewing or rehearsing information or questions, and scheduling enough time to travel to the interview with adequate time to find parking, locate the interview room, and relax before the interview. Mapping out your route and driving to the organization before the scheduled time will provide information on the amount of time it will take to get to the interview in a timely manner. Arriving early allows time to park and observe employees at work. Employers will be looking for dedicated, timely, organized, and prompt employees.

When planning for dress, think conservatively. Cleanliness and neatness in your personal appearance are essential for the interview. Dressing for success is important and being dressed professionally is a must. Choose an outfit that makes you feel confident and positive. A suit works well for men or women. Other dress

---

Box 3-6 Are There Websites with Job Openings?

Many professional organizations post job openings and career opportunities on their websites, in professional journals, and in newsletters. Other websites that post job opportunities include *www.monster.com, www.nurse.net, www.headhunter.net, www.medcareers.com, www.miracleworkers.com,* and the National Health Service Corporation (*http://nhsc.bhpr.hrsa.gov/*).

options for women include wearing a dress, slacks, or skirt with a blazer. Dress shoes with neutral hose or socks that are clean with low heals and a briefcase or purse is appropriate. Accessories are fine, but should not be flashy and distracting. Avoid heavy perfume or aftershave; light makeup is appropriate. Uniforms, lab coats, and scrubs should not be worn. Attention to personal hygiene such as well-groomed hair, fresh breath, light perfume or cologne, and minimal jewelry is important. Gum or candy should be saved for after the interview to avoid slurring of speech, snapping of gum, or distracting the interviewers. If possible, cover all body piercings with the exception of ear piercings; a tasteful, conservative earring is acceptable. Dressing conservatively is important so that the focus of the interview is on your skills and communication, not your dress. A carefully selected professional outfit will increase your confidence and not detract from the important contributions that you can and will make for the organization.

What questions do employers frequently ask at interviews?

First impressions are lasting, so it is important to make a good impression with the interviewers by making eye contact and firmly shaking each person's hand during the introductions. Speak clearly, and slowly, being positive and confident. When walking, stand erect with your head up, making eye contact with each individual you meet in the interview process. When sitting in a chair, sit straight back with your feet on the floor and your hands in your lap. If you find it helpful, take a notepad to jot down important information during the interview, but do not write every little detail down because such activity can be distracting to the interviewer. The notepad can also contain the questions that you would like to ask at the interview. Preparing for the interview is as important to success as is avoiding negative comments and using positive behaviors in the interview (Lind, 2001). Employers are looking to hire positive individuals who can effectively engage in team building and communication. Those who can work well with others and are positive about their work and work environment have a better chance of being offered a position. Box 3-7 lists positive behaviors that interviewers evaluate during an interview.

Always be prepared for unexpected questions that may take you off guard. Potential employers may ask these questions to see how you respond under pressure. They may ask if you know how to operate specific pieces of equipment or inquire about your ability to perform specific procedures. If you have never had the experience, say so; honesty is critical and most employers will not be alarmed if you are unable to complete a procedure or two. When answering difficult or inappropriate questions, avoid a defensive posture and tone and answer concisely. Defensive behaviors can detract from the interview and decrease the possibility of a firm job offer. Box 3-8 lists defensive behaviors to avoid. If you have not listed your current manager as a reference and are questioned about why he or she is not listed as a reference, answer the query clearly and succinctly. Avoiding negative comments and criticism of a current

Box 3-7 Positive Behaviors of the Applicant

- Being prepared for the interview
- Smiling and making eye contact
- Attending to all interviewers and their questions
- Being confident and enthusiastic
- Addressing individuals by name in a welcoming manner
- Being positive about past experiences and avoiding negative comments
- Explaining the benefits of an idea
- Listening attentively
- Not interrupting a speaker
- Being truthful and honest
- Identifying others concerns and feelings
- Being flexible
- Thanking the interviewer at the completion of the interview

or past employer and steering the conversation away from the past to the current employment opportunity and challenge will enhance communication.

The interviewers will ask you questions to get to know you better, to learn about your clinical, educational, and professional experiences, and to observe your communication style in the employment setting. You may encounter several different interview formats and styles. Some employers will have an initial interview where they will bring in several candidates to consider perhaps for 30 to 60 minutes. The purpose of this interview is to screen applicants and prepare a short list, often three to four candidates, for a formal interview. In each interview you are marketing and selling yourself by letting the interviewer(s) know why you are the best candidate for the position. Some organizations will use an initial telephone interview to screen applicants and then bring in three to four candidates in for a formal interview.

There are also several styles of formal interviews including individual, group, committee, or recruitment agency interviews. *Individual interviews*

Box 3-8 Defensive Behaviors

- Inattentiveness
- Loud, terse answers
- Overreacting to questions or stress
- Failure to disclose real feelings
- Mismanagement of an issue
- Improper disclosure of ideas
- Poor use of questions
- Being disrespectful or sarcastic
- Lack of preparation for the interview
- Inappropriate gestures or piercing eye contact

often occur in private practices where the provider is hiring an individual to expand his or her practice. The individual who owns the practice takes responsibility for interviewing and making the hiring decision. *Group interviews* include key individuals in an organization who will work closely with the new employee; they meet with the applicants to ask questions and make hiring recommendations. Group interviews may last one or more hours and often both query the applicant and offer them an opportunity to ask questions. *Committee interviews* are often used in the public sector or academic environment, and are composed of organizational members who are elected or selected to represent the organization in making hiring recommendations.

Box 3-9 Potential Interview Questions

- How do you handle stressful clinical situations? (Interviewer may provide a clinical scenario, such as a client presenting with chest pain, and ask how you would respond.)
- What are your major strengths and areas for growth?
- Describe a situation in which you failed and what did you learn from this experience?
- Why do you think you would be good in this position?
- Why are you interested in changing employment? Why are you interested in this position?
- Describe a recent problem you experienced and tell me how you solved it.
- How do you deal with people who are difficult to get along with?
- What leadership responsibilities have you had?
- What qualities would your coworkers say that you have?
- Do you work well with doctors, physician assistants, nurse practitioners, and staff?
- How assertive are you? Provide an example of the use of assertiveness in a clinic setting.
- Why have you applied for the position with this health center?
- Describe how you best work in terms of individual initiative or team work.
- What types of extracurricular activities do you enjoy?
- What do you consider the most important aspects of a job to be?
- What types of procedures do you feel comfortable performing?
- Are you prepared to share on-call duties?
- Do you have expertise in caring for a specific patient population?
- Why are you the best candidate for the job?
- What is your scope of practice?
- What type of physician collaboration will you require?
- Do you have a DEA number?
- Do you have prescriptive authority?
- How can an NP improve the quality of care in our practice?
- How can an NP improve our practice financially?
- What is the difference between a nurse practitioner and a physician assistant?
- What is your major weakness or area for growth?

Box 3-10   Examples of Interview Questions for Employers

- May I see an NP position description?
- May I see the organizational chart?
- Are there guidelines for the allotted time for office visits?
- Request a tour of the facility if it is not offered.
- On the tour, speak to support staff and providers.
- What are the hours of clinic operation?
- Does each provider have a dedicated medical assistant or are these shared positions?
- What type of client appointments (acute, chronic, complete physical examinations) do you anticipate scheduling for the new NP?
- Who triages phone messages?
- What is the mission of the organization?
- Are charting and diagnostic test results computerized?
- Is there feedback on quality performance indicators?
- Are educational sessions and feedback provided on coding and billing?
- Do nurse practitioners receive feedback on client satisfaction measures?
- Do providers meet to discuss office operation and client care issues?

Recruiting agencies may also be employed to make hiring recommendations for the most qualified applicants. In any interview type or situation, do not let the number of interviewers intimidate you. Answer each question by addressing the individual who asked the question and be open to each interviewer. You may be asked a multitude of questions. Box 3-9 lists potential interview questions. These questions can assist you in preparing for the interview.

What questions should I ask at the interview?

During an interview, time is often provided for the interviewee to ask questions of the employer. This is an important opportunity for you to ask key questions to determine your interest and desire for employment in the agency. Questions that you may ask potential employers include those involving the reporting structure, clinical responsibilities, hours of employment, and on-call schedule (Beach, 2001). Examples of questions you may wish to pose are listed in Box 3-10.

How should I follow up on a job interview?

It is important to thank and acknowledge the interviewer following your interview. Writing a simple, one-page letter demonstrates your professionalism and interest. The letter should be composed, typed, and mailed within one to two business days. Make sure you include the title of the position you are applying

| Box 3-11 | Example of a Follow-Up Letter |

March 11, 2005

Mrs. Tifany Lexis
Director of Recruiting and Retention
Central Health Care System
1717 Nifty Lane
Aztem, AZ 27778

Dear Mrs. Lexis,

Thank you for interviewing me yesterday for the adult nurse practitioner position in the Central Valley Rural Primary Health Care Center. I enjoyed meeting with you, Dr. Nosert, and Jill Nexic, FNP, and discussing the Central Health Care System mission emphasizing quality care.

My enthusiasm to join the Central Valley Health Care Team has been strengthened by the interview. The emphasis on quality patient care fit well with my philosophy of nursing. My educational preparation and clinical experience match the job requirements and, if offered the position, my skills would complement those of the health care team.

I continue to have strong interest in working for Central Valley Health Care as an adult nurse-practitioner. Please call me at (813)555-9921 for further information.

Thank you for your time and consideration.

Sincerely,

Sam Rekus, RN, APRN-BC

for, your continued interest, and your skill match, and politely thank the individual(s) for his or her time. An example of a follow-up letter is shown in Box 3-11.

SUMMARY

During your job search, make sure you acknowledge all employer correspondence promptly. This promptness provides concrete data to employers that you are reliable, dependable, and follow up on important tasks. To land your dream job, use a variety of sources such as the Internet, professional organizations, networks, mentors, clinical preceptors, and faculty to ensure a quick and successful search. Begin your job search during your clinical rotations. Many NP students have landed a job based on their excellent clinical performance and impression on their preceptors. Once you have successfully secured a nurse practitioner position, cancel remaining interviews and inform potential employers of your decision.

References

Beach, P.A. (2001). Interviewing 101. *Family Practice Management.* Retrieved from *www.aafp.org/fpm/20010100/38inte.html*

Harper, D.S. (1999). A professional curriculum vitae will open career doors. *Clinical Excellence for Nurse Practitioners, 3*(1), 43-49.

Hauri, C.M. (1994). Maximizing your value and worth, or: "Gerta says you're great!" *Nurse Practitioner Format, 5*(4), 233-237.

Hinck, S.M. (1997). A curriculum vitae that gives you a competitive edge. *Clinical Nurse Specialist, 11*(4), 174-177.

Hobins, V. (July 8, 2003). *How to write a CV.* Retrieved from *www.nursingtimes.net*

Lind, E. (2001). Get that job. *Chemistry and Industry,* pp. 439-441.

Meredith, P. (2001, January). Landing your first NP position: Your RN experience does count! *Advance for Nurse Practitioners,* pp. 73-74, 94.

O'Conner, S. (1999). Your curriculum vitae is a snapshot of you. *Association of Operating Room Nurses Journal, 69*(2), 398-401.

Restifo, V. (2002). The successful interview: How to market yourself in career advancement, *NSN/Imprint,* pp. 37-41.

Teasdale, K. (2002). Taking a flexible approach to career planning in nursing. *Professional Nurse, 17*(5), 309-311.

Tools You
Will Need
to Get
Started

Preparing for NP Practice: Certification and NP State Recognition

Maureen Ryan

Introduction: First Steps

Just as you graduated from a state board of nursing–approved school, passed the NCLEX-RN, and met the specific requirements in the state you practiced in as a registered nurse, you must follow a similar process to use the title and practice as an NP.

What steps do I need to take to practice as a nurse practitioner?

The following steps are necessary for beginning your career as an NP:

- Graduate from an NP program that prepares and makes you eligible to take a national certification exam.
- Apply and take the national certification examination in your specialty area. Become familiar with the recertification period and requirements for your NP certification.
- Apply for NP recognition in the state in which you wish to practice. *NP state recognition* is the legal designation conferred through a license, certificate, or other legal designation for

the title NP. The rules and requirements for NP state recognition and practice vary by state. You will need to learn the state regulation on prescriptive authority and state requirements to apply and use a federal DEA number. You should also review any other state requirements for practice such as a specific formulary, continuing education, protocols, or documentation of an agreement with a physician.

- Learn about the practice requirements of your employer. These may differ and some employers may require a credentialing or privileging process. *Credentialing* is a process by which an employer or agency gathers educational, licensure, and other information on a practitioner to determine if, in their judgment, the practitioner is able to provide satisfactory care to clients. *Privileging* is a process used by an employer or agency to certify that a practitioner has the knowledge and training to perform specific procedures or care to clients.
- Understand third-party payer requirements because the ability of the NP to bill and receive payment for services rendered is an important aspect of the process. Third-party payer requirements vary.

This chapter will assist you in understanding the process to follow when applying for certification, obtaining state recognition as an NP, and learning about the common practice requirements of employers.

Certification

What is certification?

Certification is a voluntary process to recognize professional achievement, clinical skills, practice, and knowledge (Flarey, 2000). Certification is a way of demonstrating competence in a specialty area. It is a symbol of excellence, an indicator of the ability to deliver quality care based on national standards, and it provides a mechanism for being professionally recognized for the achievement of excellence. It is a way of demonstrating advanced knowledge beyond that of the beginning registered nurse and promotes continued competency through recertification.

NPs have been practicing and delivering care for more than 40 years, but their education and certification have not always been standardized according to national guidelines. Some practicing NPs do not hold graduate degrees, and certification has not always been required by all states.

Numerous organizations offer specialty certification examinations for NPs. Certification agencies that offer NP exams include the following:
- American Academy of Nurse Practitioners
- American Nurses Credentialing Service
- American College of Nurse Midwives Certification Council
- Pediatric Nursing Certification Board
- Oncology Nursing Certification Corporation

The American Association of Colleges of Nursing (AACN) in 1995 called for all NPs to hold a graduate degree and be certified; in addition, the AACN recommended that standards for certification be developed and administered by a separate entity, to avoid multiple bodies offering certification (Anonymous, 1995). Because some states may not recognize all of the certifying bodies, or specialized categories (i.e., acute care nurse practitioner vs. adult nurse practitioner), it is important to be familiar with state law prior to taking a national certification exam.

Generally, for NPs, these certification exams are based on the knowledge needed to practice safely in NP specialty areas. The exams themselves are quite comprehensive and cover topical areas such as health promotion, disease prevention, diagnosis and management of acute and chronic illness care, client education, evaluation of care, and professional issues. Table 4-1 lists certifying agencies and specialty exams offered by each. Criteria for exam eligibility are determined by the individual certifying body, but most certifying bodies now require a master's degree to be eligible for the exam.

How do I apply to take the certification exam?

The process of applying for the certification exam can be complicated and at times confusing. The first step in the process is to obtain the correct forms from the certifying body, many of which are available on the Internet. These forms may be downloaded from the Internet or you may request a paper copy from the certifying body. Once you have the application, fill out the forms. This may seem tedious, but by following the instructions you will not have to spend time resubmitting required information. As part of the certification application, your school will need to fill out a verification of education form and prepare an official transcript to demonstrate that you have graduated and that the program you attended provided the required didactic and clinical hours. If your state board of nursing (SBN) requires direct verification of your passing the certification board, make sure to enclose the SBN form and/or complete the SBN verification form in the certification application. By enclosing the verification form in the initial certification application, the certifying body will automatically send the SBN a verification of your results. This will facilitate the timely processing of your NP state recognition.

The application process may take several weeks, so complete the required forms for the certifying body before you graduate. After you graduate and all of the forms are completed and submitted, you will receive notification that you may sit for your national certification exam. Depending on the organization, you may choose between a paper-and-pen or computer test. The certification organization provides an outline of information that will be covered on the exam. This assists you in preparing for the examination. It is important to study, and attending a review course prior to taking the exam is an excellent idea, as is buying or checking out from your library any one of the numerous

Table 4-1 Certifying Agency Information

Organization	Website or E-mail/ Specialty Exams	Paper-Pen/Computer Title	Address	Telephone
American Academy of Nurse Practitioners	www.aanpcertification.org	Computer NP-C Recertify every 5 years	Certification Program Capital Station PO Box 12926 Austin, TX 78711	(512)442-5202 FAX: (512)442-5521
American Nurses Credentialing Service (National)	www.nursingworld.org/anc/ certification/index.html Acute care NP Adult NP Adult psychiatric mental health NP Advanced diabetes Management NP Family nurse NP Family psychiatric & mental health NP Gerontological NP Pediatric NP	Computer APRN, BC Advanced practice Registered nurse Board certified Recertify every 5 years	American Nurses Credentialing Center 8515 Georgia Avenue Suite 400 Silver Springs, MD 20901-3492 Application: ANCC PO Box 791333 Baltimore, MD 29279	(800)-284-2378

Organization	Website/Email & Specialty	Certification Details	Address	Contact
American College of Nurse Midwives Certification Council	info@AAC.midwife.org Nurse midwives	Paper-pen/computer in 2005 CNM Recertify every 8 years	ACNM Certification Council 8201 Corporate Drive Suite 550 Landover, MD 20785	(301)459-1321 FAX: (301)731-7825
Pediatric Nursing Certification Board (offers pediatric acute care, PNP primary care)	www.pncb.org Pediatric NP	Computer Paper-pen CPNP-PC CPND-AC Recertify activity every year	800 South Frederick Ave Ste. 104 Gaithersburg, MD 20877-4151	(888)641-2767 FAX: (301)330-1504
The National Certification Corp. for Obstetric, Gynecologic and Neonatal Specialties	www.nccnet.org Women's health NP Neonate NP	Computer RN-C Recertify every 3 years	PO Box 11082 Chicago, IL 60611	(800) 367-5613 (312) 951-0207
Oncology Nursing Certification Corporation	www.oncc.org Advanced oncology certified NP	Computer RN, AOCNP Recertify every 4 years	125 Enterprise Drive Pittsburgh, PA 15275	(412)859-6104 Toll free: (877)-769-ONCC

exam review books available for your specialty area. Table 4-2 provides a sample of review courses and books available.

The results are generally available within 2 to 3 weeks after completing the certification examination. After successfully passing your national certification exam, you will be one step closer to being able to call yourself an NP. After graduating and passing the certification exam, you are now ready to petition the state to be recognized as an NP. Each state, by statute, will have its own process that will need to be followed and it is best to start the process as early as possible. Generally, you will need to obtain a packet of information and forms from the state board of nursing that will need to be filled out. Your college or school of nursing will need to send proof of graduation, and your scores from the national certification exam will need to be sent directly from the certifying body.

In many states, you may fill out the application to practice as an NP at the same time you are applying to take the certification exam. By completing the applications simultaneously, you often streamline the process of obtaining your NP credential. Application fees vary by state and must be submitted with the application. It may take another several weeks for the state to process your application, and then finally, you will receive your NP state recognition documentation in the mail. Display it prominently at work. You have earned the right to call yourself an NP.

What do I need to do to become recertified?

Each organization that grants certification will also have criteria for recertification. This may include a minimum number of clinical hours, as well as a combination of continuing education credits, professional publishing, precepting of NP students, or teaching. Although each certification body has its own criteria, certification generally takes place every 2 to 8 years. Make sure to review the amount and type of continuing education that is acceptable and what is not acceptable. It is important to retain records of continuing education and other relevant experiences for the recertification process. A percentage of applicants will be randomly audited and will be required to submit documentation. The certifying body will also determine the credentials that you may use after your name.

Nurse Practitioner State Recognition and Practice Requirements

What do states require for NP recognition and practice?

It is important that you investigate thoroughly and understand the specific regulations for recognition and practice in the state in which you plan to practice as an NP.

Table 4-2 Nurse Practitioner Review Courses

Organization	Website	Books/Live Courses	Certification Concentrations	Telephone
Health Leadership Associates	www.healthleadership.com/	Book and live review courses, study questions books	Midwifery, pediatric, acute care NP, women's health, gerontology, family nurse practitioner, adult	(800)435-4775
Barkley and Associates	http://npcourses.com/	CDs or Live review courses	Family nurse practitioner, acute care, adult, pediatric (acute and primary care), gerontology, women's health	(310)652-1120
Advanced Practice Education Associates	www.apea.com/courses.html	Audio tapes or CDs, live reviews, and online testing	Family and adult	(800)899-4502
Oncology Nursing Society course	http://onsopcontent.ons.org/education/AOCNSreview/	Live review	Oncology nurse practitioner	(866)257-4ONS
Fitzgerald Health Education Associates	www.fhea.com/	Live review, books, online seminars, audio tapes, and online tests	Acute care, adult, family, women's health, gerontology, and pediatrics	(800)927-5380

NP State Recognition. States differ in their processes for legal recognition and authority to use the title NP. Some states will grant a certificate, license, or other legal designation. See Box 1-2 for specific NP state designations. It is important to access the most current state requirements because changes may occur over time. Appendix 1-3 provides a listing of state-by-state contact information for NP state recognition, or you can access the National Council of State Boards of Nursing at *www.ncsbn.org/regulation/boardsofnursing_boards_of_nursing_board.asp*.

Regulations by States for NP Practice. Each state will have its own specific laws, rules, and regulations for NP practice, and each NP must be clear about what constitutes legal practice in his or her state. Box 4-1 lists some important areas of knowledge that NP should have regarding your state regulations.

What are the common requirements needed for NP state recognition?

Common requirements for an applicant for state NP recognition include the following:
1. Be licensed as a RN in the state in which you are applying to practice as an NP.
2. Submit evidence of completion of an educational program (approved by the state) designed to prepare NPs. Many states are now specifying that to be recognized as an NP, the applicant must be prepared at the master's level, although some states will grandfather applicants who graduated before 1998.
3. Submit evidence of professional national certification by an agency identified in the state laws or statues.

Box 4-1 Important Areas to Have Exact Knowledge about NP State Regulations

- *Unit or department of state government that regulates NP practice.* This is often the Board of Nursing/Nurse Examiner, but may be the Medicine, Pharmacy, or other administrative divisions.
- *Prescriptive authority.* Investigate your state requirements for federal DEA numbers and formularies or protocols (if required).
- *Practice requirements that might dictate physician collaboration or supervision.* Box 4-2 discusses the level of physician involvement in diagnosing and treating aspects of nurse practitioner practice (by state).
- *Requirements for NP state recognition renewal.* Such requirements include evidence of participation in continuing education, for instance, pharmacology.

Box 4-2 Nurse Practitioner Practice (by State): Requirements for Physician Involvement in Diagnosing and Treating

Placement of each state is based on the predominant relationship required. States vary in the level of requirement and may use collaboration, delegation, direction, or supervision to describe NP/physician involvement.

States with autonomous practice: Alaska, Arkansas, Colorado, District of Columbia, Hawaii, Idaho, Iowa, Kentucky, Maine (after initial 2 years), Michigan, Montana, New Hampshire, New Jersey, New Mexico, North Dakota, Oklahoma, Oregon, Rhode Island, Tennessee, Utah, Washington, West Virginia

States requiring delegation may be with protocol: Georgia, South Carolina, Texas

States requiring collaboration: Arizona, Connecticut, Indiana, Pennsylvania, Minnesota, Wyoming

States requiring supervision may be by procedure, protocol, guideline, or agreement: California, Florida, Massachusetts, Nebraska, North Carolina, Virginia

States requiring written collaborative practice agreement, arrangement, protocol, or guideline: Alabama, Delaware, Illinois, Kansas, Louisiana, Maryland, Mississippi, Missouri, Nevada, New York, Ohio, South Dakota, Vermont, Wisconsin

Data from Pearson L.J. (2005). The Pearson report: A national overview of nurse practitioner legislation and healthcare issues. *American Journal for Nurse Practitioners* 9(1), 9-136.

4. File the required application; for some states, applicants must pass a criminal background check and in some states, like Florida, must even be fingerprinted.
5. Pay the application fee.

What do I need to do for continued NP state recognition?

Just as each state board determines the time period for renewal of the basic RN license, they determine the time period for renewal of NP state recognition. States may require continuing education to maintain the registered nurse license, additional continuing education requirements to maintain NP recognition, and maintenance of national NP certification (Yoder-Wise, 2005). For information on the annual update of state requirements for continuing education and competency, review Yoder-Wise's (2005) editorial and table on survey results of state boards of nursing and selected national professional certifying associations.

Because the state and national certification agencies each have their own renewal time frame (which often differ) and continuing education requirements, you will need to track your renewal dates and continuing education hours to fulfill both requirements. The state board of nursing or other regulatory body will send the renewal application to the last known address of the applicant, and the applicant must renew by filling out the necessary forms and submitting an application fee. For NP state recognition, separate fees are often associated with the RN license and NP recognition.

While some states only require that NPs maintain the continuing education requirements to maintain their national certification, some states require additional hours, and some specify a minimum number of hours in pharmacology. For example, Maine requires 75 hours per 2 years for renewal of an NP license, whereas Nebraska requires 40 hours per 2 years with 10 hours being in pharmacology.

Prescriptive Authority

What do I need to do so I can prescribe medications through prescriptive authority?

All NP programs have didactic and clinical experiences that include courses on advanced pathophysiology and pharmacology, which enables NPs to assess, diagnose, and treat clients, including treatment by pharmacological interventions within their specialty. This provides the foundation for the nurse practitioner's ability to prescribe. It is essential that NPs gain and retain the right to prescribe, because restrictions on prescriptive authority challenge the NP's ability to deliver quality care.

On the state level, most, but not all, states grant NPs prescriptive privileges, either independent privileges or those delegated from a collaborating physician. Box 4-3 lists the level of physician involvement in prescribing aspects of NP practice (by state). Prescriptive authority is the responsibility of the individual states, so each state may differ in its requirements for NP prescriptive authority. Some states grant independent prescriptive authority, including prescription of controlled substances; some states grant prescriptive authority, including prescription of controlled substances with some degree of physician involvement or delegation; and yet other states grant prescriptive authority, excluding controlled substances with some degree of physician involvement or delegation (Pearson, 2005). Individual states may have formularies or protocols that will also impact the NP's ability to prescribe, and some states require written prescriptive collaboration agreements. States may also require documentation of education in the basic NP preparation or continuing education in pharmacology, pathophysiology, or other specific content areas.

How do I obtain a federal DEA number?

Obtaining a DEA number from the federal government is a two-step process. State law grants prescriptive privileges, including the right for NPs to write prescriptions for controlled substances, but it is the federal government that grants DEA numbers. As mentioned in the previous section, most states have granted the NP the ability to write prescriptions for noncontrolled drugs either by independent or delegated prescriptive rights (some states have a formulary

Box 4-3 Nurse Practitioner Prescribing (by State): Level of Physician Involvement

Placement of each state is based on the predominant relationship required. States vary in the level of requirement and may use collaboration, delegation, direction, or supervision to describe NP/physician involvement.

States with autonomous prescriptive privileges: Alaska, Arizona, District of Columbia, Idaho, Iowa, Maine, Montana, New Hampshire, New Mexico, Oregon

States requiring physician collaboration: Wisconsin, Wyoming

States requiring guidelines or agreement: Louisiana

States requiring a collaborative practice agreement, protocol, arrangement, guideline, or plan: Alabama, Arkansas, Colorado, Connecticut, Delaware, Hawaii, Illinois, Indiana, Kansas, Kentucky, Maryland, Mississippi, Nevada, New Jersey, New York, North Dakota, Ohio, Pennsylvania, Rhode Island, South Dakota, Utah (only requires collaboration for Controlled Substances II-III), Vermont, Washington (only requires collaboration for Controlled Substances I-IV), West Virginia

States requiring delegation by protocol or agreement: Michigan, Minnesota, Missouri, South Carolina, Texas

States requiring procedures, protocols, guidelines formulary, or agreements: California, Florida, Massachusetts, Nebraska, North Carolina, Oklahoma, Tennessee, Virginia

Data from Pearson L.J. (2005). The Pearson report: A national overview of nurse practitioner legislation and healthcare issues. *American Journal for Nurse Practitioners* 9(1), 9-136.

of allowable drugs). Not all states allow NPs to prescribe controlled substances, and some states limit the classes of controlled substances that may be prescribed. Some states require that NPs receive a state-issued license for controlled substances prior to applying to the DEA for a number. Appendix 4-1 describes the five categories of controlled substances and gives the complete listing of drugs as well as the DEA form with instructions.

On the federal level, NPs may apply for a DEA number, but will receive one only if they are in compliance with state law. For a listing of regulations by state, see *www.deadiversion.usdoj.gov/drugreg/practioners/index.html.* Before applying for a DEA number from the federal government, contact your state licensing authority or board of nursing to appraise the status of prescriptive authority, as well as the prescription of controlled substances.

The DEA now offers forms that can be filled out online and submitted to the DEA agency. Access the website *www.DEAdiversion.usdoj.gov* and go to "Drug Registration." Select and complete form DEA-224. You will need to furnish the DEA with your Social Security number (taxpayer ID number). The form has a total of eight items, along with a list of drugs under controlled substances I through VI. You must submit all required information, along with an application fee. DEA numbers must be renewed every 3 years; as of 2005, the original application cost and renewal cost totaled $390.

Initial registration will last at least 28 months, but not greater than 39 months. The federal government will mail a renewal application to the last known address 45 days prior to the expiration date; this application will not be forwarded to a new address. Therefore, any changes of address must be reported to the DEA. The fee must accompany the application. It takes between 8 and 12 weeks to obtain the DEA number after the application is filed. Some states may require a separate filing procedure for controlled substances, with a separate filing fee.

Employer Requirements

What are common employer requirements for NPs?

Employers and organizations (hospital, clinic, health provider group) have a direct and independent legal responsibility to take reasonable steps to ensure that the providers that it employs or allows to practice at its site are qualified to give care to clients, and that they are practicing within the scope of their practice and expertise. Before being allowed to practice in most acute care agencies and in many primary care or outpatient clinics, NPs often need to go through either or both a credentialing process and application for clinical privileges.

Employers or organizations in which NPs provide care may have a credentialing committee, which decides if the NP receives privileges, what the scope of privileges will be, and whether or not they will be renewed (Klein, 2003). This process will ensure that NPs hold the professional degrees, certifications, and experience needed to deliver safe care. The credentialing process is in place to protect the public from charlatans and unsafe practitioners, and to safeguard the hospital from liability. The credentialing process signals that you have met the qualifications needed to practice in your area of specialty, and demonstrates that the hospital administration has reviewed your expertise, education, and skills, and deems you competent to deliver care.

For the process of being credentialed at a clinical site, you will often have to fill out many required forms. Each clinical site may have different requirements, but generally you will need to produce the following:
- Curriculum vitae
- Diploma
- Transcript
- State license as a registered nurse
- Documentation of NP state recognition
- Proof of national certification
- Proof of malpractice insurance
- Professional references.

You may also be required to produce verification of other certifications such as basic life support or advanced cardiac life support (BCLS/ACLS). After the clinical site receives all of this information, the credentialing board, made up of several members of the staff, usually physicians and NPs, will decide if you are qualified to practice at their institution. These boards often only meet once a month, so it is important to have all of your information organized beforehand to avoid delays.

Privileges may be granted in combination with credentialing, or they may be granted as a separate process. This is done to protect the public from practitioners doing procedures or delivering care outside their scope of practice or expertise. Clinical privileges are granted by an agency where the NP is granted the right to perform certain clinical procedures in the agency, or to care for a certain client population. Common procedures and activities that NPs may receive privileges for include the following:

- Performing history and physicals
- Ordering and monitoring X-rays and lab tests
- Suturing
- Incising and draining wounds
- Removing foreign body in the eye
- Inserting IUDs
- Prescribing medications
- Prescribing treatment evaluations
- Initiating referrals and consults
- Sharing on-call responsibilities
- Admitting and discharging clients
- Engaging in other procedures that the NP has the education and experience to perform.

It may be wise to document all significant experiences and procedures that you perform for the purpose of documenting your experience for your annual or biannual privileges review.

Collaborative Agreements and Protocols

What is a collaborative agreement?

Collaborative agreements help define and operationalize the relationship between an NP and a physician delivering comprehensive health care in specified practice site. The content of the collaborative agreement will depend on the requirements of the state's regulations, but the agreement should be written in a way that maximizes each practitioner's unique skills in accordance with state practice laws. Some states require that an NP have a collaborative agreement in place prior to practicing, while other states require this for Medicaid reimbursement. A collaborative practice agreement will be based on the state law governing NP practice in the state in which the agreement is made. Nursing is considered an independent profession, based on its own body of knowledge. In some states NPs have independent authority, and are not considered a subset of medicine. If an NP is practicing under the scope of practice for NPs in that state, there is no need for supervision or delegation. The NP should be careful to define collaboration, and not specify supervision or delegation in situations where it is not needed.

The collaborative agreement should be developed by both the physician and the NP, should be acceptable to both parties, and should include input from other practicing NPs. Key elements of a collaborative agreement are listed in Box 4-4, and Appendix 4-2 provides an example of a collaborative agreement.

Collaborative agreements are legal documents, and the NP and physician can be held legally responsible for the relationship and duties specified by the agreement. Collaborative agreements should be acceptable to each party, and both the physician and NP must agree to its terms, and be willing to put forth the energy needed to fulfill the agreement. Therefore, if your collaborative agreement states that you will review charts once a month, then this needs to be done, and should be documented for future reference.

If you are in a state that requires a collaborative agreement with a physician, it is important to find one who supports the role of NPs, who is available on a timely basis for consultation, and who is agreeable to abiding by the mutually written collaborative agreement that will specifically spell out the responsibilities of both parties. If a physician is not abiding by the written agreement, and the issue cannot be resolved, then it is imperative that the NP end the agreement and seek other collaboration.

Careful thought should be exercised prior to entering into a collaborative agreement with a physician. Sharing similar values and approaches to client care is an important basis for a collaborative agreement, as is the ability and willingness to live up to the spirit of the agreement. NPs should have knowledge of a physician's practice style and work ethic before drafting the collaborative agreement. Physicians and NPs who have worked together and are familiar with each other will enter into collaborative agreements, as will

---

Box 4-4 Key Elements of a Collaborative Agreement

(Specific elements are state specific.)
- The agreement is written.
- Services to be provided (well-child exams, complete history and physicals, acute illness care, management of chronic illnesses) are clearly described.
- Clinical parameters for referrals and consultations are detailed.
- The agreement should be signed, dated, and available for review. It should be reviewed for necessary changes on a regular basis and at least annually.
- It includes a description of the formal evaluation of care process such as frequency and minimum number of chart reviews.
- It includes a description of frequency and types of quality reviews.
- Recognition is given to the scope of practice in the state in which the agreement is written.
- It covers delegation of prescriptive authority when needed.

members of a health care group. If a collaborative physician is not available, interview other NPs for recommendations.

Most collaborative agreements generally do not cost money. This is especially true when the NP has a collaborative agreement with a physician working within the same group or practice. However, there are times, such as when an NP is a solo practitioner, when a physician may be hired to engage in a collaborative agreement. The physician would be hired to fulfill the terms of the collaborative agreement, including being available at specific times for consultation, chart review, and if needed by state law, for prescriptive privileges. Payment would be tied into community standards for physician payment, but be prepared to pay at least $100 to $150 dollars per hour for the physician's services.

What are protocols?

Some states require a written practice agreement with a physician for NPs to legally practice (Likis, 2003). These written agreements will include a written description of the scope and restrictions of the NP's practice, and the relationship between the NP and the physician within that particular practice. Although these are often called collaborative agreements and refer to practice in broad terms, some clinical models use protocols, which can be very specific for the many conditions encountered by the NP. An example of a protocol may include diagnosis and treatment of bronchitis, otitis media, acute pharyngitis, scabies, or acne.

Protocols can be written in many forms, including narrative, algorithm, or use of a branching logic tree (Hawkins, 1984). Protocols differ from things such as standing orders since protocols will specifically include guidelines for the assessment of data that will help establish a medical diagnosis, while standing orders simply give instructions to be followed after the diagnosis is made. Protocols may also cite authoritative texts that may be used as the basis of practice, or books that are a series of protocols. In some states, this broad definition may fulfill the state requirements for protocols. If so, a broad approach is preferable because it gives the NP greater flexibility in clinical decision making.

Many protocols are disease specific, and include the major points of the history and physical that must be present to establish the diagnosis. After the diagnosis is made, the protocol includes specific treatment plans that specify medication, interventions, and follow-up. Many protocols will also include specific directions on when consultation with a physician is mandated (such as with a diagnosis of meningitis or other potentially serious medical problem). The government has published some protocols, such as the clinical practice guideline on otitis media with effusion (OME), which was developed by the Agency for Health Care Policy and Research (now the Agency for Healthcare Research and Quality) which provides evidence-based recommendations on diagnosing and managing otitis media with effusion in children. Many of these protocols are available for reproduction and can be accessed at *www.ahrq.gov.*

Protocols are based on evidence-based medicine, thereby supplying the NP with the latest and most effective treatments. They may be developed by the NP and physician collaboratively, or they may be cited as following the recommendations of a particular publication. Protocols will need to be approved through an established administrative process and therefore it may be difficult to immediately apply research or new clinical guidelines to a specific practice. One of the positive aspects of protocols is that all clinicians in a practice will be using the same guidelines based on evidence medicine, rather than using personal preferences.

Another benefit of protocols is seen during the evaluation process. By using established guidelines based on evidence-based practice as the core of the protocols, evaluation of care can be carried out by assessing whether or not the guideline was followed by the clinician as well as whether or not client outcomes were achieved. Each NP using a protocol needs to continue to read and critique the protocol and develop a strong clinical network to help keep the protocol current with the latest research findings.

However, specific protocols may be difficult to follow given a variety of clinical presentations (i.e., client has no insurance, is allergic to many medications) and may also be used against the nurse practitioner in court if there is a negative outcome and the protocol has been deviated from in any substantial way. For this reason, many clinicians advocate use of protocols that are stated in broad terms. If an NP is working with specific protocols, documentation should include justification for deviating from the stated standard. If a practice uses protocols, it is important to have input from the NPs on staff into the development and maintenance of the protocols at routine specified time periods. One way of achieving this is to have NPs volunteer to serve on the protocol committee. Appendix 4-3 gives an example of a sample protocol.

SUMMARY

There are several steps in the process of becoming a nurse practitioner. After graduation from your program, you will take a national certification examination in your specialty area, and then apply for NP recognition in the state in which you wish to practice. NP state recognition is a legal designation conferred through a license, certificate, or other legal designation for the title NP. Because NP practice is regulated by the state in which you practice, it is important to be familiar with state requirements for NP recognition including requirements for renewal.

References

Anonymous (1995). AACN urges standard for advanced nurses as enrolments climb. *Public Heath Reports, 110*(2), 229.

Flarey, D. (2000). Is certification the current gold standard? *Journal of Operative Nurses Association Law, Ethics and Regulations, 2,* 43-45.

Hawkins, J.W. (1984). Developing family planning nurse practitioner protocols. *Journal of Obstetric and Gynecology, 13*(3), 167-170.

Klein, C. (2003). The scoop on credentialing. *Nurse Practitioner, 28*(12), 54.

Likis, F. (2003). A novel model for collaborative practice agreements. *Nurse Practitioner, 28*(7), 54-56.

Pearson, L. (2005). The Pearson report: A national overview of nurse practitioner legislation and healthcare issues. *American Journal of Nurse Practitioners 9*(1), 9-136.

Yoder-Wise, P. (2005). State and certifying boards/associations: Continuing education and competency requirements. *Journal of Continuing Education in Nursing, 36*(1), 3-11.

Additional Reading

Buppert, C. (2002). Billing for nurse practitioner services: Guidelines for NPs, physicians, employers, and insurers. *Medscape 4*(1), 2002. Retrieved from http://www.medscape.com/ viewarticle/422935?src=search, May 12, 2005.

Exstrom, S. (2001). The state board of nursing and its role in continuing competency. *Journal of Continuing Nursing Education, 32*(3), 118-125.

Fitzpatrick, M. (2003). Certified practice: We owe it to our patients and ourselves. *Nursing Management, 34*(3), 6.

5

Negotiating an Employment Contract

Thomas H. Ryan

Personal Assessment

Negotiating that first contract is an exciting, but often difficult, experience for a nurse practitioner who may not feel knowledgeable enough to bargain effectively. Having knowledge about financial and legal aspects of managing a practice is necessary to successfully negotiate an employment contract.

The first hurdle for many new NPs is the feeling that they will be a financial burden on the clinic during their first 6 months of practice. As a new NP you should feel confident in your negotiations because not only do you have knowledge and skill as an advanced practice nurse, you have many skills and talents from your practice as a registered nurse, which makes your practice valuable to potential employers. True, you may need to consult more with your colleagues during your orientation period, but this is a process all practitioners go through, including new physicians. Remember, the first contract you negotiate will set the stage for all contracts that are to follow, so it is important to achieve the best terms possible when starting. Do not underestimate your value, and do not feel bound if a predecessor has undervalued his or her worth.

To mentally prepare yourself and overcome doubts you have about your practice, make a list of all the skills and talents that you will bring to the position. Perhaps you will offer health promotion, or diabetes classes, make home visits, or see clients who have a medical condition in which you have a special interest (obesity, diabetes, heart disease, depression). Your specialized practice can be extremely profitable for a practice. Nurse practitioners strengthen the clinic's financial picture by increasing the practice (client volume) in which they are often working from 80% to 90%, and receive back in salary and benefits less than one-third of their revenue. In other words, for every dollar you bring in, you get back 33 cents, but you almost double the volume for the practice.

Experienced clinicians consistently bargain for additional salary and benefits. Bargaining is influenced by experience, assertiveness, willingness to take risks, and has been shown to be much easier in practices in which NPs have already been employed.

What is a personal assessment?

Before beginning a search for a position, you should do a "personal assessment," but what does that mean?

It is important that the position you accept is a good fit for you, and that you are a good fit for the position. The position may pay a lot, but if you have to work night shifts and this disagrees with your circadian rhythms, then that is not the right fit. To make sure that you pick the right job for you, it is important to do some soul searching before setting out to find a position as an NP.

The personal assessment starts by brainstorming all of the job characteristics that you may encounter, and then choosing which ones you *must* have versus those that you would *like* to have. Examples might include some of the following areas.

Commute. How long will it take you to get to your practice location? What are the parameters for the longest commute you would be willing to drive? How much will it cost to commute, and how will the commute affect your personal life? While at first glance that "hour drive" to work doesn't seem like much, every week it will equal an extra 10 hours on the road. Can you accept losing that much time?

Financial Culture. If you are an elitist you may find it difficult to work with an impoverished client load; conversely if you are a social reformer you may find it difficult to be confronted daily with clients taking the day off from the golf course to present you with trivialities. In short, make sure that the clientele you will work with is one with which you can be comfortable. Again, is there a fit between you and the practice?

Practice Style. Is the environment of the practice structured, or is it more laid back? Is the pace frenzied because extra clients are being added to everyone's schedule? Do the practitioners follow national guidelines or are the practitioners more into the "art of care."

Location (Rural, Urban, or Inner City). The location of a practice will usually affect the client population that you will be seeing. In a rural environment, clients may have more industrial-type accidents, or suffer from a lack of resources such as education, money, or transportation. However, it may also be the environment in which you get to care for families and use all of your clinical skills. In an urban environment as well you might encounter clients who have few resources and have many chronic diseases.

Potential for Personal and Professional Growth. Will you be allowed to expand your role and develop new skills, or will you be part of an assembly-line process? Is developing professionally important for the practice you are considering entering? Will you have the ability to increase your salary and benefits if and when you are clearly expanding the practice (and pocketbook) of your employer? Will you have the ability to work in areas you find important? In short, what are the long-term consequences and possibilities?

Diversity of Practice. Some NPs are now choosing to go into specialty practices, such as orthopedics, dermatology, or acute care. It is important to think about how much diversity you will want in your practice. Are you comfortable becoming an expert in a specialty, or do you want to remain a generalist? Will a specialized focus become too repetitive such that you lose interest?

Client Population. Will you be working with a group with whom you have empathy? Will you be verbally abused by the clients? Will every client be a problem? If you don't enjoy caring for children, would you want to get into a practice where you are required to work extensively or exclusively with this population?

Types of Health Conditions Treated. Are you going to be entering a practice that presents a client population that has health problems you are willing to work with? If you don't routinely like to manage intense emotions, is a hospice job really the type of work you are willing to perform? Will you be required to manage complex cases on a regular basis, without any assistance from others? Will you only be assigned to manage and treat simple problems and perform wellness care?

Personal Expectations. What do you want for yourself in life? Will this job tend to help or hurt your chances of achieving your goals? Conversely, will you be expected to handle cases far beyond your comfort level? What do you want, and what is required by the job?

Family. Will you be able to maintain relations with your friends and family? If you are working from midnight to 8 a.m. and your spouse is working from 9 a.m. until 5 p.m., will you be able to sustain the relationship, or are your priorities career before family? If the job is going to destroy your relationships with family and friends, is the cost too great regardless of the pay? Your decisions will impact others.

Job Security. This has become a more important issue in the current culture of cost cutting and downsizing. To assess job security, you will want to know how long the practice has existed and the total number of clients served. Has there been a rapid turnover of prior practitioners? Look at the overall health of the organization before making a commitment. Even when you are employed, however, it is a good idea to continue to remain in a network where you will be privy to new opportunities and develop network connections in the professional area. If this is the only possible job prospect available for you, what would happen if you are let go after a year? By maintaining your network connections you increase your value by increasing the choices available to you. Take time to assess each opportunity and evaluate the benefits and weaknesses of each employment offer.

Child Care. More and more employers are developing in-house child care. Is this available, or even a possibility? Child care costs can be tremendous. If a family member gets sick, will you be able to make provisions to deal with that without causing hardship for the practice? What if your child is sick and you can't send her to a sitter? If you have to stay home on occasion, what will the actual effect be on your job security? If you are salaried but are missing days to care for sick family members, this might be a serious issue.

Continuing Education. Will you be encouraged to keep your education current? Will the employer sponsor some or all of the attendant costs? Are there methods in the practice for sharing newly acquired knowledge among the members of the practice? Who is going to pay the costs of continuing education?

Multiple Locations. Health care is rapidly expanding geographically. Clinics and alternate sites for care are becoming routine. Will you have one home base? Will you be required to travel from site to site? If you are expected to travel to more than one site, and the other sites are a significant distance apart, will you receive mileage for travel? If one site has a significantly lower client population and your income is based on productivity, are you going to find yourself limited in your ability to treat a larger number of clients and if so are you going to be financially penalized for a new placement at an alternate site? If your pay is based on the number of clients, what if you get sent to a clinic 30 miles away that has no steady stream of clients?

Management Structure. "Who's the boss?" Is there a particular person or group to which you will answer? Where will you stand in the chain of command? If an employee tells you to do something and you disagree, is there a designated person to whom you can address such problems? If there is an informal chain of command, what is it?

Hours. Will you have a set schedule or not? Are you protected against shifts that you simply cannot meet (to have a family, some fun, or a social life), or will you be required to work different shifts or weekends.

Care Emphasis. Whether we want to admit it or not, some practices are more focused than others on the quality of care. Will you be expected to provide care where numbers are more important than the quality of care? Are you comfortable with the type of care your practice will provide?

Practice Limitations. Are you going to have to practice far in advance of your comfort level and competency? Will there be help if you need it? Are you going to have the opportunity to develop new skills or will you be limited in your practice? Are there qualifications you must meet to fully engage in a developing practice?

Resources. Are resources available for you to access? Where are they? Do you need a password, and who takes care of that? If libraries are available for your use, you must know where and when those resources are available to you. Will you get current literature? Keys? Passwords?

Strategies and Goals. In addition to brainstorming all of the aspects of the job characteristics that you would like, you also need to do research on the practice that you will join. Before negotiating your contract or accepting any offer, it is wise to make sure that the practice itself is a good fit with your personal needs. To accomplish this, you will need to match your personal skills, interests, and experiences with practices that share your philosophy of care and career objective.

One way to achieve this is by spending time in the practice, generally at least one full day, to observe and evaluate before proceeding to negotiations. During the day of observation, you can observe if there is an adequate number of staff for the practice load, observe how the staff treats one another, and the attitude of the support staff toward the role of the NP. The receptionist is perhaps the most powerful individual in the informal power structure of any office; so make sure you interact with the receptionist to get a feel for what your long-term relationship may be like.

What are the types of practice?

Another aspect to consider is what type of practice it is. We now address some of the many types of practice that may be available to you.

Private Practice. This may involve working in collaboration with one or more providers in an area of practice. Often such practices are in specialties, such as family practice, the emergency room, or obstetrical or gynecological care. Or you may be joining a small rural general practice. There are so many opportunities! Seek them out. Don't wait for them to find you.

Corporate Practice. This may be a practice in industrial health at a factory, or development of practices for the employees of a large company. It might be reviewing records or quality assurance compliance. These positions may involve far less client contact that you are used to. Is this the type of practice you prefer? You may also inquire at a private surgical center; some of these types of organizations are hiring NPs to do preoperative screening and post-operative care management.

Public Health. The scope of practice can range from instructing and educating to blood draws and physical examination to management of health care issues of the general population. If you have never done so, consider going down to your local public health department to see what goes on there. This can help to start your understanding of the various possibilities that are available in public health centers.

The Employment Contract

Once you have completed your personal assessment and have found a job you are interested in securing, you are ready to begin negotiations for salary and benefits as an employed NP. To be prepared for negotiating your employment terms, it is necessary to understand what an employment contract is and what you would like to include in this written contract. It is important to be knowledgeable about employment contracts because many of the NP positions you will apply for involve negotiating and signing one.

What exactly is an employment "contract"?

A *contract* is an agreement between two or more parties whereby you do something for the other (such as examining clients and treating illness and managing chronic illnesses) and the other does something for you (like sign a paycheck and provide you with the equipment needed to do your job). Each party has respective rights and obligations under a contract. If there is a valid contract, it is a legally enforceable agreement. Consequences are associated with breaking a contract or agreement, and there are methods to terminate a contract that carry with them effects of termination. More often than not, the contract itself will deal with what happens if one or the other breaches the contract.

For practical purposes a contract is often beneficial for both the parties because it spells out the obligations of each party (I work, you pay me) and the term of the agreement and the consequences of a termination of the agreement. Because it is a legally binding agreement (as long as it meets the law's requirements of a valid contract, such as signature and terms of agreement), it is important for you to have an understanding of what a contract may look like in general terms and to be knowledgeable about items that can be negotiated in a contract. Then, when negotiating, you can carefully review how each item in the contract benefits one or both parties. The purpose of an employment contract is to answer any questions that might arise and to prevent recourse in court. The fewer open questions the better.

It is possible to create an oral contract. However, if there is a written contract it will generally state that none of the written terms and conditions can be changed except in writing. If there isn't a written contract, issues will always arise that are subject to more than one interpretation. Oral contracts are often based on a handshake and time and changes in personnel can fade memories. Many practitioners have accepted employment offers only to be disappointed with bonuses that were calculated differently than they remember in the employment interview or to learn that changes were made in continuing education reimbursement or that there are limits to—or the absence of—supposedly negotiated benefits.

A written contract establishes the terms of employment and is constant over personnel changes and time. It protects you as the employee and the employer. The contract should be written and signed by both parties, and it should at least provide the amount of compensation in an intelligible and understandable statement. If you don't understand a term of the contract, you are accepting the possibility of ambiguity, and you increase the risks subject to litigation because they aren't spelled out clearly. Internet Resources at the end of the chapter provides a sampling of resources for contracts.

What things usually are included in an employment contract?

A few things are pretty basic here: the names of the parties to the contract, the dates during which the contract is in effect, how it can be renewed, and a general description of what is being exchanged ["Sole Employment of Employee John Doe" "the sum of Fifty Thousand (50,000.00) dollars"]. The effective period of the contract ("From the 1st day of January 2005, until the 31st day of December 2005) and methods of renewing the contract (written notification in the event of cancellation at some period before the end of the period, which lets both parties make accommodations for the change that will be experienced during the period of transition out of the practice), together with circumstances under which termination of the contract can occur (firing, layoffs, etc., whether you are an employee "at will" who can be fired for any reason or no reason whatsoever without advance notice).

What types of items should be included in the contract?

Compensation Package. The types of items to be included in the employment contract include base salary and any bonus or productivity opportunity; if part time either a salary or per-hour pay rate; overtime pay rate and situations; if appropriate, employer retirement contribution and personal retirement contribution options, continuing education monies, and paid time off; amount of time off for vacation, personal days, holidays, and sick time; profit sharing; life insurance, short- and long-term disability insurance, health insurance for self and family; meals; clothing; and the like. The circumstances under which payment is made by the employer for the benefit of the employee (which can include life insurance, retirement contributions, stock options) are also included.

Your total compensation package is the value or cost of the job benefits such as pay, health insurance, parking fees, retirement contributions, and memberships to exclusive golf courses. Consider this: If you produce significant profits should you be entitled to share in them? And, what steps would that require (perhaps an additional contract, committee discussion, and a decision about distributions). It is important to discuss this thoroughly and get written documentation to help avoid potential disputes as to methods of computation. For example, is profit sharing based on gross or net revenues? Are all providers sharing in covering the low or no-pay clients? The specifics of profit sharing are beyond the scope of this chapter. It is, however, something you may want to consult an accountant or lawyer about for guidance in negotiating this benefit. If you will be additionally compensated by any "unit" (clients per day, complexity in client load, etc.), this should be spelled out in your contract.

Consider whether you may require time off for family leave. If your employer has more than 50 employees per day for the last 20 workweeks, then by law you get the time but without compensation. Perhaps you want compensation for such leave time. If it might be an issue, you may want to make provisions for such a leave (due to pregnancy, family emergency, health crisis) and provide for compensation during such periods. This may be considered a unique type of disability insurance; it is certainly not beyond the scope of negotiating your employment contract to make such provisions clear. All potential issues ought to be considered before solutions are needed. Your bargaining power is stronger now than after circumstances arise that require you to take time off.

Job Descriptions and Duties. Will you have a written description of your job? If there are questions about the scope of your responsibilities or duties, are these adequately addressed by the contract? Will there be requirements to get or maintain certifications and, if so, who is paying for that?

Practice Issues. These issues include such things as whether there is an employer/employee relationship or that of independent contractor. Who will pay for journals and whose journals will they be? Other anticipated issues such as money for professional memberships, medical staff dues, office space and supplies, journals, and malpractice insurance should be covered. In the event that there will be an evaluation process, who evaluates and how often, and what if any criteria are going to be used for that evaluation?

Employment. Your contract should include basics such as how long it is effective, and what the effects are of you not being employed there for some reason. Your contract generally will provide for many things, such as the effective date of the contract or the steps to take to renew the contract ("... automatically renewed unless written notice is given 90 days or more from the date this contract expires"). It should contain any limitations on your right to work elsewhere during your employment ("shall be employed by no other party") or after termination of the contract ("shall not engage in practice within 45 miles for 12 months") or whether some or any "outside pay" may be owed your employer if you do receive outside compensation for anything. To be honest, employers like the feeling of having total and exclusive employee dedication to the job.

In an employment contract, what should I look (out) for?

Many things should be considered when negotiating your contract and many means of negotiation are available. One approach is to compare what you will cost the practice to what you will produce. This approach is easy to use and can guide your negotiations.

Step 1: Determine your desired salary and benefit package. Table 5-1 provides an example of an NP salary package showing the total cost of an NP to a practice. Using this example, you can insert the salary that you would like to make, the benefits you desire, and determine the total cost of the salary package you wish to negotiate.

Table 5-1 The Cost of Your Pay Package

Salary	$76,800	WageChart
Social Security	$4,992	
401K/403B	$2,500	
Educational	$2,500	
Health care insurance	$4,608	
Paid vacation	$4,100	
Disability insurance	$1,400	
Liability insurance	$3,000	
Total cost	$99,990	

Table 5-2 What You Make Compared with Billings

		Cost and Production
Patients per day	18	
Billing per patient	$75	
Days per week	5	
Weeks per year	48	
You produce per week	$6,750	
You produce per year	$324,000	
What is the patient flow?		
What is the recovery rate on billings?		

Step 2: Determine what revenue you will generate for the practice. This is your reality check. Are you bringing in adequate revenue to pay for your salary package? Table 5-2 provides an example of a method to determine revenue projections. In this example, the NP will see 18 clients per day, 5 days per week for 48 weeks per year. This leaves 4 weeks for vacations and time off. You may choose to shorten or lengthen the amount of time that you will take off from the practice and insert this factor in your calculations. The average charge for each client, in this example, is projected to be $75. In this scenario, the NP will generate $6750 per week and bring in $324,000 annually.

Two important factors that must be considered in this projection are as follows: (1) Is there an adequate client base to generate the projected number of visits? (2) What percentage of billings will be received by the practice? (Some practices negotiate discounted visits to different insurance companies and there may be unrecoverable billings from some clients). Based on this example you can calculate your anticipated client volume, average billing, and projected total revenues for the practice. This step helps you to determine if your salary and benefit expectations are realistic, too high, or too low. It also provides information for a base salary structure and potential bonus or productivity incentive based on seeing more clients than originally projected.

Step 3. Establish a per-hour rate or determine your annual salary and benefit package. Table 5-3 identifies factors to consider when setting your

Table 5-3 May I Have an Hour of Your Time?

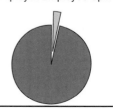

	Employer/Employee Split
How much are you billing per hour?	
What is your hourly rate?	
What is the employer gain per hour?	
How much is billed for what you do?	
What are the collection rates?	
What if you get all the non-paying clients?	
Who is at risk if the client does not pay?	

hourly or annual compensation package. It helps you sort out revenue and expense projections and factors that affect your practice and productivity.

What items should be considered in employment contract negotiation?

Certain items should be considered in negotiating your contract. If you are going to be hired as an employee, consider the following items in your negotiation for salary and benefits.

Salary. How much will you receive as paycheck income per year? This is your base salary; bonuses, productivity payouts, or profit sharing should be a separate calculation. There is abundant information on the salary ranges of nurse practitioners available on the Internet. Data from a national NP salary survey is in Table 5-4.

However, national averages may not apply to your situation. You should be able to obtain information through networking with other NPs already working to get an idea of where on the scale your locale and specialty are. Table 5-5 gives an example of salary variations in select states.

Valuable information on salary wages can be found at *www.mna3rddistrict.org, www.jobsa.com/salarysurveys,* and *www.advanceweb.com.* A good site with links to government data is *www.ga.unc.edu/NCCN/research/Salary Data Sources.htm.* The website *http://swz.salary.com* maintains current information on entire wage packages. And, of course, the American College of Nurse Practitioners is a good source for salary information for the practitioner. The ACNP web site breaks down salary in terms of vacation time, bonuses, and the like and can be a valuable tool when looking at the entire salary package. Table 5-6 lists the

Table 5-4 Nurse Practitioner Salary Surveys

U.S. National Averages	
3+ Years of experience	$62,000
First year	$57,000
Locality	
Urban	$63,000
Suburban	$64,000
Rural	$60,000
Degree separations	
PhD, administration director	$72,000
Master's	$60,000
Bachelor's	$45,500
Part-time hourly rate	$35.10

Source: Allied Physicians, Inc., Rehoboth Beach, DE. Retrieved February 2004 from *www.allied-physicians.com/salary_surveys/nurse-salaries.htm#nurse-practitioner-salares*

Table 5-5 Median Nurse Practitioner Salary by State for Selected States

Florida (31)	$57,054
New York (27)	$62,000
Ohio (26)	$62,750
California (23)	$62,000
Illinois(20)	$61,500
Texas (19)	$70,000
Georgia (19)	$65,000
Massachusetts (19)	$65,146

Source: Data from Payscale.com, Seattle, WA. Retrieved January 2005 from
www.payscale.com/salary-survey/vid-9872

results of a 2004 survey regarding the median total compensation for NPs in the United States.

Based on national averages, a graduating NP should receive somewhere around $76,000 per year in salary. Additional benefits can be determined accordingly. Certain benefits are, of course, beyond the scope of negotiation (Social Security, state and federal withholding taxes, and the like) and other benefits will be determined in part by what is already in use by the employer (contributions to retirement plan, health care benefits including deductible). And, certain benefits are clearly subject to continued negotiation (license and registration fees, reimbursement for educational expenses, and ownership of

Table 5-6 Median Compensation for a Nurse Practitioner in the United States*

Total Compensation (base + bonuses + benefits)		
Benefit	**Median Amount ($)**	**% of Total**
Base salary	68,175	73
Bonuses	163	0
Social Security	5,228	6
401k/403b	2,474	3
Disability	1,667	2
Health care	5,390	6
Pension	2,214	2
Time off	7,465	8
Total	**92,776**	**100**

*The median total compensation including benefits for a typical nurse practitioner in the United States is $92,776. This basic market pricing report was prepared by Certified Compensation Professionals' analysis of survey data collected from thousands of human resources departments at employers of all sizes, industries, and geographies. Data as of June 2004.

educational materials). Costs involved in staff privileges and the like should be covered if you will be seeing and treating clients in a facility setting.

Professional Expenses. How much will be contributed by the employer to the cost of continuing education units, attendance at conferences (including travel, meals, transportation expenses), and the time involved in attending them? How many journals, books, and professional organization memberships will be paid by the employer? Make sure to include the cost of your DEA application, licensure and certification, and lab coats in your employment contract. The amount varies considerably from practice to practice and often ranges from $1500 to $6000.

Benefits. Dental, medical (single or family coverage), and short- and long-term disability insurance are often negotiated into the contract. Sick days, jury duty, bereavement days, holidays, and unforeseen causes for missing work should be considered, together with vacations (paid or unpaid and length).

Profit Sharing. If you are increasing the profits of the practice, should you reap the benefits by sharing in those profits? And, if on the other hand the practice is not making money, should you have to contribute from your salary to make up the losses? (Believe it or not, such provisions are not uncommon in multiple-site practices where low production sites are supported by the more financially strong sites.) There are many ways to calculate and distribute bonuses or engage in profit sharing. The astute NP will be aware of these benefit opportunities and inquire about them.

A few ways that bonuses and profits may be figured include calculation of relative value units (total or worked), percentage of the total profit, percentage of the profit based on seniority, or percentage of the profit based on number of clients served and revenues generated. Some clinic operations include quality measures, on-call time, committee participation, or professional community involvement as elements in calculating or awarding bonuses or profit sharing. However, the specifics of profit sharing are beyond the scope of this treatise, because it raises questions of methods of accounting (gross versus net, etc.) and it does not fit into all practices. It is something you should be aware of and consider in negotiations. If the practice is going to generate significant funds it may make sense to further investigate this with an accountant or attorney.

Retirement. Is there an employer-sponsored retirement program in effect and, if so, will you share in it? Is the retirement plan a defined program? (In a defined retirement plan, you are guaranteed a set amount of money per specific time periods on retirement). Does the employer contribute a specific percentage of your base salary per year? Are you required to match the employer's contribution in order to participate in the retirement plan? Will your employer match dollar for dollar up to a certain percent of your salary for retirement? If so, this is a wise investment!

Retirement programs and plans vary widely from employer to employer. Some employers offer a small salary percentage match, whereas other generously fund retirement plans for their employees. Take the time to investigate this important employment benefit because the salary match can be as little as 1% to 2 % of base salary to 17% or more. This is a benefit that if not evaluated carefully can be overlooked. It could help you make a decision about what employment opportunity you ultimately accept!

Other important questions relate to your ability to contribute above and beyond the employer's retirement contributions. Can you make your own contributions to the program? Are you eligible for a 401k or 403b retirement plan? Should you be establishing a Keogh account? Is a SEP-IRA appropriate for you? Decisions about retirement funds can be intricate and confusing. Financial planning warrants professional assistance. Consequences can be significant over the life of the investment. A good investment for professional advice here may easily pay for itself many times over. If you ever plan on retirement, you had better plan on setting up your finances now. Unless you are planning on Social Security as your only source of retirement security, you will have to provide for your own retirement. Your retirement should be funded now. Do not overlook the importance of retirement saving. Starting your retirement early will assist you in securing a comfortable retirement for the future.

Malpractice Insurance. Employers are responsible for the claimed negligence of employees, but you should never leave malpractice coverage in question. If you are covered, ask for documentation of that fact. Make sure you are covered for malpractice insurance. If you are not, you will either need to negotiate this with the employer or purchase your own. These premiums, depending on your specialty and geographical location, can be costly.

It is important to understand that most malpractice insurance policies purchased by your employer will only cover clinical practice (decision making and treatment) that occurs while you are seeing clients at your place of employment. If you volunteer or provide advice to neighbors or friends, employer-purchased malpractice policies probably won't cover those types of management and treatment decisions. In these cases, it is critical for you to purchase an individual malpractice insurance policy.

Practice Evaluation. Will your practices be evaluated? How often? By whom? According to what standards? What if there are negative findings?

What is a noncompete clause?

A *covenant not to compete* is an agreement that an employee will not engage in the same or similar practice, usually for a set period of time and a set geographical area. This is to prevent a practitioner from entering a practice, establishing relationships with the clients, and then leaving that job and taking those clients and consumers with them. There are surely some circumstances under which an employer might be in need of such restrictions, but isn't it much more likely that there is room for the two of you in town if you are terminated?

A covenant-not-to-compete agreement is generally enforceable if it is reasonable in scope (time, distance). Should you sign the contract with this provision, you are agreeing to not practice or engage in gainful employment for a specified period of time in a specific geographical area. This provision can be enforced in court. Is this beneficial to you? How can such limitations after you've left your current job be a good thing for you? If you aren't supposed to take clients, spell that out in the agreement, but be very careful in contracting away your right to earn money doing what you have chosen to do. These agreements very regularly appear in employment contracts; these provisions are likewise often waived (are not a part of the contract) with successful negotiation. Demonstrate, with examples of the unfairness that may result. If you are told to take it or leave it, you better think long and hard about what it is you are considering taking before agreeing to do so. Have your eyes open, and open your employer's eyes, by demonstrating the many ways in which these agreements can cause a bad result even if entered into for the most legitimate of reasons. Propose agreeing that you won't steal clients if you leave the practice, and set time limits on that.

What about severance pay?

If and when your contract ends, you want to have some security for your future, and this should include severance pay to tide you over between jobs, as opposed to your filing claims for unemployment insurance! This should be nothing new to employers, and something you should pay a bit of attention to when entering into your contract. In considering the amount to ask for, it is reasonable to consider the effects unemployment claims would have on the employer, the length of time for which you would receive unemployment, how much you were earning before severance, and how much notice you were given before paychecks ceased to flow into your account. At its best, severance pay means that you leave with a window of opportunity; at its worst, it means you are able to survive between jobs.

Legal Issues

Is my contract legally binding?

Your contract is indeed legally binding, just like your mortgage or lease, or your agreement to pay the paper boy for your nightly paper. But keep in mind that the contract may provide for methods of changing its terms (and that should be in a writing signed by each party to the contract). For example, if your job is terminated because of a lack of client load, any provision that might seem to block your continuing on with your normal life (at another place of employment), like a covenant not to compete as just discussed, should be discussed between you and your employer to determine if the employer will waive that part of the contract. Your contract should explain how to modify its terms, which is almost universally accomplished by spelling out the changes in writing and signing a document.

What are the advantages and disadvantages of having a written contract?

The disadvantages are that it makes it more difficult for one party to deny benefits to the other over ambiguities and questions about what the real terms might be. The advantages are plentiful: clarity, questions answered, terms set out, proof of understanding and agreement (signature), agreement about what happens if the relationship comes to an end, etc. Most employment contracts clearly provide that oral modifications to the contract are not enforceable. There isn't any good reason to prefer an oral contract unless you enjoy being an employee at will who can be told on a Friday not to return to work on Monday and you don't care whether your family has that health insurance that someone mentioned at some time.

Should I have my contract reviewed by an attorney?

It would seem that since your employer has had the contract reviewed by an attorney, you should likewise have that right. An expense is associated with having an attorney look at it, so when it looks like you are going to be faced with a contract in the near future, get a lawyer on the phone and ask how much a contract review will cost—and don't sell your value short here! Peace of mind alone may be worth a couple hundred dollars. Maybe that review will pay for itself 10 times over. At worst you are out a small amount for certainty and clarification of questions; at best the visit will pay for itself over and over again. A risk-benefit analysis suggests that it might be a good idea for you to get a lawyer to look it over for you. Ask members of your network whether they know of an attorney knowledgeable in such matters. And if you feel very bold indeed, you can insist that the expense be paid for by the employer in the event you ultimately sign the contract.

How do I negotiate my contract?

The first step in the process of negotiating a contract is to become knowledgeable about NP practice in your area, scope of practice, and the benefits to a practice for hiring an NP. You will need to be prepared to present facts, and make a case for what you are worth. Remember that you are often negotiating with someone who has little to no experience in hiring personnel or dealing with contracts, so you will need to be prepared to guide the process.

Practice beforehand what you will say. Prepare a 2- to 3-minute opening statement on what you personally can add to the practice, and how the practice will benefit financially by your being hired. Know which contract issues are negotiable and which are not negotiable before starting the negotiation process. Practice in front of a mirror or videotape yourself and ask for feedback from people who will give you constructive criticism. Be aware of your language use and body language so you will project a powerful image by making eye contact, by sitting up straight, by making clear and concise statements, and by avoiding saying "Ummm" and fidgeting in your chair. Look and act business-like and professional.

Dress for your salary range. This may mean purchasing your first business suit, but it will be worth it, since every subsequent contract that you negotiate with that employer will be based on your first contract. Groom for your salary range, even if this means going out and having your hair styled and cut. While these may seem like superficial strategies, appearance does count in the business world.

Negotiation is a process, and compromise is a part of that process that needs to be developed. The goal is to create a contract that is beneficial for each party, and so you will need to have an explanation and justification for the things that you are asking for in the contract. The NP and the employer need to understand each other's point of view, and feel like they are being treated fairly. Do not become emotional during the negotiation process; if you feel you are losing control, it is better to reschedule than try to continue in an unprofessional manner. Actively listen, and ask for clarification especially if unfamiliar terms are being used. An example of this is if you are told that you will need to log "32 client units each day" and you do not understand the term. You deserve to know what you have to do to get paid. Do not be afraid that you may look ignorant by asking for clarification; instead be afraid of what you may be agreeing to if you do not understand the terms of the contact!

You may want to bring some written notes with you to jog your memory. Do not confuse organization with fear. It is not unreasonable for you to bring notes, particularly if your employer has had the contract typed up. The employer's attorney is not working to protect your rights. Your employer has an advocate. Be your personal advocate. That reasonably means you can take the time to review the contract outside the work environment. Again, you can rest assured that someone reviewed what you have been handed, so don't feel unreasonable in asking for the same courtesy.

SUMMARY

For you to achieve the most advantageous contract, you must do your preliminary work and consider as many issues as come to mind that may be subject to negotiation. You must not rely on oral promises. If it is important enough

Internet Resources

University of Minnesota School of Nursing. Negotiating an Employment Contract: Guidelines for the Newly Graduated Advanced Practice Nurse
www.nursing.umn.edu/professional/negotiating

BizHelp24.com: What Is an Employment Contract?
www.bizhelp24.com/business_law/employment-contract-3.shtml#9

'Lectric Law Library: Employment Agreement Form
www.lectlaw.com/forms/f161.htm

'Lectric Law Library: Employee Non-Compete Agreement Form
www.lectlaw.com/forms/f019.htm

FormsGuru.com: Employment Agreement
www.formsguru.com/forms/legal-forms/emplcont.html

LawDepot.com: Employment Agreement
www.lawdepot.com/contracts/employ/?pid=findwhat-employ-generic

for someone to make an oral promise, then they should not balk at putting it into writing. Make a checklist of important issues, and research the issues. Practice negotiating will help actual negotiating. And remember that in any negotiation the other side wants to come out the 'winner' so make sure you are able to present issues favorable for the other side as you seek what is important for you.

6

Third-Party Reimbursement

Katherine J. Dontje
Kathy M. Forrest

Understanding Third-Party Reimbursement

Traditionally nurses have not found themselves involved with insurance contracting. As staff nurses in a hospital setting, nursing care is bundled into a package charge, hidden within the entire client bill. This hides both the value and real expense of nursing care, often setting nurses up as an "easy target" to reduce costs in an environment where reimbursement for services is dwindling. As nurse practitioners in independent practice, we need to be familiar with insurance contracting as it affects reimbursement and the viability of our practice. As a group, NPs are becoming more aware of the need to bill independently for their services to capture revenue, build a service database, and enhance their professional standing in the health care arena. The problem comes when insurance companies either do not recognize NPs as providers or reduce reimbursement to a percentage of that allowed to physicians for the same services. Because of these issues, it is important for the NP to understand sources of revenue, types of insurance, and reasons why it is important to request an independent provider number or to become paneled with a health maintenance organization (HMO). Once the steps for reimbursement are in place, a marketing plan to spread the word of their services can be accomplished.

Why should a nurse practitioner become enrolled in insurance plans?

NPs have been providing primary care services for more than 30 years but have very little visibility. One of the primary reasons this is true is due to the fact that most NPs do not directly bill for services. Most of the data collected on physician practices comes from billing and collection data. By having their services billed through a physician, NPs have set up a situation in which the individual data for services provided to clients is not retrievable.

One of the most important issues for NPs in practice is to seek out the opportunity wherever possible to have their services billed directly under their name and provider number. This has been a challenge for NPs because of many of the restrictions that are placed on providers by insurance companies in terms of who qualifies as an independent provider. The systems were set up initially to accommodate physicians only. As NPs have grown in their role, they have sought the opportunity to become listed as primary providers. This has been met with a mixture of success. The goal is for NPs to get direct reimbursement because that not only influences professional value but also the ability to track quality of care measures (Letz, 2002).

What are the different mechanisms of payment that insurance plans offer?

Most of us don't remember a time when insurance was not available to individuals in the United States, but in reality health insurance is a relatively new concept. The first insurance plans have only been in effect since the early 1900s (Robinson & Kish, 2001). The health insurance agencies have been heavily regulated at both the state and federal levels. The primary responsibility for health insurance regulation lies with the states. This has been delegated to the states due to their responsibility for ensuring the public health of their citizens. The reason this is important to the NP is because health insurance rules and regulations can vary from state to state. The exception to this is the federal regulation related to Medicare. Medicare is a federal program with rules and regulations developed by the Center for Medicare and Medicaid Services (CMS). These federal rules are interpreted at state and regional levels, so NPs need to be aware that reimbursement for their services can vary from state to state.

Five major categories of third-party payers exist (Buppert, 2004). They are Medicare, Medicaid, indemnity insurance companies, managed care organizations that often use capitation programs, and businesses that contract for specific services.

Medicare. Medicare is a federal program administered nationally by the CMS and locally, or in regions, by Medicare agencies. Coverage is available for clients 65 year of age or older who are enrolled and pay premiums, and for individuals with disabilities who qualify according to Social Security disability guidelines.

Medicaid. Medicaid is a federal program administered state by state to mothers and children who qualify based on poverty, and for adults who may either be disabled on a short-term basis or who qualify according to their poverty status. Within these types of insurance there are various payment plans. Some of the major categories can have several options for payment; for example, Medicaid can be either a fee-for-service indemnity plan or a health maintenance organization (HMO) or managed care organization (MCO).

Indemnity Plans. Indemnity plans pay for services to providers on a per-visit, per-procedure basis according to the insurance plan's fee schedule, policies, and procedures. This type of plan was the primary source of insurance payments in the past. The problem with this type of reimbursement, however, was that there was no incentive for limiting services—the more services provided the more money you were reimbursed.

Capitation Basis. In response to growing health care costs, *managed care organizations* were developed. In this type of organization the insurer provides both health care services and payment for services within a network. *Primary care providers* (PCPs) are typically responsible for the client's coordination of services, directing them to specialty providers and related services as needed. Payment in these systems is often on a *capitation basis*, which is prepayment of a certain amount per enrolled member per month. This entails a certain amount of risk to the provider in terms of payment for services. If you have a large number of members who require extensive services (often individuals with chronic disease conditions), the resulting payment may not cover the cost of providing service. In contrast, if you have members who do not require any services, you would have a positive cash flow. The goal is to have a mix of clients, and a focus on wellness and disease prevention, to equalize the cost. This type of insurance also encourages the utilization of specific guidelines of practice and limitations on referrals unless proven necessary as a way to "manage care." Appendix 6-1 provides an example of per-member, per-month cost considerations.

NPs may be considered PCPs within the network, but they often are not paid as physician providers, even though they are providing the same service. Medicare has indicated that NPs can provide care but will be reimbursed at 85% of the normal physician rate even if the service is identical. In addition, not all MCOs will allow NPs to be considered paneled providers. A paneled provider is a practitioner (NP, PA, or physician) who has been approved by a health plan to provide care to their insured members and to receive payment by the health plan for approved services that were rendered. This has become a problem with Medicaid specifically. Federal and state rules may allow NPs to provide primary care services, but if the HMO with which the state contracts will not consider NPs to be PCPs, the NPs cannot get reimbursed for these services. This creates an unfair advantage to physicians who not only can provide the service, but also are reimbursed for the service.

Contracts. This is a payment mechanism that works well for NPs. They can work out a defined set of services, such as health screenings or education for work-related injuries, and then be paid directly to provide those services. This eliminates the third-party insurer rules and regulations and allows the NP to negotiate directly for their services.

What are the advantages and disadvantages for NPs regarding contracting for the different payment mechanisms?

NPs need to understand the various types of payment mechanisms in order to decide what types of clients they will see, how many of each type they will see in their client load, and how much they project they will be reimbursed. These issues are particularly relevant when you are looking at job possibilities. The NP needs to consider the types of reimbursement and how this will affect the type and number of clients they will be seeing as well as the salary the NP will generate. Different health insurance plans will reimburse at different rates (Abood & Keepnews; 2002). We are all aware that the private health insurance plans typically pay more than a Medicaid plan. But, if NPs choose not to take Medicaid clients because of the rate of reimbursement, they will need to fit that within their practice philosophy. In contrast, for a clinic or practice to survive, you need to have a reasonable income and means to pay for the overhead that is part of the practice.

Each of the types of insurance has pro and cons for the NP. One of the main problems is enrollment issues, which are discussed later in this chapter. Decisions about which health plans to apply for are related to the type of plan, payment method, and eligibility requirements.

An advantage of the indemnity plan is the ability to plan for reimbursement on a fee based system and get reimbursed for each time the client has an encounter with the provider. The advantage of the managed care type plans is that you will have constant income generated by its per-member, per-month reimbursement payments, but if the client is seen multiple times in one month, the reimbursement may not equal the cost of services. One of the strategies for the managed care plans is to enroll a number of clients and have a mix of healthy and ill clients so that they will offset one another. This is not always easy to do and is one of the reasons why straight per-member, per-month payment has not been attractive to providers. Capitated client populations may be "diluted" in a practice with other fee-for-service client populations as a means to control the unpredictable.

Provider Status and Insurance Contracting

For which insurance plans do you hope to get provider status?

Obtaining provider status with insurance plans allow services to be provided and reimbursed according to the plan's own reimbursement policies and fee schedules. You may hear this process referred to as *credentialing*. Except for a small minority of clients who pay their own health care bills, every encounter between a NP and a client has a third party, or insurance, carrier to act as the payer of services. It is imperative that NPs have provider status or be credentialed with these payers to receive reimbursement for services, otherwise the service will be provided at the expense of the NP's practice or result in an out-of-pocket expense to the client. (Client satisfaction is not enhanced by having to pay unexpected out-of-pocket expense. This could result in the client leaving your practice and/or spreading negative comments to other potential clients. Not exactly what you need to build your practice!)

To determine which insurance plans to participate with as an NP, you must know the client base you wish to serve and which payers represent them for your reimbursement. If you are joining an established practice, find out what types of clients comprise the current client base and what types of clients you wish to attract for your services. You will need to know what insurance plans are prevalent in the area and specifically which plans will allow NPs to credential with them and their rules for NP billing. You will also need to know the types of services you anticipate providing to this group of clients. Slager (2004) points out that clinicians are faced with three payment scenarios: payers who credential and reimburse at 100% of the physician rate, payers who reimburse at some fraction of the physician rate (Medicare at 85% for example), and payers who do not credential nonphysician providers at all. A careful analysis of the anticipated client base, considering insurance plans and their payment policies for NP services, will provide information imperative to your practice and its financial stability. Your practice is dependent on revenue for rendered client services to offset its expenses. The information you receive in advance of providing services is key to a financially successful practice.

In practice, providers typically seek provider status with the insurance plans/companies that reach a majority of clients in their geographic region. Medicare, Medicaid, and Blue Cross Blue Shield plans are prevalent across the United States. Regional variations of preferred provider organizations (PPOs), HMOs, and other fee-for-service insurance products may be sought as well. Once the client base of the practice is established, insurance plans that cover the lives of those clients can be sought to cover services provided. Each geographic region has its unique complement of third-party insurance payers. One option to identify these carriers is to contact a local medical insurance billing service for information about insurance plans/companies serving your area.

What does insurance contracting mean?

Insurance contracting denotes an agreement between a provider of health care services and an insurance plan to provide care to its subscribers and dependents. Employers typically provide health insurance to their employee groups according to the insurance plans available in their geographic region, costs associated with these plans, and the employer's size in terms of employees. Providers of health care services choose to seek or not seek provider status with insurance plans within their geographic region based on the plans' credentialing and reimbursement policies.

When providers (or groups of providers) agree to a contract with an insurance plan to provide services, they agree with the contract's terms, which follow the insurance plan's governing policies. Once the contract is in place, the provider of care has an obligation to the insurance plan, as well as to the clients for services rendered according to the plan. Clients have an obligation with the insurance plan to uphold their portion of the insurance plan, including copayments and payment of deductible amounts. It is imperative for the NP provider to know the terms of the insurance contract for both themselves and the client. This will enhance the potential reimbursement to the practice and avoid poor relations between the provider and client.

Contract agreements include many pieces of information that are important to the provider. They specify which services will be reimbursed and which will not be considered covered by benefits. The contract will also disclose information about the process of billing and who is eligible for payment. It is important to note whether NPs are included in this eligibility and at what rate. A list of services and their corresponding reimbursement may be obtained as part of the contracting process. It is important to note the method of payment: fee for service, capitation, or a combination of the two. Requirements for provider participation are also included in the contract, noting the difference between in-network and out-of-network status. Reimbursement typically differs between the categories, with resulting increases of the client's out-of-pocket costs. Provider requirements often include national board certification, malpractice insurance coverage, and professional references verifying credentials and client care quality.

Contracts with insurance carriers typically outline the process of subscriber benefit verification. Member services and provider services are often provided as resources as part of the contract with the insurer to guide both groups. Members require a resource to learn about their benefits and how to access care. Providers require assistance to ensure the client has current coverage with the insurance plan and the service rendered is covered under the plan.

Insurance contracts with provider offices also include a quality component. This is evident in the process of enrollment, in the application questions and verification of information, and in the follow-up after the contract is established. Typically office audits and/or site visits are conducted by individuals representing the insurance plan to ensure compliance with the plan's policies and procedures as well as national quality standards that guard client safety.

What is the process involved with insurance contracting?

The process of insurance contracting involves many steps and a considerable amount of time. The first step is to complete an application for the insurance plan you wish to contract. Buppert (2004) notes a complete listing of information requested in a typical application in Appendix 9-A of her book. Provider name and a wide variety of demographic information are requested. Licensure information, specialty certification, employment history in the profession, and educational preparation and ongoing education are requested. Current privileges at health care facilities (hospitals specifically) are requested with specific periods of privileges, the type held, and any leadership positions held as part of the affiliation. Professional liability coverage is requested with proof of the type, duration, and dollar amount, specifically. Professional sanction details are also requested. The application requests a list of professional reference names and contact information to attest to the NP's current level of clinical competency, technical skill, and medical knowledge. Attachments to the completed contract often include licenses, liability coverage documents, diplomas, certificates of specialty completion, board certification, delegation of prescriptive authority, and physician collaborative agreements.

The contract will also request a list of the types of services the NP is planning to provide and to what age range of clients. A plan for provision of care across the health care continuum is also commonly requested. For example, a PCP would be requested to specify which individuals in his or her practice will be providing after-hour professional coverage to clients, how clients could access this care, and what hospitals client admissions would be directed to. Hospital coverage arrangements and after-care need to be specified as well.

Once the application is submitted to the insurance carrier, the carrier's process of verifying information begins. Each professional reference, educational institution, employer, and health care institution is contacted for primary verification. Professional sanctions are investigated and all application information is verified as accurate and complete. This process of verifying application information often takes 2 to 3 months.

Notification of provider status is sent with insurance billing numbers and a letter indicating the NP has successfully completed the application processing for that insurance. A site visit of the clinical area often follows before seeing clients to ensure that a safe environment exists for the provision of client care.

No billing and reimbursement for services can be done during the application process; billing and reimbursement occur only after notification of provider status. Insurance plans may, however, allow for retroactive billing. This is not always the case so careful consideration of this factor is advised.

Many similarities exist in required application information among the different insurance plans, so even though insurance-specific forms are time consuming to complete initially, you will save some time with subsequent applications because you have already compiled the required information and documents. Audrey Alflen at Grand Management Group has developed a useful tool that can aid you in compiling all of the information necessary to start the credentialing process (see Appendix 6-2).

How do you become a Medicare or Medicaid provider?

Enrollment as a provider with Medicare and Medicaid is done by completing an application as described in the preceding section. The CMS website is an extremely useful tool for accessing both an application and obtaining information pertinent to the process of application, reimbursement for services, provider resources, billing follow-up, medication formularies, and a variety of other services.

A Medicare provider enrollment application is completed on CMS Form 585R. The PDF file is located at *www.cms.hhs.gov/providers/enrollment/forms/cms855r.pdf*. Medicare Part B provider status allows you to bill Medicare directly for your services. Services you provide will be included in the Medicare database depicting the extent and level of services provided to Medicare beneficiaries. Medicare is administered regionally by Part B carriers. The CMS website is helpful in locating regional carriers to assist you.

As mentioned earlier in this chapter, Medicaid is administered on a state-by-state basis and, hence, variations are seen in how clinicians may practice according to their particular state's rules and regulations. Individual states also regulate billing for services and enrollment of providers. Contact the provider relations department of your state Medicaid agency for a provider application as an NP. Become familiar with your state's Medicaid regulations for NP services and billing.

Both Medicare and Medicaid services are billed on CMS Form 1500 using the client's name, common procedure code, and diagnosis code format. You should become familiar with the documentation guidelines for CMS services for both Medicare and Medicaid programs as they pertain to NPs.

Once you have provider status, how do you market your services?

Marketing an NP's services can make the difference between a successful practice and one that is unsuccessful. A lot of practices have NPs as part of the core group of providers, but their names do not appear on the outside of the building. Establishing and maintaining a practice can be a challenge for the NP. No matter how good you are, unless people know you exist, your practice will not grow. Different marketing strategies will need to be employed depending on whether you are entering an already established practice or are starting up a new practice. With either type of practice, however, you will need to remember some essential components of marketing. One of the key concepts is to know to whom you are marketing; this will help you devise the best marketing strategy for that group. This can be accomplished through a market analysis, which is part of your business plan (see Chapter 7).

Letz (2002) talks about several simple strategies that an NP can use to bring in new clients and keep existing clients. The first is to ask your clients for referrals—often person-to-person referrals are the best. You will need to have business cards to share with your clients as well as information packets that you can give them to share with others. If you do receive a client referral, you need to acknowledge that referral with either a note or phone call or by talking with the individual who made the referral at his or her next visit. Some people even suggest a small gift as a thank you.

Most NPs will want to develop a business card that they can give to clients and other providers to advertise their services. Figure 6-1 is an example of a NP business card. This can be developed with minimal cost by utilizing your computer. It is important to think about how the card will look; considering what type of market you are trying to reach will help determine the design. The essential information would be your name and title, address, phone number,

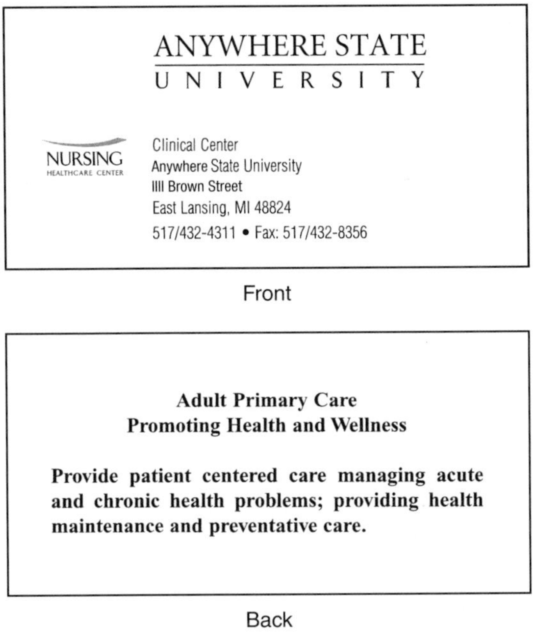

ANYWHERE STATE
U N I V E R S I T Y

NURSING
HEALTHCARE CENTER

Clinical Center
Anywhere State University
IIII Brown Street
East Lansing, MI 48824
517/432-4311 • Fax: 517/432-8356

Front

Adult Primary Care
Promoting Health and Wellness

Provide patient centered care managing acute and chronic health problems; providing health maintenance and preventative care.

Back

Figure 6-1   Example of a nurse practitioner business card.

fax number, and e-mail address. This will allow people to contact you easily. Consider carefully what number you want to give. For instance, if you choose to give out the main office number, is there a way individuals can leave you a message and how efficient is the staff in answering phone calls?

The third strategy is to develop an orientation packet that covers what a nurse practitioner is and what types of services you provide. This packet should be handed out to all new clients and possibly even be available to be given out in the waiting room and at community events. In addition to the orientation packet, Letz (2002) also suggests a marketing résumé, which includes your picture and your credentials as well as some personal information to provide to clients and colleagues.

A similar strategy for presenting this material would be to develop a website for your clinic. This will appeal to a particular population of clients and may be an option for recruiting new clients. The disadvantage of this type of marketing tool is the cost and time involved with initiating the website—determining what type of information you want to provide and then more importantly making sure the website is maintained over time. This is an additional duty that would need to be negotiated with your office because ongoing maintenance of the site takes significant time; checking links, answering client questions, and being aware of types of issues that would impact the site including HIPAA rules and regulations.

The next suggestion is to have your name on the stationary and other materials in the office and also in telephone book ads or newspaper ads. It is important to list your name in the phone book because a surprising number of clients still utilize this resource as a means of identifying a health care provider. It would be important for you to work with the business manager of the clinic to determine where ads can be most effectively placed. Taking an interest in this aspect of marketing a practice will add to your client base.

The fifth strategy is one that your entire office can implement: a reminder system for clients and a follow-up system if clients do not show for appointments. This is important for continuity of care, liability, and client satisfaction. Simply implementing a system that sends a reminder either personally, through the mail system, or electronically helps clients remember their scheduled appointments and decreases your no-show rates. It is important that you make sure clients are receiving appropriate follow-up care as well. Having the staff call individuals who do not show so they can reschedule indicates to clients that you feel their visits are important. You will also need to have some sort of system to identify and follow up on abnormal labs and tests so that clients are aware of results that have been received (see Chapter 11). This can be done by support staff but is important in providing quality care.

The final suggestion is that NPs need to develop more networking with colleagues. Networking within the community provides the NP not only with potential referral sources but also with a support system to discuss issues and concerns. This can be done through identifying a mentor or becoming part of a NP local network group. Such a group can provide opportunities for you to discuss client issues as well as to let people know you are available to take new clients.

One of the difficult things for NPs is dealing with the reality that provider status can affect whether or not you can accept clients. With many HMOs, for instance, you may not be able to be paneled independently, which then makes it difficult for the client, as they cannot select you as a paneled provider on their insurance plan. They will need to select your physician collaborator as their provider and hope they will be able to see you. This just emphasizes the need for NPs to fight for independent provider status and to become credentialed with insurance plans whenever possible.

SUMMARY

Contracting for third-party reimbursement can be a complicated process for NPs; it is time consuming and often wrought with multiple steps, barriers, and frustration. But contracting, although complicated, is a process that all NPs need to become more familiar with to streamline third-party reimbursement for their services. In order for NPs to receive payment for their services, insurance contracting with third-party payers is essential. In the past, many nurses have relied on physician billing or grant funding as a means of supporting a practice. In the current climate of increasing competition for services, NPs need to have a means of sustainability for their practice and the services they render. This chapter has provided an overview of the process of insurance contracting, how to determine what plans to consider when enrolling, an outline of different mechanisms of payment, and how to market services to clients once the payer mix is known.

 Internet Resources

Center for Medicare and Medicaid Services
www.cms.gov

American College of Nurse Practitioners
www.acnpweb.org

American Academy of Nurse Practitioners
www.aanp.org

Medicare Federal Health Care Reassignment of Benefits Application

(Application for Individual Health Care Practitioners to Reassign Medicare Benefits; Center for Medicare and Medicaid Services)
www.cms.hhs.gov/providers/enrollment/forms/cms855r.pdf

References

Abood, S., & Keepnews, D. (2002). *Understanding payment for APN service* (Vols. 1-4). Washington, DC: American Nurses Association.

Alflen, Audrey. Grand Management Group, Grand Rapids, MI.

Buppert, C. (2004). *Nurse practitioner's business practice and legal guide* (2nd ed.) Sudbury, MA: Jones & Bartlett Publishers.

Letz, K. (2002). *Business essentials for nurse practitioners.* Fort Wayne, Indiana: PreviCare, Inc. Publishing Division.

Robinson, D., & Kish, C. (2001). *Core concepts in advanced practice nursing.* St. Louis: Mosby.

Slager, J. (2004). *Business concepts for healthcare providers.* Sudbury, MA: Jones & Bartlett Publishers.

7

Starting Your Nurse Practitioner Business

Jean Nagelkerk

Getting Started

Nurse practitioners have many choices when planning their careers. When making an informed decision about owning a business or choosing to be employed in an established organization or system, each NP must:

- Evaluate his or her career trajectory.
- Determine the type of lifestyle he or she aspires to and enjoys.
- Identify the level of financial resources required.
- Evaluate his or her retirement goal, and examine career options.

Once the NP has determined that the best choice is to establish a new business venture, several steps must be taken to establish a successful business and maintain financial sustainability.

What steps do I take to determine if my business idea is realistic?

Business planning is a key element to a successful business operation. Careful planning, analysis, and research are essential when engaging in business venture development. Business planning is a careful and deliberate process of collecting data, networking in the community, and consulting with business associates.

NPs are in unique positions to assess, evaluate, and develop independent business opportunities and partnerships because they possess special skills and knowledge in nursing and have insights into current and emerging consumer health care needs.

Surveillance of health care and business environments to develop an awareness of consumer needs, wants, and desires provides opportunities for NPs seeking to fill the consumer product or service void that exists through intrapreneur and entrepreneur ventures. Identifying business opportunities that represent future potential growth or changing health care practices enhances financial viability of the business operation.

What community resources are available for starting a business?

Community resources that are available for business planning can assist a new business by helping the NP make key connections and identify important stakeholders critical to successful operations. Community organizations that offer expertise in business planning include:

- Small business center agencies
- Financial and business faculty at universities
- Local community business organizations
- Retired business owners
- Bankers
- City mentorship programs.

Chambers of commerce and local community organizations in the city where your business will operate can often provide resources to assist in business development. Cities encourage the establishment of new businesses, because businesses create new jobs and increase tax revenue. To enhance financial viability, nurse entrepreneurs who want to establish a business should seek professional assistance and utilize available community resources and services when planning that business. Nurses often work with few resources and overextend themselves, leading to burnout and frustration. Obtaining resources and community support increases the likelihood for a successful business operation.

The Business Plan

What is a business plan?

One of the first elements of successful business planning is the development of a written business plan. A business plan is key in evaluating the market forces and financial feasibility of the proposed venture. A business plan is a written document that maps out the business proposal in a logical and organized format. The business plan becomes a template that guides a business's overall operation and expenditure of resources based on the written marketing plans, product or service delineation, and revenue and expenditure projections, and it is often used to secure financial investments or resources.

A business plan requires careful and detailed planning and development. It is a document that is a blueprint for the business and covers a period of 1 to 5 years of operation and evaluation plans. It clearly states what services or products will be developed and sold. In the business plan, timelines for service or product development and distribution with clear revenue projections, expenditures, and a market plan with target goals for sales progress are clearly delineated. The business plan is based on collecting data and analyzing the information for the geographic area where the business will be located and the area it will serve. As the business idea crystallizes and is developed into a viable option, simultaneous data collection, network building, referral source identification, and partnerships begin to emerge. Relationship building is central to community and business connections and the success of a fledgling operation.

Should I seek legal or accounting help when planning a business?

Before consulting an attorney or accountant, make sure you have a clear idea of the type of business and product or service that you will initiate. By beginning your business plan, you will clearly identify the goals and objectives of your business and determine what market exists for your product or services.

Once you have completed the groundwork, an attorney who is familiar with state and federal laws regarding the type of business you are starting can be helpful with business laws and practices in your geographical area. To find an attorney with the skill set that you need for your business, contact friends and business acquaintances for referrals or contact the state bar association for their referral service. Attorneys can help you determine the business structure, such as a partnership (general or limited), corporation (professional or nonprofessional), or sole proprietorship, and the licensing laws and insurance policies.

Accountants can be helpful in describing the financing options, bookkeeping systems, and organizational structures that best meet your company's needs. Depending on your business needs and the complexity of your business you may decide to hire an accountant to set up your financial system. For a fee the accountant will do monthly, quarterly, and annual statements and perform any other accounting function that your company requires. Contacting friends, peers, or business acquaintances who have knowledge of accountants in your geographical area is one method to secure an accountant; another method is to contact a professional accounting organization for their referral service.

What are the elements of a business plan?

The business plan clearly states the purpose or mission of the proposed organization. A mission statement helps clarify and crystallize your thoughts and informs other people of the purpose of the proposed venture. It identifies and targets the market that will be served. The business plan communicates a shared understanding of key aspects of the business.

The business plan document is composed of several sections and includes pertinent data for initiating, tracking, and monitoring resources. Box 7-1 identifies the major elements of a business plan, and Appendix 7-1 provides a sample of a basic business plan for a community-based family health center. The business document typically consists of a *cover page,* which introduces the title of the new business venture; the *table of contents,* which provides a map of the business plan content; and an *executive summary,* which is 1 or 2 pages and concisely provides a description, marketing plan, and revenue projections.

The length of a business plan will vary depending on the complexity and nature of the type of business proposed, but often will be 15 or more pages in length. A good business plan is explicit and clearly describes the product, management, market, structure, cash flow projections, and exit plan. The business plan will provide a map for the organization for a period of 1 to 5 years and will establish goals, standards, and targets.

The main body of the document includes the following components:
- Vision, mission, and value statements of the venture and the industry
- Market survey research, assessment, analysis, and plan
- Detailed description of the product or services
- Design of the facility and space with equipment requirements
- Operational plans, management team, and master calendar with detailed schedule and assignments
- Cash flow analysis, revenue projections, performance targets, and measures
- Pricing for products or services
- Organizational structure and governance and communication with internal and external communities
- Risks and assumptions, exit strategies, and appendices.

The Executive Summary. The executive summary serves the purpose of setting the stage for individuals reading the business plan by providing an

---

Box 7-1 Major Elements of a Business Plan

- Executive summary
- Vision, mission, and value statement
- Market analysis
- Product design
- Operational development
- Marketing plan
- Organizational plan
- Development schedule
- Financial plan

introduction to the key elements of the proposal. The executive summary is short but powerful. It is a document that must convince potential investors, loaning agencies, and potential partners of the urgency, necessity, and viability of the proposed business venture. It clearly provides a description of the nature, goals, objectives, and outcomes of the business. A well-written business plan will catch the attention of the reader who will then read the entire document, whereas a poorly written plan will often be doomed to failure by not piquing the interest of the reader.

Strategic Planning. *Strategic planning* is a process of determining what your business will accomplish and how the business resources will be used to meet the plan (Barry, 2001; Johnson, 2004). In contrast, *operational planning* consists of the day-to-day decisions and management of the work plan and budget. Both types of planning are important, but to emerge as a leader in a viable business operation, the strategic planning process is important to develop a shared vision and set the direction for your organization in order to capitalize on the strengths and opportunities in the environment. Benefits of strategic planning include improved organizational focus and direction, evaluation and goal setting for critical organizational problems, enhanced communication and team commitment, and greater influence.

The Wilder Foundation has developed a five-step model to guide nonprofit organizations in strategic planning processes (Barry, 2001).

Step 1: Getting organized. Getting organized entails the selection of a group of knowledgeable and committed individuals to work on the development of a plan. Key people in your internal and external environment should be included. These people could include consumers, administrators, staff, consultants, and professional personnel. Selected individuals should be given educational materials or attend a workshop to familiarize themselves with the strategic planning process.

Step 2: Analyzing the situation. Assemble the organizational data, necessary literature, and worksheets to begin planning. At a planning meeting, distribute the data (organizational reports, assessments, budgetary worksheets), which illustrates the organization's health, and identify the most critical issues. During this stage a discussion of the history of the organization as well as recent progress or trials and the current mission should be reviewed. In the context of the economic, political, and social climate, a discussion of strengths and weaknesses, opportunities and threats, competitors and allies, and customer and stakeholder needs are undertaken. From this stage, the critical issues for the organizational future are identified.

Step 3: Setting the direction. Critically analyze each important issue, develop a plan or solution for the issue, and match resources. By setting organizational priorities, resources can be earmarked for these opportunities with support and evaluation plans. At this stage the group drafts the strategic plan. Specific attention should be paid to the mission and value statements, goals, strategies, implementation plan, and evaluation process.

Step 4: Refining the plan. Refinements are made through critical reviews and comments by staff, board members, business owners, and key external constituents. After these considerations are thoughtfully weighed, the plan is ready for implementation.

Step 5: Implementing the plan. Goals, checkpoints, individual and group assignments, and resource assignments for work will assist you in implementation of your plan. Establishing checkpoints for monitoring and evaluation is important for success and enables adaptation or refinements in the plan as indicated.

Vision, Mission, and Value Statements. The vision, mission, and value statements are important to establish the culture, purpose, and direction of the organization, and they play important roles in conveying the organizational philosophy to customers. A *vision* is what the organization is committed to doing. It describes the long-range goal, often a 5-year trajectory, for the organization. It creates a goal to work toward and strive to accomplish, thereby establishing a target for the organization to meet.

The *mission* describes the organizational business. It is a one-sentence statement that is central to the purpose, goals, and work of the business. It is a critical cultural element that explicates the organization's nature and main reason for existence. The mission statement describes the essence of the organization and may describe special populations or functions it serves. The mission provides employees and stakeholders, those individuals who have an interest in the company, with a clear message of organizational business direction.

The *value statements* are information about what the organization believes. They describe the assumptions or ethical relationships that provide direction for governance in the organization. The value statements explicate in a more detailed fashion a description of the vision and mission statements.

What is a market analysis?

The *market analysis* maps out, with specific facts and numbers, the potential market share for the service or product. It sets forth and illustrates how the business will succeed in the competitive marketplace. The market analysis addresses questions such as these:

- Who will purchase the product or service?
- How often will the service be purchased?
- What geographical area will be served by the business?

The marketplace, the size of existing and potential markets, and the extent and type of competition in the marketplace are all clearly identified. This analysis is important to convince investors of the ability of your company to secure a substantial market share in a competitive market to maintain financial viability. The market analysis should include the four elements or the four "P's":

- Product
- Place

- Promotion
- Price.

One framework that is often used to address marketing issues is the SWOT analysis. This analysis assesses the internal environment, management operations (strengths and weaknesses), and the external environment (opportunities and threats), that is, the marketplace. "SWOT" stands for:

- Strengths
- Weakness
- Opportunities
- Threats.

By including a SWOT analysis, potential strengths as well as weaknesses are assessed and methods of strengthening them are presented. This allows investors and the management team to capitalize on strengths to improve sales and to be aware of weaknesses and threats and address them in a proactive manner. Opportunities that are identified can be capitalized on and the market share and service orientation can be improved.

What is product design?

The *product design* and development section of the business plan describes the following in detail:

- Product or service
- Timeline for development and distribution of the product or service with specific assignments and checkpoints for completion of assigned tasks
- A resource statement that includes equipment needs, staffing, facility costs, and consultant or attorney fees
- Quality control plans
- Potential problems with creative strategies to address the concerns.

Charts are often used to illustrate tasks, checkpoints, and assignments and to easily identify the flow of work and activities to accomplish the product or services provided to the client(s).

What is operational development?

The *operational development* plan is a description of how the business will operate in a competitive environment and succeed. This element of the business plan includes details about the following:

- Structure and function of the business
- Description of the chosen location
- Type of staffing required for operations
- Other resources such as equipment needed for quality services.

Detailed financial costs of these essential expenses are identified and become an essential component of the financial plan.

How do I develop a marketing plan?

The *marketing plan* is a step-by-step description beginning with the mission, the goals, objectives, and cost of marketing. Based on the mission of the business, the market research is presented, goals and measurable objectives are identified, and a marketing mix is presented that depicts a variety of marketing strategies, which are linked to specific measurable objectives. For each objective, the costs in terms of staff, equipment, and other resources for the marketing strategies mix are delineated in a financial plan.

What is the organizational plan?

The *organizational plan* provides a snapshot of the people who will manage the day-to-day operations of the business. It includes:
- Executive(s) and staffing pattern, with the numbers and types of individuals needed for a successful operation
- An organizational chart that creates a picture of the lines of direct and indirect authority and communication channels, and an illustration of departments that provides a visual representation of the business
- Job descriptions of key personnel (often included in the proposal appendix).

What is included in a development schedule?

A *development schedule* is a master plan for the organization and identifies the necessary steps for planning, developing, implementing, and evaluating the product or services. A development schedule is a management tool that ensures that the work at all stages of business development is completed in a timely fashion. Activities that are listed include the following:
- Planning, program, and policy development
- Designing and developing the facility
- Purchasing equipment
- Marketing, hiring, and orienting staff
- Scheduling daily operations
- Coordinating quality management and evaluation plans and processes.

A master plan that identifies what needs to be accomplished, who will be responsible for the activity, the time frame in which the activity needs to be completed, and reporting lines is often included in the proposal appendix.

What is included in the financial plan?

Many investors will be extremely interested in the *financial plan* for the proposed venture. The financial plan includes short- and long-term projections of revenues and expenses. Questions that are answered in the financial plan include these:
- How long can you stay in business with the resources you currently have?
- How long before a profit is made?

- What is the break-even point?
- How much will be reinvested in the company?
- How will plant and human resources be maintained?
- How much are fixed costs?
- How will debts be repaid and over what time period?

Financial statements (balance sheets and cash flow projections) and capital costs must be included with detail in the financial plan. This section is important and requires details regarding volume projections for products or services, direct and indirect costs, product pricing, and collection procedures. The cost of the service or product multiplied by the number of services or products sold will provide a picture of whether revenues will cover costs and whether a profit will be made. Details regarding debt sources of financing and working capital assumptions are important in determining short- and long-term profitability.

The Nurse-Managed Center

What is a nurse-managed center?

Nurse-managed centers have been in existence since 1965, providing a unique approach to primary care. Historically, nurse-managed centers have served disadvantaged populations and a disproportionate number of low-income clients, hence limiting their financial stability (Anderko & Uscian, 2001; Hansen-Turton & Kinsey, 2001; Oros, Johantgen, Antol, Heller, & Ravella, 2001; Swan & Evans, 2001; Vonderheid, Pohl, Barkauskas, & Nagelkerk, 2004). Other factors that contribute to instability of nurse-managed centers include the following:

- Limited business planning
- Inability to obtain a variety of revenue sources
- Difficulty becoming credentialed by health plans
- Employers not offering plans with advanced practice nursing coverage
- Failure of health plans to list advanced practice nurses as primary care providers
- Multiple problems with prescriptive authority.

What are the issues facing nurse-managed centers?

The focus/emphasis of nurse-managed centers is to provide holistic, client-centered care to individuals, families, and communities. Given the increasing competition for scarce resources in the nation's health care delivery system, it is critical for nurse entrepreneurs to understand the financial challenges facing their businesses and to implement sound and innovative business practices aimed at self-sustainability. Failure to procure multiple funding sources and initial grant funding to establish nursing centers often leads to difficulties with securing operational capital and long-term viability (McIntosh, Nagelkerk, Vonderheid, Dontje, & Pohl, 2003; Vonderheid, Pohl, Barkauskas, Gift, & Hughes-Cromwick, 2003; Vonderheid et al., 2004).

Developing consortiums, organizations, and alliances has been one strategy used to improve nurse-managed center viability, pool scarce resources to affect policy, and share valuable information to enhance business operations. Acquiring multiple revenue sources and engaging and targeting untapped markets strengthen financial sustainability. Enhancing revenue streams and securing a financial base by charging a reasonable fee for services, collecting fees promptly, consulting with billing and financial experts, creating a financial advisory board committee, and developing a strategic marketing plan to increase the client base are successful strategies to attain financial sustainability. By increasing the number and visibility of nurse-managed centers, the public will become aware of this unique approach to health care. NPs and nurse-managed centers will become a preferred provider network for individuals seeking health care and will institutionalize nursing centers as part of the mainstream health care system.

What are the nuts and bolts of planning to open a nurse-managed center?

The first step of the journey in starting a nurse-managed center in a community is to use innovative approaches and creativity in shaping your practice and determining the best model of care. A key aspect of developing your business is to engage in sound business practices, because with no profit margin there will be no mission and you will be unable to provide your community with valuable services. Your business plan will provide the direction and outline the resources required for successful business practices and provide the direction for planning, managing, and communicating. During the development of your business plan, you will identify the benefits and barriers of your new business. The benefits may include offering a service that does not currently exist, offering a different model of care, offering services that are more convenient for clients, or offering access to care. Barriers to services may include financial obstacles, risk management issues, contract negotiations, engaging stakeholders, hiring staff, and securing appropriate facilities.

What type of partnerships should be formed?

Internal and external partnerships should be explored, created, and nourished to help develop referral sources, finance business operations, hire loyal, effective employees, assist with business operations, and serve as consultants to the business. Internal partnerships help create positive work environments and encourage personnel to work in a positive, professional manner. External networks entail working with insurance companies to credential the NPs in your practice; developing collaborative relationships with health departments, schools, community organizations, and business agencies; and creating collegial relationships with health care professionals and organizations.

Identification of stakeholders—those who have an interest in the organization—is important to increase the likelihood of success for your practice and develop strong referral bases and financial support. One successful strategy that businesses employ to network with community members is to develop a community advisory board (McIntosh et al., 2003). These boards often include influential members in the community, financial advisers, individuals who are connected to the community, individuals who will be using the services provided, and representatives of the practice. The community advisory boards engage in structured discussions and brainstorming. The advisory boards provide contacts for business ventures and meet on a semi-annual or annual basis.

Will I need to negotiate contracts?

Contracts are an important component of business negotiations and help develop partnerships, develop binding agreements, establish value for services, assist with maintaining sustainability, and provide visibility. A contract is a promise or agreement that is legally binding and is one method of communication. Even though some oral and written contracts are legally binding, in most cases a written contract is preferred in order to clearly outline the terms of agreement.

When reviewing and evaluating a contract, it is often advisable to consult an attorney. Attorneys can provide information to determine if the contract contains acceptable elements. When evaluating capitated contracts it is important to analyze the potential benefits versus potential financial risks in detail and calculate the financial implications on your practice. In some capitated managed care contracts, the practice, upon signing the contract, is liable for services that are provided above the reimbursed amount. Through careful negotiations, such provisions or elements in the contract can be deleted in order to eliminate or limit the financial liability for the practice. Chapter 6 provides detailed information about insurance contracts.

What are key physical and environmental facility issues?

One of the most important management decisions is the location of the facility for your practice. The location of the practice will, in part, determine the client load based on the geographical location and proximity. Once the location is established for the practice, a facility must be built, purchased, or leased. Your business plan should include the costs of renovation, property and facility purchase, or leasing costs. Another aspect of physical and environmental issues is the set of licensure and code regulations.

- Occupational and safety requirements, administered through the Occupational Safety and Health Administration (OSHA), must be met.
- You must apply for a clinical laboratory improvement amendment certificate for any laboratory procedures you plan on performing in your clinic.

- Fire and building codes must be met and posting of fire exits and equipment must be done, as well as conducting periodic drills.
- A hazardous waste license and disposal system should be implemented.
- A blood-borne pathogen process with a policy and procedure and annual updates for employees should be documented.
- A space should be prepared for pharmaceutical storage with a locked cabinet and a documentation system for signing out medication samples.
- Should you establish a partnership with the local health department to offer free immunizations for children in your clinic, proper forms and refrigeration standards must be implemented.

What types of decisions should be made about the organizational structure?

The development and distribution of an *organizational chart* is important for a pictorial representation of the direct and indirect lines of authority and communication channels. Developing and implementing a *community advisory board* is also an important strategy to provide resources, support, contacts, and partnerships. The creation of *policies and procedures* is important for consistency and compliance purposes. These should be kept in a central location in a notebook so that annual reviews and updates can be completed in a timely fashion. *Personnel policies* need to be in place and accessible to all employees. *Personnel records* such as CPR certificates, immunizations, current license and certifications, insurance numbers and PIN numbers for Medicaid and Medicare, continuing education records, and attendance at mandatory clinic meetings need to be maintained centrally. *Marketing materials*, such as brochures for the nurse-managed center, should be developed and distributed and a procedure for periodic review and update should be put in place.

How do I obtain start-up capital for the nurse-managed center?

Identifying and securing initial capital and consistent revenue streams are very important tasks that can make or break a business. Your business plan is a key document for obtaining loans from banks or investors for initial start-up money. Other potential sources of capital for starting your business include grants from local organizations, federal agencies, or foundations interested in access and quality health care issues that are willing to invest in alternative models of care. Personal finances also provide a way of infusing capital into a new business and then repaying the money to yourself as profits are earned. The cost of initial capital must be calculated to include interest and the time frame for repayment. Maintaining a consistent revenue stream is important, as is establishing contracts with companies for specific services such as health maintenance exams, smoking cessation sessions, DOT physicals, new employee physicals, and work-related injury or wellness programs.

What staffing issues should I anticipate?

Personnel policies and procedures (hiring, dismissal, and grievance) are important to establish and disseminate to employees to provide guidance and rules of operation. Orientation procedures should be implemented to cover the details of each position and provide staff members with the organizational philosophy, mission, goals, role expectations, tour of physical facilities, introduction to coworkers, and organizational culture.

Providing an orientation that fosters an organizational culture that makes work interesting, fun, and fulfilling helps motivate employees to be productive and collegial. The most effective orientation programs are performance based and incorporate regulatory requirements while assisting the individual to become familiar with new role responsibilities and responsibilities within your organization.

The following strategies can be used to incorporate the different learning methods of individuals :
- Group sessions
- Competency-based educational programs
- Role modeling
- Analysis of case scenarios
- Discussion or lecture
- Guided activities such as tours
- Completing forms and business requirements for employment.

Job descriptions should be developed and reviewed during the interview process and be kept in a central location, because these documents provide guidelines for each position and inform the employees of job expectations and evaluation criteria for salary adjustments and satisfactory performance. Documentation should be maintained for all contractual arrangements with physicians or other individuals or organizations. Protocols should be in place for the physician collaborative agreement, delegated functions, and guidelines for prescriptive authority for narcotics and scheduled medications. All employee records such as licensure and CPR and other certifications should be maintained and updated at regular intervals.

What types of quality assurance activities should be implemented?

Standards need to be set for the assurance of quality care provided in your practice through a quality management system. Key indicators should be established for monthly or quarterly chart audits. Examples of possible indicators include up-to-date adult and pediatric immunizations in all charts, smoking cessation discussed at every visit, annual mammograms for women 40 years of age and older, blood pressure screening for hypertension, and fasting blood glucose screening for clients with diabetes. Incorporate quality outcome measures for client response to the treatment plan. In addition, a process of collecting client satisfaction surveys, either in the clinical setting or mailing format, should be established to review and institute improvement plans to enhance quality client care in the clinic.

Coding and billing audits can be conducted internally by the manager or by hiring a consultant who can use this information in a feedback session with nurse practitioners to assist them in accurately billing services. These audits provide valuable information for capturing the revenue that is essential to the financial viability of the clinic.

Staff development activities on coding and billing, health care updates, fire safety, OSHA requirements, and other activities should be recorded and documented for each employee. Record maintenance is essential for audits and quality assurance activities. Examples of records include employee health records, equipment maintenance records, and the pharmaceutical sample log.

How do I become credentialed?

The first step in becoming credentialed is to determine what types of insurance coverage are available to potential clients who reside in the community in which you will be establishing your practice. The next step is to target the insurance companies that have the most potential clients in your community and set up an appointment to review the credentialing process, determine the average time needed to process the application for credentialing, and obtain the application for credentialing.

Complete the application form as soon as possible, because the credentialing process is often lengthy and fraught with obstacles. To complete the credentialing application process, you may be required to have a physician collaboration agreement. Nurse practitioners have negotiated many different types of collaborative agreements for a variety of compensation packages, which may include monetary incentives and/or preferential referral patterns. In addition, referral networks need to be established for hospital admitting if you choose not to admit and manage clients in the hospital. If your specialty is family practice you will need to negotiate pediatric, obstetric, and adult admission networks.

What are the financial implications?

It is important to identify initial investment capital either through grant writing or revenue sources, whether personal or from investors, either partnerships or loans with repayment schedules. *Contingency funds* are also critical for financial viability during economic downturns. Establishing an *endowment* for funding uninsured clients' office visit charges, capital improvements, equipment updates, and renovations can assist with financial expenses. Endowment funds may come from fund-raisers such as golf outings, named rooms, equipment, or raffles. Careful review and evaluation of revenues and expenses on a weekly, monthly, quarterly, and annual basis are important to identify financial trends and make any necessary corrective steps to ensure financial success.

How do I develop community partnerships?

In the broadest sense, identify the community of interest for your clinic. Identify key organizations, community members, and employers in the community and meet with them or invite them to a luncheon to distribute information about your practice. Make sure you distribute flyers and health information for them to post at their organizations or to give to neighbors or other individuals interested in health care. Place an add in a local community newsletter and community newspaper and list your practice in the local telephone directory and Yellow Pages.

Your *community advisory board* can assist you in getting the information about your practice out into the community. Providing free health care seminars at your office or on a radio program about topics that are interesting and important to the community, such as breast care, colon cancer, or skin care, can attract interest and clients to your practice. Listening to community members' concerns and needs and being responsive to them can help establish long-term community partnerships.

What evaluation activities are important?

Establishing a *systematic evaluation plan* that identifies those activities that should be carried out routinely is an important task. The evaluation plan not only identifies the important tasks, but also has checkpoints for collecting data and timelines for staff review, as well as any correctional actions. The plan includes the following types of items:
- Client satisfaction tool distribution
- Financial status report
- Community advisory board review and update of members
- Marketing plans and activities
- Staff development activities and orientation plan
- Assessment of quality indicators

What improves practice success?

Improving practice success may benefit from the following:
- *Developing clear benchmarks.* Benchmarking is a process of comparing and evaluating your services, practices, or outcomes with other practitioners

working in similar practice settings (Tran, 2003). To establish benchmarks, select those measures that you feel will improve your practice and enhance the quality of care. Examples of benchmarks include comparing types of services offered in your clinic, number of client encounters per provider per day, cost of services per provider, or immunization rate by provider against a similar clinical agency in your geographical region.

- *Creating systems that support financial viability.* Some practices have found that in order to remain financially viable they must collect direct, full payment for services at the time of the visit. Another important strategy is to develop and implement an aggressive marketing plan. Obtaining contracts with employers, community agencies, and insurance companies enhances sustainability.
- *Creating clear financial reports.* Nurse-managed centers that are able to develop clear financial reports on a routine basis assist in securing their future. By reviewing daily, weekly, monthly, and annual financial data, managers can implement strategies to ensure financial viability.
- *Maintaining strong partnerships.* Client, business, and community partnerships should be established and nurtured. Strong partnerships can provide client referrals, community networking and resources, and business partnerships.
- *Diversifying the case mix.* An important dimension of business practice is to diversify the client insurance mix. Without a diverse case mix, the business is at risk for financial hardship if a single insurance panel is changed. The diverse client mix also provides a direct marketing link in the community for your business enterprise.
- *Increasing client volume.* A strategic plan should be developed and marketing activities engaged to enhance the client volume. Specific marketing activities should be budgeted to continually increase volume.
- *Implementing timely billing and monitoring of collections.* A major step to financial sustainability is to collect the copayments of individual clients at the time of service. Electronic billing with complete and accurate information (i.e., CPT and ICD9-CM coding) increases reimbursement levels and speeds the claim process. Immediate review and correction with resubmission of rejected bills helps increase reimbursement.
- *Developing a strategic plan.* Strategic planning helps to identify what the organization intends to accomplish and how resources will be allocated. Strategic planning helps develop a vision for the organization and provides direction for future activities. This type of planning moves the organization by means of a concerted effort and provides an avenue to capitalize on emerging opportunities.
- *Obtaining money for specialized programs or equipment through successful grant writing.* Grant money may be available for programs aimed at specific population groups such as those who have asthma or diabetes or for screening activities (cancer screenings) or for initiatives for vulnerable individuals (children, homeless).

What are common problems that new nurse-managed businesses encounter?

New primary care nursing businesses will encounter many problems. Table 7-1 identifies some of the common problems that nurse-managed centers may encounter in their attempts to maintain financial sustainability.

Health Insurance Portability and Accountability Act (HIPAA)

What is HIPAA?

HIPAA was initiated by the federal government and passed in 1996 to promote the portability of health insurance, to protect against fraud and abuse, to improve efficiencies in health care systems, and to promote the use of electronic transactions. HIPAA is a federal law designed to safeguard clients' protected information. To ensure enforcement of the HIPAA regulations, the appointment of a privacy officer for each organization is federally mandated. The *privacy officer* has these responsibilities:

- Effects organizational HIPAA compliance.
- Answers employee questions regarding privacy matters.
- Assists in establishing and implementing HIPAA-related policies and procedures.
- Resolves any external or internal privacy complaint.

Noncompliance results in sanctions for the organization and may include fines and, in severe cases, criminal sanctions. A major goal of the HIPAA legislation is to protect the privacy and security of health information.

The Health Insurance Portability and Accountability Act include several components: privacy, security, and electronic data interchange. Not only does this legislation affect health care agencies and systems, but it affects vendors who supply materials and resources or services to health care institutions as well as individuals engaging in research and development activities. The HIPAA regulation has had a major impact on health care providers because it delineates responsibilities in protecting personal health care information, gives clients additional rights for reviewing and amending their health records, extends more authority to the government to regulate the client privacy issues, and promotes electronic business transactions.

Privacy. An important aspect of a client's care is the documentation in the medical record, the diagnostic test results, and medication records. The privacy regulations address issues of access to clients' protected health information. *Protected health information* is defined as the information and data directly related to the treatment plan, sensitive health information, and processing of payment for services rendered that could reasonably identify an individual.

Table 7-1   Common Primary Care Nursing Business Problems and Strategies to Avoid Them

Common Problems	How to Avoid the Problems
Employee role confusion and conflict	Develop clear job descriptions and communication channels.
Inadequate telephone triage procedures	Develop a protocol for who is to respond to a telephone query and the time frame in which the response should be made as well as documentation of the action.
Incompletely filling of provider schedules	Establish clear guidelines for length and type of appointments.
Slow revenue flow periods	Create a rainy day fund for emergencies and slow periods.
Documentation that does not support the billings	Educate providers about coding and billing and encourage medical assistants to document laboratory and other tests performed to maximize reimbursement for services provided.
Facilities not maintained adequately	Set funds aside to maintain, upgrade, and replace equipment and facilities.
Lack of courteous, happy, and friendly employees	Orient employees to proper office etiquette and encourage a positive, enjoyable, and supportive work environment.
Inadequate revenue flow and sources	Become a panel member of many insurance companies. Diversify revenue sources.
Lack of marketing	Develop and implement a marketing plan
Does not seek specialized legal or business expertise	Hire those activities or obtain consultation on areas where you do not have the expertise (i.e., legal or business skills).
Not part of a business network	Join a small business group to share information.

Examples of *client identifiers* include name, address, birth date, phone numbers, Social Security numbers, medical record numbers, account numbers, full-face photographic images, e-mail address, and fax numbers. Examples of *sensitive health information* include test results, procedures, medications, diagnoses, and health care provider name and location.

In health care settings, it is often important to communicate sensitive client information and identifiers to effectively address and develop therapeutic treatment plans. HIPAA regulations permit the disclosure of client information to those providers or individuals who need access to provide care, however, it is necessary for compliance to differentiate the type and amount of information based on the person's job description. The new standard for privacy is to provide the minimum protected health information possible for employees to do their job. HIPAA has developed new language in relationship to the sharing of protected health information in terms of use and disclosure. *Use* is the sharing of information within an organization and *disclosure* is the sharing of information with individuals external to the organization. An example of use, which is internal to the organization, would be the sharing of medical record information for the purpose of treating a client's illness or providing preventive health care. An example of disclosure, which is sharing the information with external individuals, is transcription services.

There are many examples of different types of uses and disclosures, but most of them involve the assessment and development of the therapeutic treatment plan, payment for services rendered, or administrative operations. Other types of uses and disclosures include marketing activities and reports to public health departments, law enforcement agencies, life insurance companies, service vendors, and medical forms for employers and other agencies.

Providers are responsible for maintaining privacy for clients by using individual client rooms when possible, but at times this option may not be possible. In such cases, reasonable effort should be employed to protect the client's health care information. Client information should not be discussed in lounges, hallways, meeting areas, waiting rooms, or any other public place where conversations may be heard and sensitive information unknowingly disclosed. Reasonable measures should be instituted to ensure the privacy of protected client information. Simple measures include placing computers, printers, and fax machines in unobtrusive, low-volume areas, instituting stringent policies for use of passwords, instituting automatic log-off procedures if no activity has occurred for a preset amount of time, using a security screensaver, and verification of identity of persons requesting personal health information. HIPAA applies to all volunteers, student, employees, and other temporary workers—in fact, it encompasses all individuals who work within the organization whether it is for pay or not.

Security. The security regulations have not been finalized and the compliance deadlines have not been established. This regulation will deal with how health information is protected and will define safeguards for protected health information.

Electronic Data Interchange. The aim of the electronic data interchange regulation was to encourage electronic transactions in such mediums as claims processing to improve efficiency and cost savings in the administration of health services.

What are the benefits of HIPAA?

The new HIPAA regulations have many positive aspects for clients, providers, and organizations. HIPAA established a public policy on client confidentiality. This federal law protects client information and has devised a mechanism for client disclosure. Clients now have additional leverage and the right to review their medical records and amend, not change, items contained within this document. This new legislation will require innovations in information handling, technology, and policies and procedures. Electronic payment processing will undoubtedly increase technical expertise and expand individual comfort and experimentation with electronic health records and systems.

How are clients informed about HIPAA regulations?

The federal law requires that businesses not only elicit a written authorization form describing the HIPAA regulation and their rights, but also post a notice of privacy practices in a prominent location in the facility. Care cannot be withheld if the authorization form is not signed. Explain to the client that the form only acknowledges that they have seen and had the opportunity to read the written authorization. If the client refuses to sign the authorization form, document in the health record that you made a reasonable effort to acquire their signature.

What are the HIPAA client rights?

The HIPAA regulation has developed a set of client rights to protect and inform them of their rights regarding protected privacy information.
1. Each client has the right to receive a Notice of Privacy Practices.
2. Each client has the right to review and obtain their protected health information and receive this information in a timely manner.
3. Each client has the right to amend their protected health information.
4. Each client has the right to restrict the use and disclosure of their protected health information
5. Each client has the right to authorize or refuse the use or disclosure of their protected health information that does not include treatment, payment, or operations.
6. Each client has the right to obtain a copy of the uses and disclosures of their protected health information for activities that fall outside of the treatment, payment, or operations.
7. Each client has the right to direct how and where confidential communications regarding their protected health information are made.
8. Each client has the right to contact the privacy officer in the organization or to contact the Secretary of Health and Human Services to lodge a complaint regarding the use of their protected health information or a violation of the HIPAA regulations.

Grant Writing

Many business owners have written grant applications to obtain money for specific programs, equipment, or material resources. Successful grant writing is a skill. By taking the time and energy to review potential granting agencies, the agency priorities, and funding patterns as well as making key contacts with grant agency personnel and completing a detailed application, your success at obtaining a grant award will increase.

How do I get started in grant writing?

A grant proposal involves good written communication skills; it provides an opportunity to sell your idea and to secure resources. Grants are often written to attain equipment or fund program development and implementation, quality improvement activities, and research projects. Your first job is to put your ideas in written format and sketch out your plan. Once your idea is clearly stated, you can document why it is important for the granting agency to fund your project. Identify what currently exists, the gap, and then the compelling reasons for funding this project. To document the need for your proposed project, use current statistics and relevant literature to demonstrate that you are knowledgeable about the specific project area. Documenting what you propose to change, implement, or test in simple, but measurable terms with your proposed plan, budget, and evaluation process assists in successful grant application reviews.

One of the most important parts of your grant application is the abstract or summary. In the abstract, the title is identified, the author(s), and a brief, but concise discussion of the proposed plan with purpose, measurable objectives, and evaluation plan is documented. In the body of the grant application it is important to detail what currently exists and why this is inadequate, then identify what should exist and give a rationale, and finally create a sense of urgency for your project. This will increase the priority score and likelihood of successful funding.

How do I find the right granting agency?

First, you must identify "key words" that describe your grant proposal. Key words are typically the subject area of your grant. You also may want to indicate your constituency groups. Governmental agencies have grant programs at the federal, state, county, and city levels. Many nonprofit organizations also provide grant opportunities. Many computerized programs list and describe a multitude of funding agencies. These programs can help determine an appropriate funding agency that matches your project needs.

A commonly used program is the sponsored programs information network or *SPIN*. SPIN is a database of thousands of national and international funding opportunities from both the government and private sector. Many universities and businesses have this program available to their faculty, staff, and students. If you do not have this resource available to you, a contact name and number is InfoEd International at (800)727-6427 or check *www.infoed.org/products.stm*. GrantSelect is another large database program that is available on the Internet. GrantSelect is a compilation of governmental and nonprofit funding agencies. To get more information on GrantSelect, contact Oryx Press at (800)279-6799 or visit *www.grantselect.com*.

What are successful tips in grant writing?

Successful tips for grant writing include the following:
- Follow the guidelines and criteria that are written by the granting agency.
- Contact the granting agency to obtain technical assistance or discuss your idea(s) with the program officer. This can be helpful for determining the appropriateness of your "idea" for the funding agency and to learn what types of grants are being funded.
- When completing the grant application, paying attention to detail such as font size, number of pages, and the date applications are due can prevent your application from being returned without review.
- Complete your grant application a few weeks before the deadline to provide an opportunity for colleagues to read and critique your proposal with adequate time for revisions.

When writing the grant application, use simple sentences that clearly communicate your proposed activities. Your first sentence in each paragraph should provide a summary of the paragraph and pique the interest of the evaluator. Your writing style should be simplistic, but not offensive to the evaluator nor should you state the obvious or downgrade the writing. The style of writing should be "user friendly" so that the attachments and references can be found quickly and conveniently. Each section should be labeled according to the criteria required by the granting agency. The table of contents should clearly identify the major criteria with salient subheadings for ease of review. Evaluators tend to rate well-organized, clear grant applications higher. Formatting the text with judicious use of bullets, italics, graphs, and charts can increase the ease of reading for evaluators and highlight important information or points, hence making reading and scoring your grant less work. Directions should be carefully followed for completing the grant application in order to prevent an ineligible funding status. Granting agencies often look at the legibility of the grant application as well as the accuracy of information when determining eligibility and scoring status.

Do take the time to research the granting agencies' past funding practices, values, mission, and grant funding cycles. Granting agencies have a mission and philosophy that guides their granting decisions. Specific foci are often determined for funding cycles, and grants received by the agency that fit their granting cycle are awarded higher scores and are often funded. By using specific language that the funding agency has written and by incorporating the funding foci, your grant application will have a better chance of being funded.

What are the components of a grant proposal?

Each granting agency may have slightly different criteria for their applications. Some independent agencies require only a letter with a brief description of the project, while other agencies require a full proposal. However, *most funding agencies require common components for a grant proposal, which are identified in Box 7-2.*

The *title* should be explicit, but brief. It should be comprehensive enough to describe the nature of the proposed work. The author's name and credentials and the organization that will be responsible for grant activity are also indicated on the title page. The *abstract* provides the first impression to the reviewer and is often the single most important aspect of the grant proposal. The author has an opportunity to make a strong case by developing a compelling needs statement, specific objectives, plans, and measurable outcomes for the proposed project.

The *table of contents* is the guide or map of the proposal and should include major divisions with subcomponents specifically aimed at outlining the grant application criteria into understandable and easy to find components. The *introduction* provides a capsule of what is proposed and introduces the subject to the grant reviewer. The *background* section provides relevant information about the current state with statistical data and references highlighting the need. The *project description* outlines the plan in clear measurable terms.

Supporting letters can be included to show interrelationships with agencies, to demonstrate individual qualifications, to show employer support, and to show consultant commitment. *References* that have strengthened the proposal should be complete and presented in alphabetical order with author, year, title, journal, volume, and page numbers. A brief, but concise *description of personnel* who will work on the project, their credentials, and their job activities for the

---

Box 7-2 Common Components for a Grant Proposal

- Title page
- Abstract
- Table of contents
- Introduction
- Background
- Proposal description
- Supporting letters
- References
- Description of project personnel
- Budget

grant should be listed. The *budget* is an important document to show the costs such as personnel, equipment, supplies, and consultants. Appendix 7-2 provides an example of a basic grant application.

What activities should I avoid when writing a grant?

One activity to avoid is the development of a generic grant for multiple funding agencies. The second activity to avoid is sending the generic grant application electronically to as many granting agencies as possible without reviewing the guidelines for each of the organizations and without seeking a match between the grant proposal and the granting agency. By using this shotgun approach to grant funding, you will probably experience a high rejection rate and may begin to develop a negative position with granting agencies (Bauer, 2003). This may jeopardize future grant applications, decreasing your chances for funding opportunities.

Avoid using terms that imply that you deserve the funding; instead make a case for the need or compelling reason that your program should be awarded the funding to improve specific outcomes. Describe what currently exists, the gap that you plan to fill, and then carefully lay out what you envision should be the end product. By mapping out your ideas, the granting agency will be able to clearly envision the program or project that you are seeking funding for and be able to make an informed decision about your grant.

SUMMARY

NPs who decide to start their own practices must be familiar with business planning. Learning the community resources, developing a business plan, and consulting with business and legal experts improve the sustainability of the new business. Engaging in strategic planning, developing a marketing plan, complying with HIPAA regulations, negotiating contracts, and writing grants are also important aspects of business planning and development. NPs who are innovative and open to risk and rewards have many opportunities to design and own health care businesses.

References

Anderko, L., & Uscian, M. (2001). Quality outcome measures at an academic rural nurse managed center: A core safety net provider. *Policy, Politics & Nursing Practice*, 2(4), 288-294.

Barry, B.W. (2001). *Strategic planning workbook for nonprofit organizations*. Saint Paul: Amherst H. Wilder Foundation.

Bauer, D. (2003). *The "how to" grants manual: Successful grantseeking techniques for obtaining public and private grants* (5th ed.). Westport, CT: Greenwood Publishing Group and American Council on Education.

Hansen-Turton, T., & Kinsey, K. (2001). The quest for self-sustainability: Nurse-managed health centers meeting the policy challenge. *Policy, Politics, & Nursing Practice, 2*(4), 304-309.

Johnson, D.E.L. (2004). What is strategic management, planning? *Health Care Strategic Management, 22*(2), 2-3.

McIntosh, E., Nagelkerk, J., Vonderheid, S., Dontje, K., & Pohl, J. (2003). Financial viability of nurse managed centers: Role of the financial advisory committee. *Nurse Practitioner 28*(3), 40, 46-48, 51.

Oros, M., Johantgen, M., Antol, S., Heller, B., & Ravella, P. (2001). Community-based nursing centers: A model for health care delivery in the 21st century. *Policy, Politics, & Nursing Practice, 2*(4), 277-287.

Swan, B.A., & Evans, L.K. (2001). Infrastructure to support academic nursing practice. *Nursing Economics, 17*(1), 20-28.

Tran, M.N. (2003). Take benchmarking to the next level. *Nursing Management,* pp. 18-23.

Vonderheid, S., Pohl, J., Barkauskas, V., Gift, D., & Hughes-Cromwick, P. (2003). Financial performance of academic nurse-managed primary care centers. *Nursing Economics, 21*(4), 167-175.

Vonderheid, S., Pohl, J., Barkauskas, V., & Nagelkerk, J. (2004). The safety net: Academic nurse managed center's role. *Policy, Politics, & Nursing Practice, 5*(2), 84-94.

Vonderheid, S., Pohl, J., Schafer, P., Forrest, K., Poole, M., et al. (2004). Using FTE and RVU performance measures to assess financial viability of academic nurse-managed centers. *Nursing Economics, 22*(3), 124-134.

8

Coding and Billing for Nurse Practitioners

Ramona Benkert
Audrey Westdorp
Mary P. White

Coding for Nurse Practitioner Services

Coding and billing for nurse practitioner (NP) services can be a complex and overwhelming task. At times it seems a diversion to the "real work" of an NP. Yet, understanding coding and billing for NP services is essential to employment security and is a daily function performed by NPs. Medical practices, facilities, and agencies have found that NP/physician teams are key to providing high-quality and cost-effective care (Flanigan, 1998; Neveleff, 1999). However, the problem of deciphering how federal and state law and diagnostic coding rules apply to a specific practice situation can deter groups from fully utilizing NPs.

Although coding and billing for NP services overlap, this chapter begins with a discussion of coding because it is more straightforward than billing and likely to be more familiar to NPs. Numerous authors have discussed the various issues of billing for NP services (Abood & Keepnews, 2000; Buppert, 2004) and their work will be used as a guidepost for discussion. In addition, a nonexhaustive list of common terms and definitions used in the coding and billing process is included in Appendix 8-1.

What does "coding" for NP services mean?

Coding for NP services is a process of documenting the nursing and medical diagnoses and procedures for all of the services rendered by an NP in the course of a day's work, including the clinical judgment process. NP services are currently coded using the same manuals as physician providers: *International Classification of Diseases, 9th Revision, Clinical Modification* (ICD9-CM) (Hart & Hopkins, 2004), *Current Procedural Terminology,* fourth edition (CPT-4) (American Medical Association [AMA], 2004), *Health Care Financing Administration Common Procedure Coding System* (HCPCS Level II) (Centers for Medicare and Medicaid Services [CMS], 2004), and also nursing-specific coding manuals.

Psychiatric NPs, psychologists, social workers, and psychiatrists use the *Diagnostic and Statistical Manual for Mental Disorders–IV* (DSM-IV) (American Psychological Association, 1994) for the diagnostic coding of their services. Mental health care providers can use the CPT coding manual; however, it is limited in its applicability for these types of services. For example, Medicare Part B payments for mental health services are limited to CPT codes 90801-90802, 90804-90899, central nervous system assessments (96100-96117), health and behavior assessments (96150-96155) (CMS, 2003b).

Nursing diagnoses and nursing intervention classification systems have been developed to support the "nursing" work of NPs (Dochterman & Bulechek, 2004; North American Nursing Diagnosis Association [NANDA-I], 2004). In addition, nursing outcomes classification manuals exist for coding the outcomes of NP care that are nurse sensitive (Moorhead, Johnson, & Maas, 2004). Although these classification systems may be less familiar to practicing NPs than the medical diagnostic classification systems, they are important for documenting the nursing interventions and outcomes that are often invisible to the providers, payers, and health care community. Research has indicated a sharp increase in the use of these classification systems by colleges of nursing, nursing departments in health care settings, and nurses (Keenan, Treder, & Clingerman, 2001).

What is an ICD9-CM code?

Billing for client encounters and other procedures must be accompanied by a diagnostic code. Diagnostic coding for health care dates back to the 17th century. By 1948, the World Health Organization (WHO) had published the *International Classification of Diseases* (ICD), which combined causes of mortality and morbidity (WHO, 2001). After the 1988 passage of the Medicare Catastrophic Coverage Act, the ICD9-CM gained great importance for the diagnostic coding of health care services. The ICD has become the standard for the coding of disease and diagnostic entities during the provision of health care. All health care providers and systems throughout the world use the ICD coding system.

Currently, all insurance carriers in the United States use the ninth version of the ICD9-CM to delineate the clinical picture of each client. The coding system uses three- to five-digit codes to classify diseases, injuries, impairments, symptoms, and causes of death. Although all insurance carriers use ICD9-CM, Medicare and the Health Care Financing Administration (HCFA) have become the "gold standard" for rules regarding coding for health care services.

What are some simple rules for coding?

A few simple rules apply to the use of the ICD9-CM code book. First, the diagnosis must justify the procedure, meaning that the procedure code or codes (current procedural terminology-4, CPT-4) to be discussed later in the chapter must be supported by the ICD9-CM diagnostic code selected for the billing process. The diagnosis (ICD9-CM) that is primarily responsible for the encounter or procedure (CPT-4) should be listed first. For example, an electrocardiogram CPT-4 code (93000) is reimbursable with the diagnosis of chest pain (786.59), but is not reimbursable for a diagnosis of bronchitis (466.0). The link between the ICD9-CM code and the CPT-4 code must be accurate and reflect accurate clinical decision-making processes. If a NP is performing or requesting a particular procedure on a client, the ICD9-CM code selected for the visit must support all of the procedures, documentation, and charting included in the bill for services. Logic and clinical acumen prevail. Second, clinicians must code only the conditions treated. In Chapter 9, the important links between documentation and coding are discussed in more detail. Yet, in short, to avoid rejected claims, rebilling, and delayed payments, the clinician can only code for conditions treated on the day of service.

Third, the principal diagnosis is the reason for the encounter with the clinician. It may seem simple, yet in the complex negotiations of a health care visit, clinicians must recall that the main reason a client sought a service must by the primary diagnosis code for the visit. Even if multiple problems are uncovered, the primary ICD9-CM must be consistent with the chief concern for the visit. If a client has acute and chronic problems, the code for the most acute or most serious condition should be listed first. Finally, when coding, be as specific as possible. The final rule is discussed more fully in the answer to the next question.

How specific do I need to be with the use of ICD9-CM codes?

Medicare and other insurers require that diagnosis codes be detailed to the greatest level of specificity. HCFA requires that each service, procedure, or supply be identified with the most exacting and specific detail using the fourth and fifth digits when indicated. Coexisting or chronic conditions should only be listed if applicable to the client's treatment. Shortcutting codes or "truncating," as Medicare calls it, will result in rejected claims and delayed payments. In addition, conditions that no longer exist should not be coded and if the diagnosis changes following a procedure, the new diagnosis should be coded. Finally, the ICD9-CM manual has specific instructions in some sections that may be indicated by additional notations such as "see…," "see also…," "see category…," and "with…." These instructions direct the clinician to look else where in the manual, look under another main term, direct you to Volume 1, or enhance the specificity of the diagnostic documentation, respectively.

How is the ICD9-CM manual organized?

The ICD9-CM is separated into three volumes for basic medical diagnostic codes. Specialized manuals also exist for other clinical settings, including hospitals, hospice, and long-term care facilities. Volume 1 of the three-volume set is a tabular list of diseases and is located in the back of the coding book. Volume 1 contains three sections: tabular listing of classification of diseases and injuries; supplementary classifications of factors influencing health status (V codes) and of external cause of injury and poisoning (E codes); and appendices for morphology of neoplasms, glossary of mental disorders, drug list numbers, industrial accidents, and three-digit categories. Volume 2 is the alphabetical index to diseases and is located in the front of the book. Volume 3 is a procedure code list for hospital use only. Volumes are to be used in conjunction with one another, with Volume 1 being the absolute source. Volume 1 may have additional instructions or clarifications. Volumes 2 and 3 should never be used as stand-alone documents.

The alphabetic index, Volume 2, is organized according to "Main Terms," which refers to the condition. The condition is often the last word in the diagnosis. For example, upper respiratory infections would be listed alphabetically under the "condition" of "infection, respiratory."

Volume 3 is a classification system for surgical, diagnostic, and therapeutic procedures and includes an alphabetic index and tabular list. These codes are used for hospital inpatient coding. While the majority of insurance companies do not require the use of Volume 3 for physician billing, in hospital settings, Volume 3 of the ICD9-CM is still used. Medicare Part B does not accept codes from Volume 3. If you use them, your claim will be denied. If you are not sure if the codes you are using are correct, check with your carrier, fiscal intermediary (FI), or billing consultant (Lash Group, 2003).

What is an ICD9-CM modifier?

ICD9-CM modifiers are often nonessential modifiers. The main term may be followed by a list of terms, or modifiers, in parentheses. For purposes of billing, the presence or absence of these terms in the diagnosis does not affect the code indicated for the main term. For example, the diagnosis of "Diarrhea, diarrheal" followed by "(acute) (bloody)" is not further clarified by using these nonessential modifiers.

What are ICD9-CM subterms?

Sometimes an ICD9-CM main term is followed by a list of subterms. These subterms do affect the appropriate code selection. Subterms define differences in etiology or location. For example, the subterms for the ICD9-CM diagnosis of "Cellulitis (682.9)" include "abdominal wall (682.2)," "anaerobic (040.0)," or "ankle (682.6)." Missing specific subterms is a common problem in office practices. Often a base code is used but falls short of being specific, and subterms can increase the complexity of a visit, thereby necessitating a higher visit code (an evaluation and management or E&M code). Missing specificity affects reimbursement rates, which affects the financial bottom line of a practice. Many practice employees are unaware of the need to update their data files or encounter forms to enhance the specificity of the diagnosis code, thereby affecting the billing process. The lack of specificity can slow the process for the billing personnel, because they will need to review the chart and possibly contact the employee to clarify the coding. In the worst case scenario, the biller will use the code defined by the employee without clarification and a lower reimbursement rate will be requested due to an inexact coding process.

What is a "V" code?

V codes are used to describe a client who may not be currently ill, but who has come to see the health care provider for a specific reason. They can also describe "routine" health care needs, such as an annual Pap smear. These codes can also be used for individuals with potential health hazards related to communicable diseases or persons accessing health services related to reproduction and development (i.e., low-birth-weight status). Formerly, many indemnity insurers, such as Aetna or Blue Cross and Blue Shield, often did not reimburse for V code diagnostic processes. Many clinicians tended to avoid V codes due to this reimbursement dilemma. With the shift toward managed care insurance plans, V codes can now be used for reimbursable services.

What is a CPT-4 code?

The CPT-4 coding system (also called the HCPCS Level I) is a systematic listing of descriptive terms and identifying codes for reporting procedures and medical services performed by physicians and other appropriately licensed individuals (AMA, 2004). A CPT-4 code is a set of five-digit codes that applies to medical services rendered in ambulatory care offices, outpatient clinics, or ambulatory surgery centers. They are categorized by specialty or service, and include office and hospital visits or consultations, preoperative evaluations, and ancillary diagnostic services. CPT-4 codes should correlate with ICD9-CM codes. For example, an electrocardiogram (93000) can be billed to an insurer for an office visit for a client with an ICD9-CM code for chest pain (786.50); however, an electrocardiogram cannot be billed to an insurer for a client with an ankle strain.

How is the CPT-4 manual organized?

The manual is rather easy to navigate. It is more straightforward than the ICD9-CM coding. The E&M codes appear at the front of the book. They are numbered in the 99000-99999 series. Following the E&M categories, all other codes fall in numeric order beginning with 00100 and continuing through 99199. The common part of the code or base code precedes the semicolon in the CPT-4 procedural description (i.e., "Catheterization, urethra; simple [53670]").

One symbol to watch for in the CPT-4 manual is the asterisk (*). The asterisk will appear in front of a surgical code, and means that the service includes a surgical procedure. It is most frequently found in dermatology procedures. The asterisk is very important because it means that the appropriate E&M service may be billed, as well as the surgical code. For example, if an NP performs an incision and drainage (I&D) (56420) on a small Bartholin cyst, he or she can also bill the insurance company for a low, moderately complex health visit, including a pelvic examination. It is not double billing; it is billing for all of the services rendered. Money can easily be lost through insufficient coding of all CPT-4 services rendered or the lack of attention to detail in the CPT-4 manual. Yet, in the 2004 CPT-4 manual, many of the items with asterisks have been removed.

What are E&M codes?

The evaluation and management or E&M codes are those numeric descriptions that are used for the client encounter with the provider. The E&M codes are divided into categories such as office visits, hospital visits, consultations, preventive medicine, and nursing home care. Each category is then further divided into subcategories. The basic aspects of the E&M codes include the level of decision making by the provider during the visit. Time is not the most relevant factor in determining an E&M code for a visit with a client; it is the level of complexity of the visit. In addition, the E&M codes are affected by the client's status as a new or established client of the practice or provider. For example, if a client is new to the NP and the visit involves problem-focused decision making, the visit is coded as a 99201. Evaluation and management (E&M) guideline definitions are included in Table 8-1.

Other components of E&M services that may affect coding and billing include counseling, coordination of care, nature of the presenting problem, and time spent face to face with the client. The most contentious part of the current E&M

Table 8-1 Evaluation and Management (E&M) Guideline Definitions

E&M Term	Definition
New client	A person who has not received any professional services from the provider or another provider from the same group (and the same specialty) within the past 3 years
Established client	A person who has received professional services from the provider or another provider of the same practice (and the same specialty) within the past 3 years
Concurrent care	Certain E&M services that are rendered by more that one physician with the same or similar specialty on the same date of service
Counseling	A discussion with a client and/or family concerning one or more of the following areas: diagnostic results, impressions and or recommended studies, prognosis; risks and benefits of management options; instructions for management and or follow-up; importance of compliance with chosen management options; risk factor reduction; and client and family education
Consultations	Examination by an additional physician or specialist, at the request of a referring physician, the client, or the client's family

coding guidelines is the level assignment for medical decision making. A simple representation of the E&M decision making process is depicted in Table 8-2.

Billing for various levels of service must be supported by adequate documentation according to published guidelines (CMS, 2003a). Centers for Medicare and Medicaid Services (2004) have set specific documentation requirements that must match the E&M code selected. White and Benkert discuss this in greater depth in Chapter 9 of this text. An extensive description of the E&M guidelines and the Medicare program is available at *www.hcfa.gov/medlearn/ pubs.htm*. In June 2000, new E&M guidelines were published. A complete listing of the requirement can be found at *www.cms.gov*.

Table 8-2 Simple Representation of E&M Decision-Making Process

Decision-Making Level	Diagnoses/ Treatments	Data Complexity/ Amount	Risk
Straightforward	Minimal	Minimal	Minimal
Low	Limited	Limited	Low
Moderate	Multiple	Moderate	Moderate
High	Extensive	Extensive	High, likelihood of death

What is a CPT-4 modifier?

CPT-4 modifiers are two-character codes (alpha-alpha, alphanumeric, or numeric-numeric) that may be added to procedure codes to better describe them. Modifiers are essential terms that follow the CPT-4 code. These essential modifiers can greatly affect reimbursement because they indicate how a procedure has been altered. For example, the modifier "-21" denotes a prolonged evaluation and management service. The -21 modifier would be used when the visit required more time than even the highest E&M code allows for the delivery of the service. A written documentation of the reason and an official report are required to substantiate any consideration for payment of these modifiers. As an aside, these modifiers are rarely paid (Westdorp, 2004b).

Another modifier, "-25" is used when the visit encompasses the primary reason for the visit, as well as an additional unexpected service. A -25 modifier is used to identify a "significant, separately identifiable evaluation and management service" by the same provider on the same day as a procedure or other service. In other words, if a person presents for a procedure such as an incision and drainage (I&D) of a Bartholin cyst, and the person also is complaining of cephalgia and pain and pressure over the sinus area, the I&D would be billed with code 56420, and the E&M for a problem-focused history, exam, and straightforward decision making regarding a presenting sinusitis would be billed with 99212 with the -25 modifier. This modifier alerts the insurance payer to the need to separate the diagnosis to the appropriate code and consider each individually for payment.

Yet another modifier, "-50," indicates bilateral procedures. So in the previous example, if the client were to receive an I&D for mole removals on both arms, the -50 modifier would be added to the E&M service code. Several modifiers are available and assigned by HCFA, AMA, and local insurance carriers. An informative resource from MedLearn (1997) provides a list of the most common modifiers used in the coding and billing process for NP service delivery.

What does "up-coding" mean?

"Up-coding" is the term applied to the use of an E&M code that cannot be justified by the documentation of the visit. Up-coding is a serious concern. According to HCFA administrators, up-coding is a fraudulent activity punishable by fines and other penalties (Abood & Keepnews, 2000; Kent, 1998). NPs should never intentionally up-code; they need to make sure the documentation of a visit matches the E&M code applied to the visit. Yet research has found that NPs can up-code in error since the HCFA guidelines for a new client encounter require more documentation than an established visit (Allen, Reinke, Pohl, Martyn, & McIntosh, 2003). According to billing and coding experts, this is not an uncommon error (Westdorp, 2003). Many providers are unaware of the degree of documentation required for new client visits. All providers require extensive and ongoing education regarding the evolving E&M documentation guidelines. The most recent educational tool was developed by the Centers for Medicare and Medicaid Services (2003c) for physician resident training, but the module is applicable for nurse practitioner providers also.

What does "down-coding" mean?

"Down-coding," although not fraudulent, has other serious ramifications. Down-coding is the process of using an E&M code that underrepresents the degree of work and the procedures involved in a client encounter. Research has found that NPs and other providers have a tendency to down-code versus up-code a visit (Horner, Paris, Purvis, & Lawler, 1991). The rationale for this appears to be a propensity to be concerned about the client's financial status and a fear of fines for fraudulent activity. Horner and colleagues found that underreporting of the number of diagnoses was substantial; the billing forms listed only 69% of the diagnoses identified in the progress notes. In 60% of visits, each diagnosis on the billing form had a matching diagnosis in the progress note. Horner and colleagues argued that this could have been improved to 78% of the visits if broad categories of disease were used. Unfortunately, many of the providers in the study were physicians. Many NPs are new to the process of billing for services and more research is needed to evaluate the coding practices of NPs.

Down-coding has ramifications for NP employment security and practice finances. Even if an NP is not the owner of a health care business, undercoding can result in insufficient productivity assessments of his or her work especially if productivity is measured by income generated. A provider's down-coding for services can seriously jeopardize a practice's long-term sustainability (Vonderheid, Pohl, Barkauskas, Gift, & Hughes-Cromwick, 2003).

Nursing Language

Can you describe the nursing diagnosis and nursing interventions classification systems?

NANDA-I is the North American Nursing Diagnosis Association International, which sets the standard for the classification of nursing diagnoses. Although the acronym NANDA-I stands for the organization, it is commonly used to refer to the language itself and is used here to denote the language. A nursing diagnosis is a crucial step in a systematic and individualized plan of care (Barnum, 1994). The NANDA-I nomenclature represents clinical nursing judgments about actual or potential health problems. NANDA-I diagnoses describe a client's reaction to disease or injury and could be compared to the medical community's ICD9-CM codes, which describe the actual disease or injury. NANDA-I currently contains 167 approved diagnoses classified into nine domains. Each diagnosis consists of a label, definition, major and minor defining characteristics, and related factors.

NANDA International is the organization that supports the use of the nursing classification system. NANDA-I (2003) is "committed to increasing the visibility of nursing's contribution to client care by continuing to develop, refine and classify phenomena of concern to nurses." Essentially, they develop, refine, and promote a taxonomy of nursing diagnostic terminology for general use by professional nurses. NANDA-I is the most commonly used method of developing nursing diagnoses. A recent survey of the 43 schools of nursing in Michigan indicated that NANDA-I usage remains consistently high at 91% (Keenan et al., 2001). The vast majority of nursing schools across the nation and abroad use and teach NANDA-I nomenclature in their curriculum. When used in conjunction with the Nursing Interventions Classification (NIC) and the Nursing Outcomes Classification (NOC), both developed at the University of Iowa College of Nursing, the NANDA-I classification system represents a complete set of languages for capturing the nursing process.

The NIC is a comprehensive listing of nursing interventions that are grouped based on labels that describe nursing activities (like CPT-4 codes). It is divided into seven domains and 30 classes. The system was created for use in various nursing and health care settings. NIC can be used with other languages such as CPT-4 and ICD9-CM. NIC is recognized by the American Nurses Association (ANA) as a data set; it is also included in the National Library on Medicine's Metathesaurus for a United Medical Language.

Few NPs have had exposure to the NIC system. In fact, NPs have resisted the use of NIC in their practice documentation; however, a recent pilot study found that NPs in primary care can identify NICs and nursing diagnoses in practice when cued (Jenkins, 2004). Jenkins believes the past resistance to the use of NIC and NANDA-I has been due to a lack of familiarity with the concepts and usage of nursing classification systems. Yet, it is expected that in the future, more NPs will be familiar with these systems (Keenan et al., 2001). Appendix 8-2 provides a case study example that merges the use of E&M coding, CPT-4 coding, NANDA-I, and NIC in a coding exercise.

What is NOC?

NOC is a taxonomy of standardized "nursing-sensitive" client outcomes, which means outcomes that nursing care can affect. The NOC system was developed for multiple recipients of nursing care and encompasses the entire continuum. NOC provides a consistent measure of client outcomes (Moorhead et al., 2004). Similar to NIC, the NOC taxonomy is a relatively unknown classification system to NPs.

What purpose do the NANDA-I, NIC, and NOC classification systems serve if I can't bill for the use of these nursing coding systems?

Multiple purposes have been identified for using a nursing classification (or coding) system (Duke University School of Nursing, 2003). The Duke University website (*www.duke.edu/~goodwill010/vocab/NANDA.html*) is worth a brief review for those who are completely unfamiliar with the nursing standardized classification systems. The rationale for use of the systems includes benefits to clients, health care, research, and education. It is beyond the scope of this chapter to discuss the numerous advantages of standardized nursing language. A review of the NANDA-I, University of Iowa, and Duke University School of Nursing websites would be worth your time if this remains a pressing question.

Most experts would site the foremost reason for using a standardized nursing language as similar to the rationale for using any classification system—they provide a simplified terminology to describe what might typically be described using various, different words or phrases. Standardized systems like NANDA-I, NIC, and NOC can describe all aspects of nursing care so that nurses, including NPs, can communicate what nurses do that differs from what other health care professionals do. Standardized languages benefit nursing practice through the provision of a clear terminology that conveys the knowledge base and the essential aspects of nursing care. As a profession, this allows nurses to articulate the unique contribution of nursing to other members of the health care team, administrations, and the public (Duke University School of Nursing, 2003; Johnson et al., 2001).

Summary

In summary, coding for NP services is a complex decision-making process with numerous tools and classification systems to assist with the process. Of course, one's own clinical acumen cannot be replaced by manuals and textbooks, yet it is advisable to become familiar with these multiple resources and the evolving rules and regulations that surround the coding for health care services.

Billing for NP Services

Billing for health care is a more recent process than the coding of disease classifications, yet even in the 18th century clients made out-of-pocket payments in cash or through barter for health services. In fact, in the first half of the 20th century, out-of-pocket cash payments were the most common method of reimbursement for health care services (Bodenheimer & Grumbach, 2002).

Billing for NP services is an even more recent process. Although a few NPs have predated medical care for similar services, the process of billing for these services has only come about with the advent of Medicaid and Medicare in the 1960s (Sheehy & McCarthy, 1998; Lindeke, 2000). Medical practices, facilities and agencies have found that NP/physician teams can provide high-quality care (Brown & Grimes, 1993). Yet the problem of deciphering how laws and individual insurers' rules apply to the NP practice situation can deter practices from the most appropriate billing for NP care (Buppert, 2002). The following are common questions asked by NP students and new practicing NPs.

Why is the billing for services so complex and confusing?

Wide variances in states' laws and significant differences in the policies of third-party payers on reimbursement for the services of NPs make the quest for payments a journey through a maze. The federal government frequently defers to state law regarding NPs. Some states' laws on NPs were enacted in the 1970s before the advent of direct payments to NPs for services rendered. Other states' laws on NPs are brand new. Each of the states has its own legislators, governor, lobbyists, medical associations, and nursing associations that influence legal language and the process (Buppert, 2002).

In addition, the wide array of client needs, providers, and payment systems make for a complex health care industry. Practice arrangements between NPs and physicians, hospitals, home health agencies, mental health facilities, and nursing facilities have different rules and provisions for the care provided by NPs. These varying arrangements are often not addressed by current rules and so providers either ask for new rules or struggle to decipher how a situation is interpreted within the existing rules. No single health care payer has a set of rules that applies to all situations and all practice arrangements.

Which third-party payers allow for billing of NP services?

The categories of third-party payers that allow for billing of NP services include Medicare, Medicaid, commercial indemnity plans, commercial managed care organizations (MCOs), and businesses and schools that provide health services to employees or students. Yet, each of these categories of payers has different rules on billing for NP services. In fact, the rules vary by type of NP, by the state and site in which the service is delivered, and by the working relationship to a physician provider.

An up-to-date, state-by-state guide in which to determine the regulatory and state rules regarding Medicaid and some indemnity health care plans can be found at the American Nurses Association website (*www.nursingworld.org*). The rules for Medicare are more consistent state to state, but the rules do acknowledge the need for NP services to be in agreement with state law. MCOs and indemnity plans are even more varied. Moreover, independent versus employee/employer billing processes vary, including whose name is on the check, amount reimbursed, and supervision/collaboration by a physician.

Appendix 8-3 summarizes the basics for each category of insurer for NPs. The basics for each category of payer are also described in subsequent questions.

What are some common terms encountered in the process of billing for NP services?

A list of common terms related to billing and reimbursement are included in Appendix 8-1. The terms were derived from a compilation of a variety of sources that are identified at the bottom of the table.

Can you describe Part A versus Part B of Medicare billing?

Medicare has traditionally consisted of two parts: Hospital Insurance (HI), also known as Part A, and Supplemental Medical Insurance (SMI), also known as Part B. A new third part of Medicare, sometimes known as Part C, is the Medicare + Choice program. In 2000, 40 million people were enrolled in one or both of Parts A and B of the Medicare program, and 6.4 million of them chose to participate in a Medicare + Choice program (Centers for Medicare and Medicaid Services, 2002).

Medicare Part A claim reimbursement is based on the provider's cost, as negotiated with the fiscal intermediary (FI). Reimbursement includes services provided by home health agencies, rural health clinics, hospitals, skilled nursing facilities, and nursing homes. Part A inpatient hospital care is reimbursed at a predetermined rate per discharge, in accordance with the diagnosis related group (DRG) and at a federally standardized payment amount that is payment in full for inpatient operating and capital costs.

Medicare Part B reimbursement is based on an established "fee-for-service" schedule for services filed to the Medicare carrier. These services include physician services, clinical laboratory, injectables, and durable medical equipment. Medicare Part B physicians are reimbursed at 80% of the lowest of three rates: the established fee schedule, a reasonable or customary charge, or their billed charge for services. Medicare Part B will only pay following satisfaction of the client's deductible. NPs are directly reimbursed at 85% of the physician fee schedule rate for the same services, which include physician (NP) services, ambulance, durable medical equipment, and diagnostic tests. Some services are reimbursed at 100% of the lower of either the established fee schedule or their billed charge for clinical laboratory services, influenza or pneumonia vaccinations, and other exceptions as defined by CMS.

What are some of the specific rules regarding Medicare billing of NP services?

Medicare has developed the most specific rules regarding billing for NP and physician services. Foremost, the NP must meet the Medicare educational qualifications and the services must be within the NP's scope of practice as defined by state law (Abood & Keepnews, 2000; Buppert, 2002). The individual must hold a state license or its equivalent as an NP and must be certified by a national certifying body. The NP must accept 85% of the physician fee schedule for direct billing or 100% for indirect billing (or "incident to" billing). The services are those typically performed by a physician and must be performed "in collaboration" with a physician. Finally the services cannot be double billed by another provider or a facility; this means that the physician collaborator and the NP cannot bill for the same service even if the physician was heavily involved in the process of care.

In general, Medicare requires that practices bill services under the provider number of the individual performing the service. However, Medicare does allow for "incident to" billing, which is described more fully next (Buppert, 2002).

What is "incident to" billing?

"Incident to" billing is billing for services delivered by a physician's employee and the care is "supplemental to" the physician's services. "Incident to" billing requires that the NP be an employee of the physician, although answers from Medicare are conflicting on this point. One consistent requirement, however, states that the physician must be "on site" at the time of service. The service is considered to be under the physician's plan, not independent of the physician's plan of care. When billed "incident to" the physician's plan, the service is billed under the physician's provider number, and the practice can receive the full physician fee, under Medicare provisions (Buppert, 2002). "The incident to rules are stated in the Medicare Carriers Manual (Part 3, Chapter II, section 2050), available online at *http://www.hcfa.gov/pubforms/14_car/3b2000.htm*" (Buppert, p. 3).

Buppert (2002) provides examples of appropriate use, unclear use, and illegal use of "incident to" billing. An example of appropriate use would be when a physician evaluates a new client to a practice, diagnoses hypertension, and initiates treatment. The NP who is employed by the physician sees the client for follow-up visits, but the physician still sees the client on a periodic basis that is defined by the practice. All services are billed under the physician's number.

Unclear use that has not been defined by CMS is the term "initial services" for new problems and "active participation" in the plan of care. No rules are set for the addition of new problems by the same established client or how participative the physician needs to be in the care delivery. These may have different meanings to various auditors, clinicians, and administrators.

Finally, illegal use of "incident to" billing would include a situation in which the NP provides care to clients at a satellite office where the physician is never present, but the services are billed under the physician's provider number.

NPs may bill for services "incident to" their care provision. An example would be the performance of an immunization by a medical assistant that is billed under the NP's provider number.

Does the physician need to cosign an NP's documentation in order to ensure payment for billed services?

No, unless specifically required by state law, physicians are not required to sign NP notes to secure reimbursement. For a state's requirements, an NP or physician can query the state board of nursing.

Are there more payer considerations with Medicare billing for NP services?

Yes, in fact, there are a multitude of other payer considerations with Medicare billing. It is beyond the scope of this chapter to describe in depth all of the rules involved in Medicare billing. Yet, a few important considerations include the definitions of "physician service" and "collaboration," prohibitions against dual payments, hospital inpatient versus outpatient NP care delivery, and finally kickback rules. Buppert (2002) provides a concise summary of these extenuating circumstances and should be referred to for further reading.

Another important resource for Medicare billing information is the resident training manual provided by CMS at *www.cms.hhs.gov/medlearn/medicare%20 resident-v2.pdf*. This resource discusses additional complex issues such as advanced beneficiary waivers and rules for Medicare secondary payer status. In most cases, Medicare is the primary payer when an individual has more than one insurance carrier; however, there are circumstances in which Medicare must be the secondary payer. The CMS training manual clarifies these circumstances. In addition, providers can obtain a waiver or signed notice from a client, if the provider believes Medicare may not cover a service, but the provider or client would like the service. The notice must be given to the client prior to the service to allow the client to make a decision regarding future payment for an uncovered service. For example, if a client or provider would like to order a screening mammogram prior to the Medicare frequency rules, the provider may request the client to sign a waiver or notice that indicates the client's payment responsibilities in the event Medicare does not pay. These and other complex situations are discussed in the manual. The manual is a required resource for any provider, but specifically for those with a large Medicare client population.

Does the location of service affect amount or type of services that can be billed to Medicare?

Yes, the location of service delivery is critical to understanding Medicare billing (i.e., Part A versus Part B); the amount billed is also affected. The three locations that encounter the greatest confusion are the delivery of NP services in the home, in a nursing home, and in the hospital (Buppert, 2002). Because NPs are authorized in most states to perform both nursing and physician services, a home health care agency, physician's office, or NP's office must be clear about the distinction when services are delivered in the home. If the billable service to Medicare is a Part B or physician service, then the NP, agency, or practice can bill under the NP's number following all of the rules described earlier. If, however, the NP is providing "nursing services" and billing Part A of Medicare as a home health service then the visit requires a physician's order and can only be billed through the home health agency. The fee schedule is based on the type of service offered and appropriate federal registers must be consulted. Home care agencies are billed under a prospective payment system and use a different set of fee schedules than the typical Part B physician services fee schedule.

An NP may bill Medicare for "physician services" performed in a nursing home under four conditions: (1) An admission evaluation can only be performed if state law or physician delegation occurs; and regular visits can be performed (2) if state law permits, (3) if a physician delegates, or (4) if the NP is not employed by the nursing facility and is working in collaboration with a physician.

Finally, in-hospital care has seen significant growth in recent years, as have the acute care NP programs (All Nursing Schools, 2004). Yet, in-hospital care is affected by the hospital cost report, the NP's employer designation, and, of course, state law. If a hospital is receiving reimbursement for the NP's salary as a component of the annual cost report to Medicare, the hospital cannot bill separately for the NP's services. If, however, the cost report does not include the NP salary or if the NP is an employee of a physician group or is a subcontractor to the hospital, then the NP services can be billed as a component of Medicare Part B physician services. However, an NP cannot take over the care of hospitalized clients on his or her own. Under federal laws covering hospital care, a hospital must require that every client be under the care of a physician (Buppert, 2002).

What are some of the specific rules regarding Medicaid billing of NP services?

Medicaid rules differ from Medicare because the Medicaid program is administered by the states and each state has varying regulations regarding billing for NP services (Buppert, 2002). The federal laws governing Medicaid mandate that states reimburse family and pediatric nurse practitioners directly, but states are not mandated to reimburse adult, geriatric, clinical nurse specialists, or psychiatric NPs. Some states have broadened their rules to include these other NPs. The American Nurses Association (2003) provides an up-to-date listing of state regulations. In addition, the *Nurse Practitioner Journal* provides an annual update in January of each year that provides the current regulatory updates for each state. According to the recent updates, most Medicaid fee-for-service plans pay the NP 100% of the physician fee schedule, but not all states reimburse at 100%. Each state's regulations must be reviewed for specific rules regarding Medicaid billing for NP services. For the exact rules by state, you can contact the state Medicaid administrator. A list of state contacts can be found at *http://cms.hhs.gov/medicaid/mcontact.asp*.

Employers of NPs may elect to bill "incident to" the physician for NP care or bill directly for NP services if covered by state law. Medicaid billing is complicated by the fact that many Medicaid recipients are now enrolled in a managed care plan as opposed to a direct fee-for-service arrangement (Buppert, 2002). The number of managed care plans varies by state. An NP or his or her employer would need to determine the Medicaid managed care rules to accurately bill for NP services. Managed care plans have distinct rules that differ from the federal and state laws; more information on managed care plan billing is discussed in the answer to the next question.

What are some of the specific rules regarding managed care organization billing of NP services?

In general, MCOs will only allow billing for those providers admitted to the plan's provider panels (Buppert, 2002): "MCOs do not admit every physician to provider panels and may or may not admit NPs to provider panels" (p. 9). The rule regarding provider panel admission for billing applies to Medicare and Medicaid managed care plans, as well as commercial managed care plans.

MCO policies on empanelment of NPs vary but the three most common policies are (1) admitting NPS to the provider panel; (2) declining to empanel NPs, but allowing NPs to service on a physician's panel; and (3) declining to empanel NPs and limiting MCO clients from being serviced by an NP in lieu of a physician. The third policy is of course the most restrictive. "A practice wishing to have an NP admitted to a managed care provider panel must query each separate managed care plan regarding its policies" (Buppert, 2002, p. 9). If a MCO is silent on the rules or specifically requires the designated provider to deliver the services, they may consider it fraudulent to delegate the authority to an NP. Each NP and/or each practice must assess the MCO rules before delegating authority or billing directly for NP services. Moreover, the practice or NP should solicit a written authorization for NP inclusion in a contract during negotiation with the MCO to ensure reimbursement for NP billing.

What are some of the specific rules regarding commercial indemnity insurer billing of NP services?

Indemnity insurers allow billing for health care provider services on a fee-for-service basis. Similar to MCOs, each company has its own policies regarding billing for NP services. The policies vary, and can include (1) direct billing for services, (2) indirect billing for services, and (3) denial of billing for NP services. The rates and physician collaboration requirements also vary. Some states require commercial indemnity plans to reimburse NPs for physician services and others do not. Indemnity plans may adopt Medicare rules or adopt their own separate rules. Each NP and/or each practice must assess the commercial indemnity insurers' rules prior to delegating authority or billing directly for NP services. Moreover, the practice or NP should solicit a written authorization for NP inclusion in a contract during negotiation with the commercial indemnity insurer to secure reimbursement for NP billing. "Practice managers may find it useful to prepare grids that track the various insurers' policies" (Buppert, 2002, p. 9).

Who sets the fee schedule for billable services?

The payer sets the fee schedule, yet due to the overarching influence of HCFA and CMS, many of the fees are benchmarked against the U.S. Department of Health and Human Services' rates. Medicare pays 80% of the client's bill for physician services and the client pays 20%. Medicare will pay the NP 85% of the physician's "usual and customary" fee of 80% of the bill. Physician services are paid through a fixed-fee schedule, charges for which are based on three key resource-based relative value units (RBRVUs). The RBRVU system fixes a national value for each procedure code (CPT-4) based on the sum of the RBRVUs associated with (1) the physician's time, intensity and technical skill required for the service; (2) the practice's overhead expenses; and (3) malpractice insurance premiums. Thus, the RBRVUs are higher for specialists and providers with higher malpractice rates (e.g., neurosurgeons).

RBRVUs are established locally to allow for variations in practice costs among geographic areas, and each pricing locality for a given state has a Geographic Practice Cost Index (GPCI) for each RBRVU. Physician fee schedules for all Medicare Part B carriers are calculated using one national conversion factor (CF). Congress determines the CF each year, considering inflation rates, claim volumes, Medicare enrollment, and other factors that may affect the Medicare budget.

The fee schedule is set by the U.S. Department of Health and Human Services' Center for Medicare and Medicaid Services. CMS publishes the physician fee schedule annually. It appears in the *Federal Register,* and Medicare providers can request copies from their local Medicare carrier (or the organization/ payer who handles Medicare billing for a particular state).

Legislators in the federal government also adjust the fee schedule as the federal budget comes under scrutiny. As health care expenses become an increasing percentage of the gross national product, the fee schedules for Medicare are adjusted to alter the burden on the U.S. economy (Bodenheimer & Grumbach, 2002). Medicare schedules then have a ripple effect on other payers.

What is a "super bill"? What is an "encounter form"? What is a "router slip"?

A "super bill," an "encounter form," and a "router slip" are typically considered the same document; they are documents completed by the clinician and then delivered to the billing or office staff for their use in billing the services rendered during an office visit. The form typically includes the client's identifying information, E&M coding choices for new versus established clients, applicable CPT-4 codes for the practice, supplies used, and in many cases the laboratory or diagnostic testing ordered during the encounter. Appendix 8-4 provides two examples of "super bills"; yet, the format and the breadth and depth of the document vary widely across practice settings.

Geomedics (2004) provides a super bill template that can be downloaded for free and is customizable for your practice. The best documents contain up-to-date codes and provide the most common ICD9-CMs used in the practice. An ideal document is easy to use; it is concise yet contains a breadth of options consistent with the common office processes. The "super bill" is the communication mechanism between the biller and the clinician; any form that creates confusion, lacks depth, or is difficult to use will affect the reimbursement capabilities of the practice. Therefore, it can significantly impact the financial "bottom line."

What is a CMS 1500 (formerly an HCFA 1500) form? And, do all NP visits get submitted on a CMS 1500 claim form?

The CMS 1500 is the claim form used by billing experts to request payment for services rendered to clients with Medicare or Medicaid. The claim form is a standardized form developed by the Centers for Medicaid and Medicare Services (formerly the Health Care Financing Administration) in 1990 to simplify the payment process.

The CMS 1500 was initially limited to claims from clients with Medicaid or Medicare. Currently, many commercial insurers and MCOs have also switched to or allow the use of the CMS 1500 form in their claims process, but they also have their own claim forms. Again, many of these insurers provide an electronic transmission process, but some offices continue to use the paper claim method of billing for services. Many practices use an electronic transmission claim process, but the CMS 1500 is still commonly used by smaller practices.

When should a practice consider computerized billing versus a billing service?

Many practices both large and small are moving to the use of billing services and/or electronic transmission due to the increasing complexity of the billing process (Westdorp, 2004a). Use of a billing service or filing of electronic claims often affords ease of use and cost savings through the use of knowledgeable experts who have expertise in this complex, ever-changing process of health care billing.

Yet, electronic transmission is not commonly performed via office-based computer systems. The Health Insurance Portability and Accountability Act

(HIPAA) regulations have created some recent complications to this process. Computerized practice management systems have hit the market with good price points and easy-to-use Windows-based software, but the new HIPPA regulations have created security issues for most companies. A billing company serves a purpose when and if the specialty is such that no office staff is required, such as emergency department physicians, radiologists, anesthesiologists, and pathologists. However, in the practices interacting with clients, point of exit data entry done accurately eliminates the need for any type of outside billing service. An outside billing service removes the communication and interaction and creates an arm's length distance that can lead to many breakdowns in communication and responsibility.

What happens if a client has more than one health insurance company?

The issues of a primary versus a secondary payer for a particular claim or bill for service are complex. A "primary payer" is the company that pays first and pays the bulk of the claim. The secondary payer covers any remaining amount not covered by the other insurance company. The type of insurance plans in which the client is enrolled further complicates the answer. When the client is under 65 years of age and has standard, employer-based coverage, the insurance plan that is assigned to the client is the primary and a family member's policy (i.e., a husband's or wife's policy) becomes the secondary payer.

When a client is over 65 and Medicare Part B eligible, the complexities of Medicare rules and regulations affect the primary versus secondary payer question. When Medicare-eligible beneficiaries continue to work after they are eligible for Medicare benefits, their medical services must first be filed to their employer's primary insurance company and then to Medicare Part B. The Medicare Secondary Payer (MSP) program also applies when services are paid by the Black Lung program, United Mine Workers, no-fault or liability insurance, disabled Veterans Affairs (VA) programs, and worker's compensations plans. Medicare is also considered a secondary payer when Medicaid programs for end-stage renal disease cover a client's health care. Moreover, even in Medicare-eligible clients, if VA, a Medicare HMO, worker's compensation, United Mine Workers, or the Black Lung program cover a service, Medicare will not make any secondary payments.

In all other Medicare-eligible client situations in which the client is not currently employed and has a second insurance, Medicare is the primary payer and the other insurance program is the secondary payer. Medicare has set up a coordination of benefits (COB) department to assist providers, beneficiaries, and others in the complexities of the rules and regulations regarding Medicare secondary benefits processes. All MSP inquiries can be directed to the contractor at (800)999-1118 or (800)318-8782.

What does it mean to "bundle" a payment or to "unbundle" a bill?

"Bundling" can be described as a bundled payment or bundled services. The two are interrelated. A bundled payment is made for services that are commonly bundled together. A bundled payment is defined as the use of a single payment for a group of related services (University of Washington, 2004). The payment system packages a group of medical services, rather than allowing for payment of each individual service. Often a bundled payment rate exists when an insurer pays a single rate for one or more of a group of different services furnished to an eligible individual during a fixed period of time. The payment is the same regardless of the number of services furnished or the specific costs, or otherwise available rates, of those services.

A "bundled service" combines closely related specialty and ancillary services. The bundle may include two or more components usually provided by different providers, each with their own unique provider qualifications, even if the components fall within the same service category. For example, preoperative care, surgical treatments, and postoperative care are commonly bundled together as a service and paid in the same manner.

When the payment or services are provided according to the insurer's rules, the process is legal. However, a provider or a health care corporation that "unbundles" the services in order to enhance reimbursement is committing fraud. "Unbundling" is the billing of each stage of a procedure as if it were a separate procedure. Medicare has defined these activities as fraudulent because the "unbundling" purposefully results in a significantly larger payment to the provider. For instance, a durable medical equipment company was found to have billed for the component parts of a wheelchair separately, thus receiving four or five times more than if the wheelchair alone was billed as a single item. Diagnostic X-ray series have also been frequently billed as separate, distinct units or procedures rather than as a series or set.

Although the intent differs, down-coding or "bundling" of E&M office codes to diminish the costs to clients is also considered fraudulent. Yet, a study by the American Academy of Primary Care Associates found the practice to be "very frequent" among its members (*www.aapca1.org/aapca1/DistrictResults.asp*).

What happens if I make an error in billing or if a bill gets rejected?

Multiple options exist for rectifying an error in billing, whereas a rejected bill may take a significant amount of work to rectify, appeal, or substantiate. The health care billing process is fraught with error risks. The complex process is prone to error because multiple distinct codes and modifiers must be accurately documented on a claim form in order to obtain a clean billing process.

Fortunately, an error can be rebilled to the insurer with a note identifying the error and the corrected item. No penalty is applied for the error when the correction is handled in a timely manner.

Claims that are not considered "clean" will almost always be rejected or denied. However, there are always going to be situations when the insurers will incorrectly deny or reduce the payment, even if the claims were billed cleanly. Therefore, you should be prepared to appeal a payment decision that you find unfavorable to your practice.

The first step in the appeal process is the appeal letter. The way the appeal letter is written is very important. The rule is "Keep it simple, factual and polite" (Lash Group, 2003, p. 51). The letter should include the following three elements: (1) State the problem, (2) explain why the service or item should be paid, and (3) tell them what you want them to do. State the problem including a description of the services that were denied along with the dates of service. The explanation for payment should include a description of its medical necessity or explain the rule used to make the determination for payment. Make sure you conclude the letter with a statement about what you expect them to do to correct the denial or error. A sample appeal letter is included in Appendix 8-5.

The Medicare appeals process is complex and subject to change (Lash Group, 2003). As of July 2003, there were three levels of appeal for Medicare claims. Effective October 1, 2002, a redetermination appeal must be requested within 125 days of the dates on the remittance payment. If you receive a denial of the redetermination review, you have 6 months from date of the denial letter to request a fair hearing from the Medicare carrier. The denial must involve an amount in question of at least $100. Three options for a hearing exist: (1) a review by a hearing officer (on-the-record hearing), (2) a telephone hearing, or (3) an in-person hearing. Should the second appeal level be denied, an administrative law judge (ALJ) hearing may be requested. An ALJ hearing is the third and final process. Specific rules also apply to this process.

Commercial insurers and MCOs do not offer all of the levels of appeal that are offered by Medicare. However, there are fewer denials due to fewer statutory and regulatory restrictions. The general steps for these appeals include clarifying the client's insurance status, appealing by telephone, and finally sending an appeal letter. As a final resort, you may contact the state insurance commission for clarification and further appeal decisions.

What is the link between documentation, coding, and billing?

In Chapter 9 of this text, White and Benkert discuss the important links between documentation, coding, and billing. In short, billing for various levels of service must be supported by adequate documentation and coding according to published guidelines and the rules and regulations of the insurer. NP providers must avoid purposeful fraudulent coding and billing even if it benefits the client.

What do I need to know in hiring a coder and biller for my practice?

Despite the necessity to acquire a working knowledge of coding and billing for NP services, the fact remains that the NP cannot do it all. An office manager who is also an experienced coder and biller can maximize collectibles in most practices. The NP needs to be aware of billing and coding, but also needs to know when and how to hire an office manager and a coder/biller. Hiring a well-qualified individual or service takes know-how, some networking, and effective hiring practices on your part. Finding a reliable coder/biller and office manager takes recruitment skills. Price and Strickler (1999) offer some expert advice. Foremost, they argue that the organization must encourage the applicant through multiple recruiting methods, such as online recruiting and telerecruiting. One of the best methods is to include a toll-free number or e-mail address and ask candidates to contact you for more information. A great resource for hiring for health care practices is *The Medical Practice Preemployment Tests Book*. It can be obtained by calling The Practice Management Information Corporation at (800)633-7467, or you can also contact Wonderlic Personnel Test, Inc., which distributes many types of employment testing books; they can be reached at (800)323-3842.

In addition to recruiting methods, an NP must know the criteria for hiring effective personnel. The major problem is that most people do not understand the complexities of medical billing. Many people are setting themselves up as medical billers with nothing more than a CD-ROM tutorial and generic billing software. Box 8-1 provides criteria for the hiring of a qualified coder, biller, and office manager. The eight tips on finding a coder and biller were adapted from Frazier's (2001) tips on finding a billing service.

What should be my working process with the coders and billers in a clinical setting?

As a medical billing consultant, one of the authors (AA) has found that the most common problems in medical or health care practices result from a breakdown in communication between the clinical providers and the coding and billing staff. Basic communications can fall apart during a busy day.

When it comes to coding and billing, a language barrier also exists; clinicians are usually thinking in terms such as "rule out" and "differential diagnosis." Coders and billing staff, however, are thinking in terms of "actual symptoms," "diagnosis," and other primary terminology from the ICD9-CM and CPT-4 manuals. Coders and billers are also working to get a claim paid, whereas clinicians are thinking about honing their clinical judgment and deciphering a client's concern toward a treatment outcome. A mutual understanding of each person's role and language calls for monitoring our "role-centrism." NPs would be best suited to work across the language barriers with coding and billing staff

Box 8-1 Hiring a Qualified Coder/Biller and Office Manager

Tips for Hiring a Qualified Coder/Biller

- Check with the Better Business Bureau for complaints.
- Check references.
- Assess knowledge and training on a variety of issues, such as compliance, HIPAA, state laws, state insurance managed laws, and electronic and paper claims submissions.
- Ask how long the coder/biller has been working in the area of medical billing.
- Ask how many clients the coder/biller has and what his or her specialties are.
- Determine the biller-volume ratio (average biller/charge receipts).
- Look for billers with certifications (i.e., Certified Professional Coder or CPC certification).
- Review the services offered such as filing claims to all private and government insurers, maintaining accounts, and sending statements.

Tips for Hiring a Qualified Office Manager

- Consult your colleagues.
- Develop an "appropriate" position description (i.e., ask colleagues and other staff to do a needs assessment of the practice).
- Check references.
- During the interview process use hypothetical or problem-solving questions.
- Do a background check (e.g., for lawsuits, illegal activity).

by developing a rudimentary understanding of coding and billing and, as with any health care communication, NPs would benefit from acknowledging the potential for miscommunication. Mutual acknowledgments of each person's expertise are called for in these situations.

SUMMARY

Coding and billing for health care services is a complex process whether the clinician is an NP or another type of provider. Two overarching rules for all providers to consider are (1) the ICD9-CM diagnosis code must justify the CPT-4 procedure code and (2) do not assume you understand the rules for NP billing. The coding and billing process is complex and evolving. An NP would do well to stay abreast of the rules and maintain a good working relationship with the biller/coder in the practice setting.

References

Abood, S., & Keepnews, D. (2000). *Understanding payment for advanced practice nursing services: Volume one: Medicare reimbursement.* Washington, DC: American Nurses Association.

Internet Resources

Centers for Medicare and Medicaid Services
http://cms.hhs.gov/

Timeline for Reimbursement legislation
www.nursing.umn.edu/professional/reimbursement/6.html

Realities of reimbursement for NPs
www.nursing.umn.edu/professional/reimbursement/index2.html

Complete resource on billing and other issues related to reimbursement for NPs
www.nursing.umn.edu/professional/reimbursement/index2.html

All Nursing Schools. (2004). Featured schools: AcuteCare Nurse Practitioner Programs. Retrieved July 2, 2004 from *http://www.allnursingschools.com/featured/acute-care-nurse-practitioner/*

Allen, K.R., Reinke, C.B., Pohl, J. M., Martyn, K.K., & McIntosh, E.P. (2003). Nurse practitioner coding practices in primary care: A retrospective chart review. *Journal of the American Academy of Nurse Practitioners, 15*(5), 231-236.

American Medical Association. (2004). *CPT 2004: Current procedural terminology: Professional edition.* Washington, DC: Author.

American Nurses Association. (2003). ANA governmental affairs. Retrieved October 16, 2003, from *http://nursingworld.org/gova/charts/medicaid.htm*

American Psychological Association. (1994). *Diagnostic and statistical manual for mental Disorders- IV (DSM-IV).* Washington, DC: Author.

Barnum, B.J.S. (1994). *Nursing theory analysis, application, evaluation* (4th ed.). Philadelphia, PA: J.B. Lippincott.

Bennett, S.L., Casebeer, L.L., Kristofco, RE, & Strasser, S.M. (2004). Physicians' Internet information-seeking behaviors. *Journal of Continuing Education in the Health Professions*, Winter, *24*(1):31-38.

Bodenheimer, T.S., & Grumbach, K. (2002).*Understanding health policy: A clinical approach* (3rd ed.) New York: Lange.

Brown, S.A., & Grimes, D.E. (1993). *Nurse practitioners and certified nurse midwives: A meta-analysis of studies on nurses in primary care roles.* Washington, DC: American Nurse Publishing.

Buppert, C. (2004). *Nurse practitioner's business practice and legal guide*(2nd ed) Boston: Jones and Bartlett.

Buppert, C. (2002). Billing for nurse practitioner services: Guidelines for NPs, physicians, employers and insurers. *Medscape Nurses, 4*(1), 1-15.

Centers for Medicare and Medicaid Services. (2002). *Medicare resident and new physician training program: A comprehensive guide designed to inform physicians about the Medicare program* (6th ed.). Available at *www.cms.hhs.gov/medlearn/medicare%20resident-v2.pdf*

Centers for Medicare and Medicaid Services. (2003a). State and Federal Medicaid Contacts. Retrieved November 5, 2003, from *www.cms.hhs.gov/medicaid/mcontact.asp*

Centers for Medicaid and Medicare Services. (2003b, March 28). *Program memorandum: Medicare payments for Part B mental health services*. Retrieved January 15, 2004, from *www.cms.hhs.gov/manuals/pm_trans/AB03037.pdf*

Centers for Medicare and Medicaid Services. (2004). Physician information resources for Medicare. Retrieved July 12, 2004 from *http://www.cms.hhs.gov/physicians/*

Dochterman, J., & Bulechek, G. (Eds.). (2004). *Nursing interventions classification (NIC)* (4th ed.). St. Louis, MO: Mosby.

Duke University. Website (2003). Accessed on 30 October 2003 Available at: *http://www.duke.edu/~goodw010/vocab/NANDA.html*.

Flanigan, L. (1998, June). Family physicians and nurse practitioners: A perfect team. *Family Practice Management*. Retrieved October 23, 2003, from *www.aafp.org/fpm/980600fm/spectrum.html*

Frazier, D. A. (2001, August). Follow these eight steps to finding a billing service. *MGM Update, 40*(15). Available at *www3.mgma.com/articles/index.cfm?fuseaction=detail.main&articleID=11864*

Geomedics. (2004). Business and productivity solutions for healthcare professionals. Retrieved August 18, 2004, from *www.geomedics.com/downloads/superbill.htm*.

Hart, A.C., & Hopkins, C.A. (2004). *2004 ICD-9-CM: Professional for physicians: International classification of diseases, 9th revision, clinical modification*. Los Angeles, CA; Practice Management Information Corporation.

Horner, R.D., Paris, J.A., Purvis, J.R., & Lawler, F.H. (1991). Accuracy of patient encounter and billing information in ambulatory care. *Journal of Family Practice, 33*(6), 593-598.

Jenkins, M. (2004, January 20). Personal communication.

Johnson, M., Bulechek, G., Dochterman, J., Maas, M., & Moorhead, S. (Eds.). (2001). *Nursing diagnoses, outcomes, & interventions*. St. Louis, MO: Mosby.

Keenan, G.M., Treder, M., & Clingerman, E. (2001). Survey indicates sharp increase in usage of NANDA, NOC and NIC. *Michigan Nurse, 74*(8) 19, 21.

Kent C. (1998, May 26). Medicare audit: Physicians improperly bill for $.59 billion. *Physician's Weekly News, 15*(20). Available at *www.physiciansweekly.com/archive/98/05_26_98/itn1.htm*

Lash Group. (2003). *Oncology coding and reimbursement for beginners*. Available at *www.procritline.com/pubs/coding/coding.jsp*

Lindke, L. (2000). Timeline for reimbursement legislation. Retrieved December 13, 2003 from *http://www.nursing.umn.edu/professional/reimbursement/6.htm/*

MedLearn. (1997). *Nurse practitioners—Evaluation & management coding*. St. Paul, MN: Medical Learning, Inc.

Moorhead, S., Johnson, M., & Maas, M. (Eds.). (2004). *Nursing outcomes classification (NOC)* (3rd ed.). St. Louis, MO: Mosby.

Neveleff, D.J. (1999, September 15). Gastroenterologists find physician extenders help improve care and income. *Gastroenterology Practice Options*. Retrieved October 23, 2003, from *www.geoptions.com/cgi-local/display_article.cgi?263*

North American Nursing Diagnosis Association. (2004). *Nursing diagnoses: Definitions and classification 2003-2004*. Philadelphia, PA: Author.

Price, S., & Strickler, B. (1999, February). Recruiting for the year 2000: Putting tomorrow's workforce in place. *Personnel Postscript/HR Issues, 14*(2). Available at *www3.mgma.com/articles/index.cfm?fuseaction=detail.main&articleID=11344*

Sheehy, C.M., & McCarthy, M.C. (1998). *Advanced practice nursing: Emphasizing common roles.* Philadelphia, PA: F.A. Davis.

The increasing impact of ehealth on physician behavior. Available at *http://www. harisinteractive.com/news/newsletters/healthnews/HI_HealthCareNews2001 Vol1_iss31.pdf*

University of Washington. (2004). *Glossary of terms. Department of Public Health and Community Medicine.* Available at *http://depts.washington.edu/hsic/resource/glossary. html#b*

U.S. Department of Health and Human Services Office of the Inspector General. (2001, June). Medicare coverage of non-physician practitioner services. Accessed October 21, 2002, from *http://oig.hhs.gov/oei/reports/a525.pdf.*

Vonderheid, S., Pohl, J.M., Barkauskas, V., Gift, D., & Hughes-Cromwick, P. (2003). Financial performance of academic nurse-managed primary care centers. *Nursing Economics, 21*(4):167-175.

Westdorp, A. (2003, December). Health care and business consultant, Grand Management Group. Personal communication.

Westdorp, A. (2004a, February 19). Health care and business consultant, Grand Management Group. Personal communication.

Westdorp, A. (2004b, August 11). Health care and business consultant, Grand Management Group. Personal communication.

World Health Organization. (2001, April 9). *International classification of functioning, disability and health. 54th World Health Assembly: Report by the secretariat.* Geneva: Author.

The Tools You Will Need to Practice

9

Documentation for the Nurse Practitioner

Mary P. White
Ramona Benkert

Documentation

Documentation is one of the most time-consuming, yet important, aspects of your advanced practice. The old adage "if it isn't written, it wasn't done" applies to everything you do as an advanced practice nurse (APN). Documentation is used to evaluate and plan the client's immediate care and to monitor his or her health care over time. It enables providers to communicate with each other and provide continuity of care. It helps with accurate and timely claims review and payment, and ensures appropriate utilization review and quality of care evaluations.

Fully documenting your client encounters, including all pertinent data and interventions, will decrease your risk for liability and also justify the evaluation and management (E&M) code used for billing. As a nurse, you have been documenting client care routinely. As NPs, you are now under scrutiny from several sources, and your professional "presentation" will depend in large part on how well you document your care and interventions.

This chapter provides documentation guidelines for the standard subjective, objective, assessment, and plan (SOAP) format, including standardized progress notes and E&M coding. It also provides guidance on writing a referral letter and a letter of consultation and discusses the advent of the electronic health record.

SOAP Note

What is a SOAP note?

A variety of options exist for organizing the data you have collected in a client encounter. One of the ways is to document the data gathered in a SOAP format. The SOAP method of documentation organizes collected data into various sections based on the type of data collected during the visit.

Subjective data includes any and all data that is client initiated. Any information *stated* by the client is considered subjective data. In other words, the information you obtain in taking the client's history is subjective, based on the client's perception of his or her problem or health status. The client responds to your questions with information that is skewed by his or her impression or recollection of the symptoms or event(s). Any component of the client's history is considered subjective data. These components are discussed in detail later in this chapter. As shown in Table 9-1, the headings of **S, O, A,** and **P** organize the SOAP note. The subjective data is listed under the **S** heading of the SOAP format.

Objective data includes all information obtained through your physical examination of the client. Any data that is directly *observed* during your client encounter is considered objective data. It can also include information obtained through a review of the client record, such as the results of previous diagnostic studies that pertain to the client's current health situation. The objective data should directly relate to the data gathered from the history. For example, if the client presents with a head cold, the objective data should include the findings from physical examination of the head, ears, nose, throat, lymph nodes, and lungs. The inclusion of findings from a pelvic examination when there is no subjective data to support the need for the exam is not appropriate. The objective data is recorded under the **O** heading in the SOAP note within the client's medical record.

Once you have collected all subjective and objective data through your history and physical examination, you review the data collected to determine the most likely diagnosis or diagnoses for the client's condition. Your diagnosis is your *assessment* and is listed in the SOAP format of the client's medical record under the **A** heading. Your diagnoses must be supported by the data listed under the *subjective* and *objective* headings. Each diagnosis should also include its status, such as "hypertension, stage I," not just "hypertension." Diagnoses, like coding criteria, can include medical (ICD9-CM) as well as nursing classifications. Chapter 8 provides a discussion of these classification systems and types of diagnoses or health care decision making that occurs during a client encounter.

The final section of the SOAP note is the *plan* (**P** heading). The plan specifies your therapeutic interventions *specific* to the diagnoses or assessment determined, or what you *plan* to do for the client. The section is divided into multiple sections. The most common subsections include diagnostic testing, referrals, pharmaceutical and nonpharmaceutical interventions, client education, and return visit.

Table 9-1 Examples of SOAP Documentation

Paragraph Format

S	Client is a 58-year-old white female presenting with 3-day history of cough. Denies fever or chills, sore throat, headache. C/O head congestion, clear discharge from nose, and fullness in both ears. Works as child care aide, and was recently exposed to multiple ill children.
O	Well-developed, well-nourished white female in no acute distress. VS: BP 120/72, P 72, R 16, Temp 97.6°F. Tympanic membranes intact without erythema; light reflexes intact bilaterally; nasal mucosa swollen and erythematous, bilateral nares patent. Frontal and maxillary sinuses both tender on palpation; posterior pharynx without erythema, and without visible mucous trails. No cervical adenopathy palpated. Lungs are clear to auscultation in all lung fields, and are resonant to percussion.
A	Viral upper respiratory infection Alteration in comfort related to head congestion
P	*Diagnostics*: none *Therapeutic*: over the counter mucolytics, decongestants, acetaminophen, or ibuprofen prn *Education*: increase fluids and humidity; reinforced importance of good hand washing, preventing spread Return to clinic as needed or if not improved.

Abbreviated Format

S	58 yo WF c/o 3 d hx cough. Cough nonproductive, worse @ noc, (+) head congestion, clear rhinitis, ear fullness. (−) fever, chills, ST, HA. (+) exposure to sick children; employed as child care aide.
O	WDWNWF in NAD VS: 120/72 72 − 16 − 97.6°F. TMs intact, (−) eryth, light reflex intact bil Nasal mucosa (+) eryth / swelling; nares patent (+) frontal/maxillary sinus tenderness R>L post pharynx (−) eryth, (−) trails (−) cervical adenopathy lungs CTA, resonant throughout
A	Viral URI Alteration in comfort d/t head congestion
P	*Dx*: none *Tx*: OTC mucolytic, decongestants, acetaminophen/ibuprofen prn *Ed*: Increase fluids/humidity Reinforced hand washing, prevention of spread *RTC*: prn / not improved

Advanced nursing education has often cited the addition of client counseling, collaboration/referral, and the evaluation criteria to achieve the expected outcomes (Robinson, Kidd, & Rogers, 2000).

In the standard documentation, the P heading begins with all of the diagnostic testing you are ordering to help further refine your diagnosis. The diagnostic testing list includes all of the laboratory tests, radiological tests, and other special examinations that you intend the client to have to confirm your final diagnosis. Second, list all medications prescribed for the client that relate to the diagnosis or diagnoses listed. The medication documentation needs to include the name of the medication, dosage, frequency of dosing, amount of medication to be dispensed, and the number of refills allowed. Documenting this information on the medical record will help eliminate confusion for the client. It will also assist other providers who encounter the client with a list of actual pharmaceutical interventions given to the client. Nonpharmacological modalities are listed next, and include but are not limited to physical therapy, external supports, home monitoring of disease (i.e., home capillary glucose testing), prescribed diet, thermal therapies, and many others.

The next item in the plan should be the health education that was provided to the client, such as instruction on diet, exercise, smoking cessation, self-care modalities, or disease processes. Many of the nursing interventions could be included in this section (Dochterman & Bulechek, 2004). Your plan must reflect appropriate medical and nursing interventions for the specific diagnosis(es) listed under the assessment. Last, the note should conclude with a time frame for the client to return for reevaluation. Getting into a habit or regimen of noting your therapeutic plan in this order will eliminate mistakes of omission in your documentation of the prescribed therapeutic regimen.

How do I keep my SOAP note concise, succinct, and complete?

It is frequently difficult for beginning practitioners to succinctly and concisely document the client encounter in the SOAP note. The tendency is to write in complete sentences, in paragraph form. Keep in mind that you are not the only practitioner who will be reviewing the client medical record. Keeping your documentation simple, concise, and to the point will allow easy readability of your note. Handwritten notes in particular are difficult to read, because penmanship varies widely and is affected by how much time is spent actually writing. Eliminating unnecessary words, such as *the, a,* and *an,* some adjectives, and some phrases such as "client states" allows the reader of your note to read only the pertinent data. A note should include only those adjectives that directly describe a finding and are critical in the differential diagnosis. Table 9-1 provides an example of an encounter documented in paragraph form and in an abbreviated form.

The use of medically accepted abbreviations also improves the conciseness of your note. Yet, a note that is too succinct can create confusion also. For example, "erythematous, well-circumscribed annular papular lesion" is more descriptive and accurate than "red, papular lesion." The general unwritten rule is to be accurate and descriptive, yet succinct. Acceptable abbreviations for use in the medical record vary somewhat from institution to institution, so check with your medical records department to get a list of acceptable medical abbreviations for use in documentation in your institution. Many physical assessment texts will provide a list of approved medical abbreviations that have wide acceptance. Appendix 9-1 lists some commonly used medical abbreviations.

How can I simplify the standardized format for documenting a SOAP note?

Numerous physical assessment textbooks provide a guide for documentation of a routine client encounter, yet there is no mandated format for documentation. The most common format is the SOAP format, but preprinted progress notes or other problem-oriented medical record forms of documentation are also frequently used. Several examples of preprinted progress notes can be found in Appendix 9-2. These preprinted notes will provide you with a guide for developing your own. In addition, a comprehensive manual developed by MedLearn (1997) entitled *The Nurse Practitioners' Guide to Evaluation & Management Coding* provides an excellent resource for the principles of documentation and provides a guide for developing preprinted notes.

Most important, the medical record should be complete and legible, and the documentation of each client encounter should include the items found in Box 9-1.

Moreover, most APNs create preprinted forms to capture the important review of system (ROS) questions for a particular disease entity. For example, the hypertension note included in Appendix 9-3 incorporates the relevant questions for a routine visit with a client who has stable essential hypertension.

Do nursing professionals have a documentation format that differs from these standard SOAP notes?

Gordon (1994) has developed a framework for organizing a nursing assessment and documentation format based on functional patterns, in order to organize the diagnostic category and standardize data collection. The functional patterns include but are not limited to a nutrition-metabolic pattern, activity-exercise pattern, role-relationship pattern, and value-belief pattern. Each of these patterns within the documentation framework was developed to provide a process of assessment that incorporates nursing-sensitive criteria that are not typically the foci of standard medical assessments. The framework is also intended to provide a basis for nursing diagnoses, interventions, and outcomes. The North American Nursing Diagnoses Association (2004) and others have incorporated the functional patterns into the newest taxonomy being used across the country. Although commonly used in undergraduate education, Gordon's work has been less frequently adapted to advanced practice education.

The OASIS and Omaha systems (Centers for Medicare and Medicaid Services, 2004; Omaha System, 2004) of documentation and assessment have been used

Box 9-1	Items to Include in Documentation of a Client Encounter

- Date
- Reason for the encounter
- Relevant history
- Prior diagnostic test results/physical exam findings
- Assessment, clinical impression, diagnosis
- Orders for:
  - Lab tests
  - X-rays
  - Other tests from ancillary services
  - Reasons for and results of X-rays, lab tests and ancillary services
- Plan of care:
  - Discharge plan
  - Client instructions
- Past and present diagnoses accessible
- Relevant health risk factors
- Client's progress:
  - Response to treatment
  - Change in treatment
  - Change in diagnosis
  - Client noncompliance
- Written plan for care:
  - Treatments and medications with frequency and dosage
  - Any referrals and consultations
  - Client and family education
  - Specific instructions for follow-up
- Intensity of the client evaluation and the treatment
- Complexity of the medical decision making
- Signature, not initials

Note: ICD9-CM, CPT-4 and HCPCS codes used must reflect the medical record documentation.

widely in extended care facilities and home health and have some overlap with Gordon's functional pattern assessment. The combined Omaha Assessment and OASIS has been particularly valuable. It provides an efficient, consistent means to ensure compliance with the comprehensive assessment requirements for skilled nursing facilities and home health care. Both of these systems, Omaha and OASIS, have been used by nurse-managed centers delivering primary care to communities (Barton et al., 2003). Similar to the Medicare E&M documentation requirements, reimbursement for services is tied to these requirements. Moreover, nursing personnel more often use these documentation processes. Unfortunately, these three systems have yet to become commonplace among most nurses in advanced practice.

Evaluation and Management Documentation

How much do I need to document for each E&M coding level?

The levels and types of E&M coding determine the amount of documentation required to verify the accuracy of the billing processed for a client encounter. When documenting E&M services, you should include these three key components: history, physical examination, and medical decision making. It stands to reason that the briefer the visit and the simpler the medical decision making, the less documentation is required. Each of these items will be discussed in detail.

History. The history includes the chief complaint (or why the client came to see you today), the history of the presenting illness, the review of systems, and the client's past health, family, and social histories (Bickley, 1999). The depth of documentation of these elements will be determined by the E&M code chosen for that visit. Regardless of the E&M level, the chief complaint must be documented. The chief complaint cannot be documented as "client here for follow-up" or "client here for medication refill" or other similar, nonspecific phrases. The *reason* for the follow-up, "follow-up of hypertension and diabetes" or "stomach pain for 2 days" is an essential qualifier for documentation of the chief complaint (MedLearn, 1997).

The second component of the history that is influenced by the level of E&M coding is the history of present illness (HPI). The HPI is a review of the illness from onset to time of presentation. The HPI must contain at least one, and sometimes all, of the critical elements. Refer to Appendix 9-4 (Evaluation Requirements for E&M Documentation) for a list of these critical elements. NPs also include the client's perception of the problem in the HPI. Although this is not "billable," it is an important element to include because numerous research studies have found that a client's belief about a disease process impacts his or her willingness to follow a treatment plan (Freund & McGuire, 1999).

A *brief* HPI lists one to three of the critical elements, while an *extended* HPI includes at least four elements or the status of at least three chronic or inactive conditions. For example, you have completed your evaluation of a client whose chief complaint is "head congestion for 6 days." A brief HPI may include "congestion worse at night," "notes chills, fever of 101° F last evening," and "relieved slightly with Pseudoephedrine 60 mg and acetaminophen 1000 mg." The three critical elements of timing, associated signs and symptoms, and modifying factors are listed and comprise a brief HPI. If your note on this same client states the following: "congestion and cough worse at night, notes chills and fever of 101° F last evening, notes nonproductive hacking cough, congestion relieved slightly with Pseudoephedrine 60 mg and acetaminophen 1000 mg, frontal headache present all day, rates as 5/10 on 0/10 pain scale," it now includes five of the critical elements: timing, associated symptoms, modifying factors, location, and severity. The note is then considered an extended HPI.

For another client, an extended HPI could include "here for an evaluation of diabetes, COPD and osteoarthritis of both knees." As long as you address the *status* of these chronic conditions, your note will be considered an extended HPI. For example, the status of these chronic conditions could state "daily blood glucose measurements are 110 mg to 135 mg, has had no episodes of increased shortness of breath or increased wheezing or cough, and uses pain medication for the knee pain only at night, walks with a cane when away from home." By addressing the status of at least three chronic diseases, your HPI becomes extended.

The next component in the history is the past health, family, and social history (PFSH) (MedLearn, 1997). The elements of the past health history, family history, and social history are listed in Appendix 9-4.

The PFSH is divided into two levels, pertinent and complete. If your history addresses at least one of the specific areas (past health, family, social), your PFSH is considered *pertinent*. A *complete* PFSH would include information on at least two of the specific areas. A comprehensive assessment of the client often includes documentation of all three areas.

The final component in the history is the review of systems. The ROS is defined as a review of the client's body systems, assessing for any current or previous signs and symptoms that the client may have (MedLearn, 1997). The ROS frequently directs the determination of necessary testing, identifies diagnoses, and provides a baseline status on other body systems. The documentation of the ROS could be obtained from a form the client completed prior to a visit, your direct interview, or a notation from your support staff. You must review the ROS from the client or staff, and make a note to that effect. The required elements of the ROS are listed in Appendix 9-4.

The ROS has three levels for E&M coding and decision making: problem pertinent, extended, or complete. The number of systems that were reviewed and documented determines the level. A ROS that is limited to the system identified in the HPI is considered *problem pertinent*. When your ROS includes 2 to 9 systems, including the one related to the HPI, it is considered *extended*. Documenting at least 10, including the system related to the HPI, and occasionally including all 14 systems, comprises a *complete* ROS. Any system with a pertinent negative or positive response must be individually documented. For example, you evaluate a client with a chief complaint of cough for the past 2 weeks. Pertinent negative responses in the ROS may include "denies chest pain, shortness of breath, hemoptysis; denies head/nasal congestion, ear fullness, sore throat; denies chills, fever; denies heartburn, acid backwash, excessive eructation/flatus, early satiety." These negative responses are pertinent in the evaluation of cough, and include respiratory, head, eyes, ears, nose, throat, and gastrointestinal systems. All other systems reviewed require a notation that the ROS was negative or they can be individually documented.

Examination. The second key component to documentation for E&M services is the examination. The examination must relate to the client's problem identified in the history. It can range from a single system to a multiple-system examination of the client, but the examination must include only those systems or components necessary to further evaluate and define the client's problem. An examination of any system not related to the problem(s) identified in the history is inappropriate. The Health Care Financing Administration (HCFA) (MedLearn, 1997) has identified seven body areas and 11 body systems (Table 9-2) that are to be used in the evaluation of the level of E&M coding as it relates to the examination.

The level of E&M coding is determined by the extent of the examination of each system. Within each of the preceding areas and systems, the Centers for Medicare and Medicaid (CMS) (2002) has identified critical data that must be documented. Appendix 9-4 (Evaluation Requirements for E&M Documentation) lists a condensed version of each system and its "bullets" or critical data. Some or all of the "bullets" must be documented to support the level of E&M coding.

Four levels of physical examination must be documented to justify a particular E&M code: problem focused, expanded problem focused, detailed, and comprehensive. A *problem-focused* examination focuses on a limited examination of the affected body area or organ system and should include one to five elements identified by a bullet in the CMS criteria (MedLearn, 1997). For example, your client presents with a sudden onset of redness in the left eye, and based on the client's history, you suspect he has conjunctivitis. Your examination of the left eye includes checking visual acuity, assessing the condition of the conjunctiva, inspecting the eyelids, and checking the pupillary reaction. You examine only one body system, because this condition rarely requires evaluation of other

Table 9-2 Body Areas and Organ Systems to Document for E&M Evaluation

Body Areas	Organ Systems
• Head (include face)	• Eyes
• Neck	• Ears, nose, mouth, and throat
• Chest (include breast and axillae)	• Cardiovascular
• Abdomen	• Respiratory
• Genitalia, groin, buttocks	• Musculoskeletal
• Back	• Skin
• Each extremity	• Neurological
	• Psychiatric
	• Hematologic, lymphatic, immunologic
	• Genitourinary (female)
	• Genitourinary (male)

Source: MedLearn. (1998). *Nurse practitioner evaluation & management coding* (p. 63). St. Paul, MN: Medical Learning Inc.

body or organ systems. Upon review of Appendix 9-5, under the body system "eye," you will note that you have included three of the bulleted elements, and the examination is considered problem focused.

When you examine the affected body area or system, as well as other symptomatic or related body systems, you have performed an *expanded problem-focused* examination. E&M criteria require an expanded problem-focused examination to address at least six bulleted elements in one or more organ systems or body areas (MedLearn, 1997). If your client presents for reevaluation of stable hypertension and has no change in his history, your examination may include a statement of general body habitus, measurement of height and weight, blood pressure readings in both arms sitting, both arms supine, pulse rate, respiratory rate, auscultation of heart sounds, auscultation of lungs, and assessment for peripheral edema. As listed in Appendix 9-5 under cardiovascular examination, you have included six total bulleted elements: (1) general appearance of the client; (2) vital signs (height, weight, pulse and respiratory rates); (3) blood pressure readings in both arms; (4) auscultation of the heart, including murmurs; (5) auscultation of the lungs; and (6) checking for peripheral edema. The examination would then meet the criteria of an expanded problem-focused visit. If, however, you did not document the assessment of peripheral edema, your documentation would be insufficient to justify this level of coding.

A *detailed* examination must include performance and documentation of 2 bulleted elements from each of six areas/systems or 12 bulleted elements in two or more areas/systems (MedLearn, 1997). For example, if your client complains of "cough for the past 2 weeks" and you complete a detailed history and suspect chronic bronchitis, your examination could be documented as follows:

> 48-year-old, well-developed, well-nourished white male with a temperature of 99.8° F, pulse of 88, respiratory rate of 20, blood pressure right arm sitting 132/85, and left arm sitting 140/88; tympanic membranes are clear, nasal mucosa without erythema or swelling, posterior pharynx with mild erythema at anterior palatine arches, no mucous trails visible; cervical lymph nodes and supraclavicular nodes are nonpalpable, trachea is midline; respiratory movement is symmetrical, nonlabored, lungs have end-expiratory wheezes heard throughout, chest is resonant all fields; heart has regular rate and rhythm, no murmurs, rubs, or gallops heard, no peripheral swelling noted; abdomen soft, nontender, normoactive bowel sounds, no organomegaly or masses noted.

The note includes at least two bulleted elements from six systems (constitutional, ears, nose, mouth and throat, lymphatic, respiratory, cardiovascular, and gastrointestinal) and would be considered a detailed examination.

A *comprehensive* level of examination requires performance and documentation of at least two bulleted elements in each of nine systems or all of the elements in a single organ system (MedLearn, 1997). To illustrate this, consider a client who presents with sudden weight loss of 30 pounds over the past month. You perform a comprehensive history and physical examination. Your documentation of this encounter is listed in Appendix 9-6.

This examination includes at least two bulleted elements from 10 systems and meets the criteria for a comprehensive examination (at least two bulleted elements in at least 9 systems). Refer to Appendix 9-4 for further review of the distinctions between the various documentation levels.

Medical Decision Making. The final component in documenting E&M services is the complexity of medical decision making. This component is frequently the most difficult to understand and evaluate. The four types of medical decision making are straightforward, low complexity, moderate complexity, and high complexity. Unfortunately, the terminology within the E&M documentation and coding manuals make reference to the decision-making process using traditional terminology; however, nursing decision making is an essential aspect of the documentation process.

Medical decision making involves consideration of three elements: the number of diagnoses or management options, the complexity and/or amount of data to be reviewed, and the risk of complications and/or morbidity or mortality (MedLearn, 1997). Referring to Appendix 9-4 under diagnoses or management options, you will note five levels of complexity: (1) self-limited, minor; (2) established problem, stable or improved; (3) established problem, worsening; (4) new problem, no additional workup required; and (5) new problem, additional workup planned. Each of these levels carries an arbitrarily assigned numerical value. For example, if you list the diagnoses of (1) diabetes, controlled; (2) hypertension, stable; and (3) osteoarthritis, controlled, for your client, you have listed three established problems in stable status. Referring to Appendix 9-4, these diagnoses would earn a total of three points. Three points places the number of diagnoses or management options in the "multiple" category.

The complexity or amount of data to be reviewed is the second element of medical decision making. Using the previous client example again, you have reviewed the lab results from the previous visit, which included a normal fasting blood glucose, a hemoglobin A1c of 6.6, a lipid profile reflecting an elevated cholesterol of 225 mg/dL, a low-density lipoprotein of 130 mg/dL, a high-density lipoprotein of 57 mg/dL, and a triglyceride of 190 mg/dL; a complete chemistry panel and thyroid panel were within normal limits. The knee X-ray you ordered at the last visit demonstrates marked degenerative arthritic changes in both knees with spurring noted on the left knee, and a carotid Doppler performed since the last office visit shows 35% stenosis on the left carotid and 50% stenosis on the right carotid. You order urine for microalbuminuria today. You have reviewed blood results, diagnostic test reports, and have ordered an additional test to establish the kidney function in a diabetic and hypertensive client. The total points (as reflected in Appendix 9-4) for this element are three, and this result merits the moderate level of data to be reviewed.

The final element in medical decision making is the assignment of risk. Decisions regarding a particular client's health care are affected by that client's current health status, chronic illnesses, risk for complications (due to the current illness, concurrent chronic illness[es], or prescribed therapies), and other factors. Risk level is assessed as minimal, low, moderate, or high. Determination of risk level involves an evaluation of the presenting problem, any diagnostic procedures, and the management options selected (MedLearn, 1997). According to MedLearn (1997), "the 'assessment of risk' of the presenting problem is based on the risk related to the disease process anticipated between the present encounter and the next one. The assessment of risk of selecting diagnostic procedures and management options is based on the risk during and immediately following any procedures or treatment." The highest risk level assigned any one category determines the final level of risk. Again using the same client as in the previous example, and referring to the table of risk in Appendix 9-7, the presenting problems were the three chronic stable illnesses (moderate level), you ordered a urine test (minimal level), and you reviewed and renewed the client's current prescription medications (moderate level). The highest level of risk is moderate, and therefore the overall risk for the medical decision making for this client is moderate.

The client encounter documented in Appendix 9-6 illustrates the entire process of documentation according to E&M guidelines and should clear any remaining confusion you may have.

How do I dictate the documentation of a client encounter?

Dictation of client encounters is an efficient method of documentation. Dictated notes are frequently more complete, thorough, and legible than handwritten notes. Dictation, once learned, takes less time to perform than handwriting the notes. It is helpful to have a consistent format for your dictation to assist you in providing complete, detailed, and concise documentation. When speaking into a phone or microphone, it is not uncommon for a practitioner to utter unnecessary phrases, or become distracted and disorganized. Having a "cue card" (Table 9-3) prompts appropriate organized dictation.

You can review your dictation, make deletions and additions fairly easily while you are engaging in the initial dictation. Check with the transcriptionist or medical records department to determine how to review and edit your dictation at your institution.

Begin each dictation with your name and title, location of clinic (especially if working in a large institution, or if your dictation is done by someone outside your practice area), and date. State the client's name, spell the client's name, and give the medical record number. The SOAP format in dictation will consist of several "paragraphs." Begin dictation by stating the specific headings prior to dictating the data under that heading. Under the "Subjective Data" heading include separate "paragraphs" for (1) the client's reason for the visit or the presenting complaint, history of present illness; (2) past health and family histories, medications, allergies, tobacco use, alcohol or other substance use, social history; and (3) review of systems or functional health pattern review. After each of the preceding sections, state "new paragraph" so the dictation service will know where to begin the new paragraph. Spell out any words that may be easily misunderstood by the transcriptionist, including medical terminology that may be unusual or unfamiliar.

Table 9-3 Dictation Cue Card

Dictation of	Your name and title
Location	Service location, if applicable
Date	Date of encounter, date of dictation (if different)
Patient's name	State it and then spell it
Patient's medical record number	State MRN #

Subjective Data

Paragraph 1	• State "presenting complaint" then list reason for visit, or the presenting complaint.
	• State "history of present illness" and then list data.
Paragraph 2	• State "past medical history includes" and list pertinent past medical history.
	• State "family medical history" and list pertinent data as appropriate.
	• State "current medications" and list them, "allergies and reaction."
	• State "social history" and list pertinent data, including smoking status, substance use, marital status, occupation as appropriate
Paragraph 3	• State "review of systems" and then list your signs and systems from head to toe (i.e., "denies headache, vision changes, TIA symptoms, no blurred vision. No syncope... . Denies chest pain, palpitations, chest tightness or heaviness. Denies cough, PND, DOE, SOB," etc.).

Objective Data

Paragraph 1	• State "vital signs" and list them.
	• State "physical exam findings" and list them in ordered fashion. List body parts for ease of information transmission (usually head to toe) (i.e., normocephalic, CN intact, HEENT within normal limits, no thyromegaly, no carotid bruits, neck supple, etc.).
Paragraph 2	• Review previous labs or diagnostic studies.

Assessment

	• State " assessment" and list diagnoses in order of priority, and their status.

Continued

Table 9-3 Dictation Cue Card—cont'd
Plan

- State "plan" and list:
  - Diagnostics ordered at this visit (lab, X-ray, Doppler, etc.).
  - Any referrals to specialists, reason, name of specialist.
  - Medications prescribed (name spelled out, dose, frequency, number dispensed, refills).
  - Nonpharmaceutical therapies (PT, OT, heat, splints, diet, etc.).
  - Education provided (disease specific, diet, exercise, smoking cessation, etc.). Document the number of minutes spent in discussion with patient and/or family.
  - Details of return visit.

Under the "Objective Data" heading, include paragraphs for (1) vital signs and physical examination findings, and (2) review of laboratory or other diagnostic testing pertinent to current visit. Again spell out any words that may be unusual or difficult for the transcriptionist to understand.

Under the "Assessment" heading, list and number the health problems diagnosed at this visit, including the status of each problem listed. The "Plan" heading should include a numbered list of proposed therapeutic interventions, which are stated in the order of (1) diagnostic testing or evaluations that you are requesting; (2) referrals to other providers, including the name and location of the provider being consulted; (3) medications you are prescribing; (4) nonpharmacologic interventions you are prescribing; (5) education you provided the client; and (6) when the client should return to the office for further evaluation and follow-up.

Remember to review all transcriptions of your dictated notes for accuracy and completeness. If you note any errors, make corrections on the typed note with your initials next to the correction(s), and sign the note with your full signature to indicate you have reviewed the transcription.

Electronic Health Record

What is an electronic health record?

The electronic health record (EHR), also known as the electronic medical record (EMR) or the computerized client record (CPR), is a computer-based version of the client's paper record, and contains all pertinent client data commonly found in a client's "chart." The overall goals of the EHR are to ensure ease of accessibility to client records, improve the quality of care provided, and improve the efficiency and accuracy of providers evaluating the client (Reider, 2003). The trend toward electronic storage of client's medical records is increasing yearly as more clinicians, providers, and institutions incorporate the EHR into their systems. EHRs are becoming more common-place due to the accelerated liability costs and the historic documentation problems encountered with standard paper recording. Documentation of clinical encounters in paper records invariably lacks the pertinent information that the providers need to access at the time of the client visit (Reider, 2003).

The EHR is still a rudimentary product compared to the complex nature of a paper chart. Barash (2001) has described five levels of functional complexity of the existing EHR systems. The first level encompasses automated medical records, which are still paper records with some automated tasks being performed. The second level involves the transfer of handwritten or dictated and transcribed data into a computerized medical record by scanning or indexing the information. This data is organized much like a paper record. The third level of the EHR incorporates the same data as the second level, but organizes it into a computerized format; this level of EHR also incorporates the ability to interact with general care modalities, such as ordering diagnostic tests, writing prescriptions, consultations, and billing. The fourth level incorporates multiple medical records on a single client from multiple settings and providers into a single EHR, producing a more comprehensive record of the client; this type of EHR requires specialized identification systems for access to ensure confidentiality, and the capability of multiple electronic systems to communicate and interact with one another. The final, and most comprehensive is the fifth level of EHR, and it is often referred to as the electronic health record (or EHR). An EHR incorporates a comprehensive collection of health information on a particular client from a multitude of health care and non–health care providers based on the client's health status.

What are the advantages of an EHR?

Having the client information easily accessible through an EHR has multiple advantages; it improves the quality of care provided and improves provider effi-ciency and effectiveness. An EHR eases the audit process for insurer standards and for research and quality improvement purposes. The use of an EHR reduces the time and labor costs associated with paper records (Barash, 2001). They assist the provider with the ability to generate referral or consultation letters, write prescriptions, interface with billing agencies, and provide easily accessible and verifiable documentation of care for billing requirements (Barash, 2001; National Health Services Information Authority, 2002). Some systems allow multiple providers to be interacting with a single client's file simultaneously.

Another advantage is the ability to set up regional networks with combined client databases, allowing for reduced paperwork at the billing level, avoiding false billing claims, and identifying the most cost-effective treatment. Remote providers, (i.e., those who are helping providers distant from the client access vital health information that will ensure appropriate and efficient provision of emergency health care) can easily access an electronic health record.

What are the disadvantages of an EHR?

No record-keeping system is without its downfalls. Some of the disadvantages of an EHR are the initial cost of acquiring the system and its software, the costs of maintenance, and the costs of updating and upgrading the system as necessary. Noncompatibility with other electronic record systems is another disadvantage, and often causes an added cost burden to the provider or system seeking an EHR (Carroll, 2000; Reider, 2003). Training costs and the need for occasional updates in training are another disadvantage. The potential for unauthorized access to the EHR is a major concern for privacy issues and a clear stumbling block in the use of comprehensive EHRs (Bergeron, 1998).

What are the privacy concerns of an EHR?

Privacy advocates note two basic concerns surrounding the utilization of an EHR. The first concern is based on a client's fundamental right to control access to information about their health status (Computer Science and Telecommunications Board [CSTB], 1997). Organizations utilizing EHRs must obtain explicit permission for the distribution of any client-related information. A second privacy concern involves the release of information to individuals not authorized to access the records. The concern centers around the potential for social or economic distress of the client if particular individuals or institutions had unauthorized access to the record (CSTB, 1997). For example, if life insurance companies or future employers had access to private health information, individuals might experience job or benefit discrimination based on information gleaned from an EHR.

How can I protect the privacy of an EHR?

The Health Insurance Portability and Accountability Act (HIPAA) of 1996 required the Secretary of Health and Human Services to make recommendations to Congress on ways to protect the privacy of medical records (Mehlman, 1999). "The basic solutions that are being proposed are, first, to require record makers and keepers to implement a set of technical steps to protect the security of medical records and, second, to impose penalties on makers and keepers of records who release them for unauthorized or inappropriate purposes" (Health Hippo, 1997).

Strict guidelines and policies must be in place in health care organizations to restrict and monitor the access and usage of any client's health record (Joint Computing Group of the General Practitioner's Committee and the Royal College Practitioners, 2000). Secure identification numbers or access codes must be used. Some systems incorporate fingerprint identification to ensure that only authorized personnel obtain access. Simple measures such as locating data entry portals in areas with highly restricted access or privacy shields are also recommended. Policies that require individuals to log on and off the computer system after each use will also help maintain limited access to unauthorized persons. Moreover, individuals should never leave an open record unattended. Many institutions have developed HIPAA policies and procedures. The future will indicate whether it is the policies or the policing of the policies that is the critical step toward protecting client's health information.

Does an ideal EHR or documentation system exist?

No, an ideal EHR or documentation system has yet to be developed. Multiple corporations and organizations are searching to perfect their "product line," but no clear winner has come forth. According to Bostrom (2004), the nurse managed center of Grand Valley State University sought input from multiple vendors for an EHR for their health center to no avail. After many reviews and consultations with corporations across the country offering the "ideal" and "flexible" EHR product, the nurse practitioner-run center still encountered dilemmas in the implementation, ease of use, flexibility, and other important aspects of documentation system.

An ideal EHR or documentation system would be easy to use and provide access for all levels of health care personnel; provide the ability to enter data, review, and process records at a single workstation; have the capability to integrate with other systems; have large storage capacity; and require minimal maintenance and updating. An ideal system would allow your "fingers to do the walking" through the client's health information, providing you with immediate availability to all the information you need to effectively and accurately evaluate the client for his or her presenting concern. You would no longer have to wade through a "pile waiting to be filed," wasting valuable time, to find the reports you need, or the lab result you ordered at the last visit. Yet, the EHR and an ideal documentation system continue to be an evolving process and an ideal replacement for the paper record has yet to be found; however, as cost and efficiency become the primary drivers in health care, a solution to the documentation conundrums of paper charts may become an item of only historical significance.

How do I know I've documented enough detail to "stand up in court"?

Concern over adequate documentation to protect you from legal action is always an issue for beginning as well as seasoned practitioners. Being complete and thorough in your evaluation and subsequent documentation is imperative to your protection from liability. Yet, notes that are too detailed can be documenting "too much information," lending itself to misinterpretation. The determination of "how much is enough" and yet "not too much" presents the NP with a fine line or gray area of health care services. Continued practice, consultation with other providers, and experience will help you define where

Box 9-2 Recommendations to Reduce Risk of Liability in Documenting Client Encounters

- Always sign the medical record documentation, even if it is dictated. Sign at the bottom of the note just like a letter. A signature and credentials, rather than initials, is always the safest way to indicate review or authorization.
- Indicate the time spent with a client regardless of the type of service rendered or if counseling was performed.
- List any referrals or subsequent services, such as X-ray, mammogram, and specialty examination.
- Initial any ancillary test results.
- Indicate where and when the client is to return for treatment.
- Document any indication that the client is not following the treatment plan or refusing to follow the practitioner's advice.
- Document any telephone conversations that occur with the client or family members.
- Document any telephone conversations that occur with other health care practitioners.
- Indicate any client allergies. Also indicate if there are "no known allergies."
- Indicate any conditions the client has now or had in the past that may affect treatment or medical decision making.

Source: MedLearn. (1998). *Nurse practitioner evaluation & management coding.* St. Paul, MN: Medical Learning Inc.

to "draw the line." Developing a routine in your documentation will reduce omissions of data, thereby reducing your risks for liability. Box 9-2 details suggestions found in the MedLearn manual (1997) for reducing your risk of liability.

As an NP, it is wise to include a statement about any consultations with physicians or related health care providers that you had at the time of the client visit. Because state and federal regulations and also insurers' rules vary by the type of payer, it is wise to document the collaborating physician or provider in one's note (American Nurses Association, 2004). Each state's practice act must be consulted to define the rules regarding physician collaboration or supervision of NPs. To avoid legal as well as liability dilemmas, NPs and the providers they work with must remain current on the state practice regulations and any required documentation.

Referral and Consultation Letters

How do I write a letter of referral?

If your assessment of a client's condition necessitates evaluation by another health care provider, you will need to write a letter of referral. Referral letters communicate confidential information about your client that will enable the consulting provider to determine an accurate assessment of the client's condition. The referral letter should include "client identity, degree of urgency, referrer identity, reason for the referral, presenting problem, past medical history, examination findings, drug sensitivities, and any other specific information relevant to the client" (Ward, 2000, p. 52). The letter needs to concisely and thoroughly provide the consulting practitioner with all of the information required to provide an accurate and prompt evaluation of your client. No consultant wants to wade through information to elicit "just the facts," but at the same time, she or he needs enough information to determine the direction the evaluation should take. Providing the appropriate information will also eliminate unnecessary duplicate diagnostic evaluations.

If the referral is urgent, you should speak directly with the consultant, explain the reason for the referral and its urgency, and give all the details necessary for the consultant to begin an accurate evaluation. You can then follow up the verbal referral with a written referral or "hard copy." An example of a referral letter used by one of the authors (MW) can be found in Appendix 9-8.

As an aside, it is imperative that you become familiar with appropriate professionals qualified to evaluate your client's particular condition. Referrals should be made to professionals in whom you have confidence. Your client will view your referral as an extension of your professional management of his or her health condition. Referral to a less than qualified professional, or a referral that is made to appease a client's demands, reflects poorly on your clinical judgment and your management of the client's health needs.

When I provide a consultation for another provider, how do I write the letter of consultation?

When you provide a consultation on another provider's client, you need to communicate your findings, diagnosis, and therapeutic recommendations not only to the client, but also to the referring provider. Your letter of consultation should be on the professional letterhead of your institution or practice and be addressed directly to the referring practitioner.

Begin the letter by listing the client's name and medical record number. Provide a review of the reason for the consultation, including the presenting complaint, then a summary of the client's history, including the history of the present illness, pertinent past health history, and your clinical findings, including results of any diagnostic testing you ordered or provided the client. The summary of the client's presenting concern is followed by a paragraph describing your diagnosis(es), your therapeutic interventions and recommendations, and when you need to reevaluate the client. Conclude your letter with a brief statement thanking the referrer for the referral. Also include your contact information should the referring provider have further questions or concerns related to the management of this client. An example of a consultation letter developed and used by one of the authors (MW) can be found in Appendix 9-9.

SUMMARY

As illustrated in this chapter, documentation of your client encounters requires careful thought to include all data that will support the billing submitted for the encounter. It must also provide a clear, succinct, yet thorough record of the client's health status and your interventions, allowing other providers involved in the client's health care to accurately and appropriately evaluate the client. Documentation guidelines for reducing liability risk have been presented and need to be considered when completing your charting. As more facilities and health care practices adopt the use of electronic health records, NPs will be challenged to adapt to these changes, and continually demonstrate the highest standard of professional performance and quality of care.

References

American Nurses Association. (2003). ANA governmental affairs. Retrieved October 16, 2003, from *http: //nursingworld.org/gova/charts/medicaid.htm*

Barash, C. (2001). Computerized patient records: Positive impact for medical practices, patients, and profit. Berdy Medical Systems. Available online at *www.berdymedical.com/White%20Paper%20Web.doc*

Barton, A.J., Gilbert, L., Erickson, V., Baramee, J., Sowers, D., & Robertson, K.J. (2003). A guide to assist nurse practitioners with standardized nursing language. *Computers, Informatics Nursing, 21,* 128-133.

Bergeron, B. (1998). Can electronic medical records really achieve information sharing? *Post Graduate Medicine, 104*(7). Available online at *www.postgradmed.com/issues/1998/07_98/dd_jul98.htm*

Bickley, L. (1999). *Bates' guide to physical examination and history taking* (7th ed.). Philadelphia, PA: J.B. Lippincott.

Bostrom, A. (2004, July). Personal communication.

Carroll, J. (2000). Electronic medical records: If not now, when? *Managed Care.* Available online at *www.managedcaremag.com/archives/0007/0007.emr.html*

Centers for Medicare and Medicaid Services. (2002). Medicare resident and new physician training program: A comprehensive guide designed to inform physicians about the Medicare program (6th ed). Available at *www.cms.hhs.gov/medlearn/medicare%20 resident-v2.pdf*

Centers for Medicare and Medicaid Services. (2004). OASIS software and data sets. Retrieved August 31, 2004, from *www.cms.hhs.gov/oasis/oasisdat.asp*

Computer Science and Telecommunications Board. (1997). *For the record: Protecting electronic health information.* Washington, DC: National Academy Press.

Dochterman, J., & Bulechek, G. (Eds.). (2004). *Nursing interventions classification (NIC)* (4th ed.). St. Louis, MO: Mosby.

Freund, P.E.S., & McGuire, M.B. (1999). *Health, illness, and the social body* (3rd ed.). Upper Saddle River, NJ: Prentice Hall.

Gordon, M. (1994). *Nursing diagnosis: Process and application.* St. Louis, MO: Mosby.

Health Hippo. (1997). Electronic data interchange. Available online at *http://hippo. findlaw.com/electron.html*

Joint Computing Group of the General Practitioners' Committee and the Royal College of General Practitioners. (2000). *Good practice guidelines for general practice electronic patient records.* Available online at *www.doh.gov.uk/gpepr/guidelines.pdf*

MedLearn. (1997). *Nurse practitioner's evaluation & management coding: A reimbursement guide.* St. Paul, MN: Medical Learning Inc.

Mehlman, M. (1999). Emerging issues: The privacy of medical records. *The Doctor Will See You Now.* InternetMedCorporation. Available online at *www.thedoctorwillseeyounow. com/articles/bioethics/medrecords_4/*

National Health Service Information Authority. (2002, July). The advantages of electronic medical records over "physical" paper records. *NHS Week.* Available online at *www.nhsia.nhs.uk/def/pages/nhsweek2002/advantages.asp*

North American Nursing Diagnosis Association. (2004). *Nursing diagnoses: Definitions and classification 2003-2004.* Philadelphia, PA: Author.

Omaha System, The. (2004). The Omaha System website. Retrieved August 31, 2004, from *www.omahasystem.org/*

Reider, J. (2003). The electronic medical record: Promises and pitfalls. *Medscape General Medicine, 5*(3). Available online at *www.medscape.com/viewarticle/460247*

Robinson, D., Kidd, P., & Rogers, K.M. (Eds.). (2000). *Primary care across the lifespan.* St. Louis, MO: Mosby.

Ward, H. (2000). Writing referral letters. *The Journal of the RCN Nurse Practitioner Association, 14*(35), 52-53.

10

Client Education

Kim Litwack

Communicating through Client Education

Client education is perhaps one of the most important skills that a nurse practitioner (NP) brings to his or her practice. The ability to explain symptoms, diagnoses, and treatment options is one of the defining characteristics of NP practice. It requires excellent communication skills that are appropriate for a variety of ages and the ability to assess a client's response to information provided.

Why is client education important?

Clients present for care because of unexplained symptoms, because of a recommendation from a friend or family member, because they have questions, or because they have accepted their role in being proactive in meeting their own health care needs. As a provider, you are in a position to explain those symptoms, confirm the recommendations, answer questions, and reinforce health-seeking behaviors (Saarman, Daugherty, & Riegel, 2000).

Don't clients simply want a prescription and to be done as quickly as possible?

Sure, it may be easier to simply write a prescription for sinusitis and to finish with the client in a matter of minutes. However, providing information about smoking cessation, influenza vaccines, use of humidifiers, and good hand-washing techniques to prevent the spread of upper respiratory infections may likely keep this client from presenting repeatedly for sinus infections.

Is there a right time to teach?

Every visit is the right time to teach, however, it may not be the right time for the client to learn. It will be important for you as a provider to assess client readiness and the need to know on every visit, and to adjust your expectations accordingly. There is a difference between need to know and nice to know. For example, a client who presents with a fever of 102° F, pharyngitis and muscle aches, and a positive rapid strep test will likely only be able to focus on the prescription instructions. A client who presents in no physical discomfort may be more ready to listen to more detailed information. The client has to be motivated to learn. Motivation may be because of symptoms, fear, pain, the desire to learn more, a suggestion of a friend or family member, aging, or injury.

Readiness to Learn

How do you assess readiness to learn?

There are two ways to approach readiness to learn. One is to look for client cues signaling readiness, and the other is to look for barriers to learning.

What are the cues for readiness to learn?

A provider can look for a number of clues in assessing readiness to learn. A client who asks questions, a client who does not appear rushed or stressed, a client that presents with no barriers to learning is ready to learn. The application of the Transtheoretical model is a useful assessment tool to determine in what stage of readiness to learn a client is presenting (Prochaska & Velicer, 1997).

What is the Transtheoretical model?

The Transtheoretical model of change is a model of behavior change that has been used extensively as the basis for developing effective interactions to promote health behavior change (see *www.uri.edu/research/cprc/transtheoretical.htm*). Change in behavior is seen as the outcome, and the model provides a means to assess readiness for change. Change in behavior, particularly as it relates to health care and illness prevention, is seen as one outcome of client education (see *www.changecompanies.net/Transtheoretical_Model.htm*).

Precontemplation. In this stage, the client is not intending to take action in the immediate future. This may be due to lack of information about the outcome of unhealthy behaviors, or because he or she has tried in the past to change behavior and was not successful. Traditional client education programs have not addressed this stage and have simply assumed, generally wrongly, that a client, by virtue of the fact that he or she is present in the office, has made the commitment toward a behavior change. Teaching at this stage is often ineffective because the provider is addressing outcomes, whereas the client has yet to see the importance or need for the change, or has yet to realize alternatives that might prove successful.

Contemplation. In this stage, the client is intending to change behavior and is beginning to be able to verbalize the pros and cons of behavior change. The balance between the two is often unclear, and the ambivalence felt is a perfect time for the provider to provide additional information supporting the rationale for behavior change and addressing the reasons against behavior change.

Preparation. In this third stage, clients are intending to take action and have begun to make plans to do so. The provider can assist by verifying plans, offering support, and continuing to reinforce the benefits of behavior change.

Taking Action. In this stage, clients take overt actions that are observable. These behaviors can be reinforced by the provider, and specific outcomes brought to the attention of the client.

Maintenance. In this last stage, the client works to maintain newly acquired health behaviors and to avoid relapse. Success builds confidence, and observed behaviors with measurable outcomes can help to reinforce ongoing and future client successes.

If the provider is able to accurately determine from which stage the client is operating, client education can be addressed accordingly, with the goal of promoting health and minimizing illness and its effects.

Is there an example of the application of the Transtheoretical model?

One example of the application of this model would be in the management of hypertension. The client may be presenting to the office for the first time for a preemployment physical exam. He is asymptomatic and has no complaints. You note an elevated blood pressure, and further assessment reveals a rather sedentary lifestyle, frequent fast-food lunches, and mild obesity. If you were to start right in with pharmacologic intervention, referral to a nutritionist, a strong recommendation to start exercising, and a request to obtain labs for cholesterol and renal function, this client may immediately consider the visit over, with no desire to return for further care. He is not considering the need for a change, has never been told of the need for a change, and has now been hit with the need for many changes by a provider with whom he has no relationship.

If, however, on this visit, the finding of high blood pressure was pointed out, with information given about the significance of this value and its impact, the client is given the chance to assimilate the information and to ask further questions. All of the previously listed interventions are certainly appropriate, and may occur with time, but the client first has to accept the diagnosis and understand the rationale for change. Perhaps at this visit, only information will be given about high blood pressure and why restoration of normal pressure is important, and additional information will be given about further risk reduction. The client may be asked to take materials home to read, and a future appointment scheduled to continue the conversation and to provide additional information. The provider can help the client prepare to take action, perhaps in the form of starting a medication, the initiation of a walking program, or diet and weight management. Once the client takes action, the provider can reinforce the behaviors as well as the outcomes to assist the client in being successful. Obstacles to success can also be problem solved. The outcome is a client whose blood pressure is controlled, with positive health behaviors and significant risk reduction.

Barriers to Learning

What are the barriers to learning?

Barriers to learning may be client related or setting related. Client-related and institutional setting barriers are listed in Boxes 10-1 and 10-2, respectively.

Are there strategies that a nurse practitioner can use to overcome these barriers?

Absolutely. The NP needs to examine his or her interactions with clients to determine the presence of client-related barriers to learning. Interventions should be targeted toward the identified barriers. For example, a client who is febrile and in pain will likely benefit from the administration of an analgesic before continuing with the remainder of the visit. A client who speaks a

---

Box 10-1 Client Barriers to Learning

Language
Educational level
Developmental level
Pain
Stress
Financial resources
Culture
Religion

Box 10-2 Institutional Barriers to Learning

- Lack of privacy
- Poor scheduling; lack of time
- Lack of provider commitment to education
- Lack of resources
- Lack of qualified support staff
- Lack of available translators

language other than the language spoken by the provider will benefit from an appropriate translator. The client who does not understand the impact of controlling asthma because he does not understand the pathophysiology of the disease will benefit from teaching focusing on the disease cause, in addition to its management.

Institutional barriers are often harder to overcome. They require an assessment and definition of the problem, and a quality improvement plan for addressing the barrier. All providers and staff in the setting must be aware of the problem, and together must make the commitment to finding solutions. Poor scheduling, for example, limiting the time a provider can spend with a client, may require adjustment in intervals between clients. Because this has an impact on revenue and the ability of the site to meet the needs of clients who need to be seen, a compromise may need to be worked out among all staff. For example, one center that provides women's health care has the provider doing the hands-on pelvic exams and diagnostic testing, but it utilizes a registered nurse to explain contraceptive options prior to the client seeing the provider and again after seeing the provider once a decision has been made as to type of contraception.

Effective use of resources maximizes the volume of clients that can be seen, and provides for quality client education. Satisfaction with the system in this situation is high for providers, staff, and clients.

The Importance of Client Education

Is client teaching cost effective and worth the investment?

In a word, yes. Assessing the cost effectiveness of any intervention, client teaching included, requires the evaluation of the costs associated with a particular intervention, in comparison with the health effect of the intervention. With effective client teaching directed toward self-management, cost savings are realized by a reduction in provider visits, treatment and pharmaceutical costs, and after-hours calls and by a decrease in hospitalizations (Eisenberg, 1989). A review of the literature identifies programs that have evaluated the cost effectiveness of teaching related to asthma, arthritis, congestive heart failure, diabetes, colorectal screening, immunizations, and advanced directives (Brown, 1990;

Henrick, 2001; Kruger, Helmick, Callahan, & Haddix, 1998; Lee, Ewert, Frederick, & Mascola, 1992; Osborne, 1999; Rickheim et al., 2002; Stoloff & Janson, 1997; Wagner, 1990).

Many health maintenance organizations (HMOs), in particular, have committed resources toward client education, often coordinated by an NP or PA, registered nurse, or certified educator, with the goal of making the organization more cost effective while at the same time improving client health and reducing disability associated with disease and illness. Physician and group practices may dedicate one NP or PA provider to the role of client education, particularly when that practice deals with one specialty population, for example, clients with asthma or clients with congestive heart failure. Being able to document the cost effectiveness of client education is data that potential employers like to see and may result in the development of a position where previously none existed. Note that client education is a billable service (Freda, 2004).

How do I become an effective educator?

First, recognize that you most likely already have the skills needed to be an effective educator because prior to becoming an advanced practice provider, you were first a registered nurse. You know how to communicate with clients and their families. What has changed now is that you are in the role of completing advanced assessments, making diagnoses, and developing treatment plans. You are developing yourself as an advanced practice provider and are learning often right along with your clients.

Is there anything I should remember in teaching?

Stay focused. Set reasonable objectives for yourself and your client. Decide again what the client needs to know. Then you have to decide how you will communicate the information.

Teaching Resources

What resources do I have in teaching?

Your first resource is your client. You need to determine what your client already knows. Second, you have a wealth of information from coursework, your experience as a nurse, and your precepted clinical experience as a student. You have clinical practice guidelines developed by interdisciplinary teams that address practice standards and the rationale for their implementation. You have journals, textbooks, and the Internet. You may be seeing pharmaceutical representatives who provide you with information. You have colleagues with a wealth of information. You also have access to the same resources that your clients do. Clients are reading the *Reader's Digest* and obtaining information about heart disease. They are watching the Discovery Channel for information about joint replacement. They are surfing the Internet to interpret symptoms and to, in some cases, determine treatment.

Are all of these resources useful?

Only with critical evaluation can you determine the value of any teaching materials. Clinical practice guidelines are evidence-based practice standards that have been compiled by interdisciplinary teams. The pharmaceutical representative's job is to get a medication into your office, so he or she may not provide you with objective data that supports a competitor's drug. The *Reader's Digest* is not a refereed journal. Textbooks go out of date. You need to critically evaluate the materials you choose to use in teaching.

How do I critically evaluate an Internet site?

The Internet can be a valuable resource for both you and clients seeking health information. However, information can be posted on the Internet by anyone with access to a computer.

When reading material on the Internet, it is important to evaluate each site for the following:
1. *Credibility*: Evaluation of the source, credentials, ability to contact.
2. *Content*: Is it accurate and complete? Are references provided? Is the site reviewed or accredited by the HON Code of Conduct for Medical and Health websites? (see *www.hon.ch.HONcode/Conduct.html*).
3. *Disclosure*: Includes information about the purpose of the site, funding, or other sponsorship and advertising. Does it acknowledge that information provided is not intended to replace the client-provider relationship?
4. *Links*: Are they current and relevant?
5. *Design*: Is it user-friendly?

Clients need to be taught how to critically evaluate materials on the Internet as well. Encouraging clients to print materials they are using to make decisions and to bring those materials with them to a visit with their provider will enable the provider to address specifics. Note that there are many very good, useful clinically focused sites that clients and providers can access in obtaining clinical information. There are also sites that are proprietary, incomplete, and unsafe (see *www2.widener.edu/Wolfgam-Memorial-Library/webevaluation/webstrib.htm*).

What about developing my own materials?

This is an excellent idea. Developing your own materials allows you to include information that you feel is important, and to develop it in such a way as to maximize its use in your setting. For example, if you see a fair number of clients with asthma, you might choose to develop a set of teaching sheets each addressing different topics related to asthma management. For an example of a client education handout on asthma see Appendix 10-1.

What should I remember when developing these materials?

The rule of thumb is that materials should be written at a fifth-grade level. Reading level can be measured by using the Flesh-Kincaid Index, the Fog Index, SMOG-testing, the Fry Formula and a number of other approaches (see *www.u-write.com/low-lit.shtml* and *www.fpd.finop.unm.edu/groups/ppd/documents/information/writing_tips.cfm*). Microsoft Word includes readability statistics as part of its spell-checking capability. (See Box 10-3 for instructions on the use of the readability function.)

What about client education for children?

Obviously, children's ages vary wildly. For children under the age of 3, most education will be directed toward the parents. After age 3, the child may have questions that require simple answers. Allowing the child to play with equipment may be one strategy that works well with children ages 3 to 7. Videos have been used as well, rather effectively with children ages 7 to 12, but require a quiet time and place. Models work well for children and adults to explain the normal functioning of a body part or injury. Written materials may be limited to coloring books for children ages 4 to 8. Older children can understand written materials that are clearly written, easy to understand, and written at a fourth-grade level.

SUMMARY

Client education remains vitally important to every aspect of health promotion and disease management. Lack of client understanding leads to increased costs, errors, complications, and treatment delays, as well as anger and frustration for clients and providers. By becoming skilled in the principles of client education for adults and children, as client load dictates, the nurse practitioner is in a position to optimize every visit, with the goal of reaching mutually set outcomes.

Box 10-3 Readability Statistics

To access this tool in Microsoft Word
1. Highlight the text you are interested in measuring.
2. Click "Tools."
3. Click "Spelling and Grammar."
4. The readability scores will appear after the spell check.

Internet Resources

www.hon.ch.HONcode/Conduct.html
www2.widener.edu/Wolfgram-Memorial-Library/webevaluation/webstrbib.htm
www.uri.edu/research/cprc/transtheoretical.htm
www.changecompanies.net/Trantheoretical_Model.htm
www.u-write.com/low_lit.shtml
www.fpd.finop.unm.edu/groups/ppd/documents/information/writing_tips.cfm

References

Brown, S.A. (1990). Studies of educational interventions and outcomes in diabetic adults: A meta-analysis revisited. *Patient Education and Counseling, 16,* 189-215.

Eisenberg, J.M. (1989). Clinical economics: A guide to the economic analysis of clinical practices. *Journal of the American Medical Association, 262,* 2879-2886.

Freda, M. (2004). Issues in patient education. *Journal of Midwifery and Women's Health, 49*(3), 203-209.

Henrick, A. (2001). Cost-effective outpatient management of persons with heart failure. *Progress in Cardiovascular Nursing, 16*(2), 50-56.

Kruger, J.M., Helmick, C.G., Callahan, L.F., & Haddix, A.C. (1998). Cost-effectiveness of the arthritis self-help course. *Archives of Internal Medicine, 158,* 1245-1249.

Lee, S.H., Ewert, D.P., Frederick, P.D., & Mascola, L. (1992). Resurgence of congenital rubella syndrome in the 1990s. Report on missed opportunities and failed prevention policies among women of childbearing age. *Journal of the American Medical Association, 267,* 2616-2620.

Osborne, H. (1999). In other words: Advance directives—helping people understand. *On Call, 6,* 1-3.

Prochaska, J.O., & Velicer, W.F. (1997). The transtheoretical model of health behavior change. *American Journal of Health Promotion, 12,* 38-48.

Rickheim, P.L., Weaver, T.W., Flader, J.L., & Kendall, D.M. (2002). Assessment of group versus individual diabetes education. *Diabetes Care, 25*(2), 269-274.

Saarmann, L., Daugherty, J., & Riegel, B. (2000). Patient teaching to promote behavioral change. *Nursing Outlook, 48,* 281-287.

Stoloff, S., & Janson, S. (1997). Providing asthma education in primary care practice. *American Family Physician, 56*(1), 1-7.

Wagner, J. (1990). Costs and effectiveness of colorectal cancer screening in the elderly. *Journal of the American Medical Association, 264,* 2732.

11

Risk Management: Tracking Systems

Lori Houghton-Rahrig

Potential for Error

Each year in the United States, more than 38 million clients are admitted to hospitals and 820 million visits are made to primary care offices (Robeznieks, 2004). According to a study by the Institute of Medicine (1999), approximately 44,000 to 98,000 medical errors are estimated to occur in the acute care setting. With many more primary care visits than hospital admissions each year, one might conclude that there is a greater potential for errors in the primary care setting; however, few studies are currently available to support this premise.

One of the few primary care studies available at the time of this writing determined that a significant number of errors could occur in the primary setting. The researchers in this study examined 351 client visits at seven primary care offices with care being provided by one or more of the 15 practicing physicians within these offices. In this study, researchers Elder, Vonder Meulen, and Cassedy (2004) defined "harm" to include "physical discomfort, an adverse drug reaction, a physical injury, progression of disease, or causing the client increased emotional distress." Elder et al. found that out of 351 client visits to a primary care setting, 117 errors or "preventable adverse events occurred" with harm occurring in 18 clients and potential harm for 53 clients.

Another primary care study (Dovey et al., 2002) evaluated 344 errors reported by 44 primary care physicians over a

4-month period. This study defined "error" as "something that should not have happened, or was not anticipated." Eighty-two percent of the 344 errors were considered to be administrative errors such as communication problems or billing errors. Thirteen percent of the errors identified in this study were errors in judgment. Four percent of these errors were deemed "adverse events."

A more recent study (Phillips et al., 2004) that evaluated approximately 49,000 malpractice claims made against physicians over a 15-year span showed that 5921 (23%) were indeed errors. Of these 5921 claims, 2003 (34%) were due to diagnostic errors. "Problems with records" made up 439 of these errors, resulting in 156 deaths. Although, it is important to note that these data are somewhat skewed in that they were derived from malpractice claims, one must wonder about the possibilities of errors in the primary care setting.

As evidenced by these studies, problems often occur as a result of a "breakdown" within or between one or more of the systems such as the office system, between the laboratory system and the office system, or between the client and the office. For instance, in the Dovey et al. (2002) study, the office received a client's biopsy report stating that melanoma was found, but there was no contact information for the client. This may be considered both a laboratory and an office system problem. Another client died as a result of not having received important information. This could be considered an interoffice problem (Dovey et al., 2002).

These are a few of many examples in which errors may occur across the health care continuum within or between systems. The Committee on Quality Health Care in America (2001) outlined a framework to assist health care providers, health care organizations, and clients in avoiding errors and promoting safety through the redesign of health care systems in its book *Crossing the Quality Chasm*. No client should be injured as a result of errors (including human errors), within and between health care systems (Committee on Quality Health Care in America, 2001, p. 62). Process improvement methodologies may be key in helping to identify actual and potential safety issues in order to effectively redesign health care systems that will support optimal care.

As noted, many errors can occur across the health care continuum. Tracking systems can be beneficial in the identification and prevention of actual and potential safety issues within and between various health care systems. This chapter focuses on the development of tracking systems and provides a brief overview of paper and computerized tracking systems. A discussion of the use of an electronic health record will be included, as well as factors to consider when establishing a computerized tracking system.

How can errors potentially occur?

As noted in the earlier examples, many potential areas exist in which errors can occur. The following case study will be used to examine the potential errors that can occur between the systems in which health care is delivered.

The systems are a series of steps, or interactions, that occur between one entity and another in order to deliver care such as the system between the laboratory and the primary care office, the system within the office, and the system between the office and the client.

> Mrs. R., a 41-year-old female, had a routine Pap smear during her annual physical examination. Her last Pap smear was 3 years ago. She was 17 years of age when she first had intercourse and has had 3 sexual partners during her lifetime. She has a 10-pack per year history of smoking and is currently trying to quit smoking. Mrs. R. denies painful intercourse or abnormal bleeding. She denies any sexually transmitted infections. She believes that she is in a monogamous relationship with her husband of 11 years. She and her husband have 3 children, ages 7, 4, and 2 years. Mrs. R. manages the local public museum.

> A Pap smear was taken and the results were sent to the laboratory. Two weeks later, the results were returned to the provider's office. The results showed CIN 1, a low-grade squamous intraepithelial dysplasia. The provider did not notify the client of the result, because the lab report was lost in the office, unbeknownst to the provider. The client, a busy professional and mother of three young children, had not contacted the provider because she assumed the Pap smear was normal—as it has always been—and assumed that the provider's office would have notified her if the results were abnormal. The error in following up with the client was found when the client came back into the office 6 months later complaining of a vaginal yeast infection. The provider then noticed that the client's last Pap smear result was not in the chart. The laboratory was contacted and another report was faxed to the office. The client was informed of the Pap smear results and was referred to a gynecologist for a possible colposcopy.

This is an example of a real-life scenario. Errors such as these may result in serious consequences such as delayed treatment for a progressive—and potentially fatal—disease. It is frightening to imagine a scenario such as this, especially as a new nurse practitioner (NP). Errors like these are unacceptable, but they can happen.

What can I do to prevent potential errors?

Examining system processes using flowchart methodology may be beneficial to ensure quality care. The flowchart shown in Figure 11-1 represents steps in the process carried out for a client with abnormal Pap smear results.

How do we interpret this flowchart?

In looking at Figure 11-1, it is amazing to see all of the numerous steps involved in this one process! Potential areas in which errors could occur are noted with an asterisk.

The following is a list of potential problems that could occur in the abnormal Pap smear process between the laboratory and the primary care office,

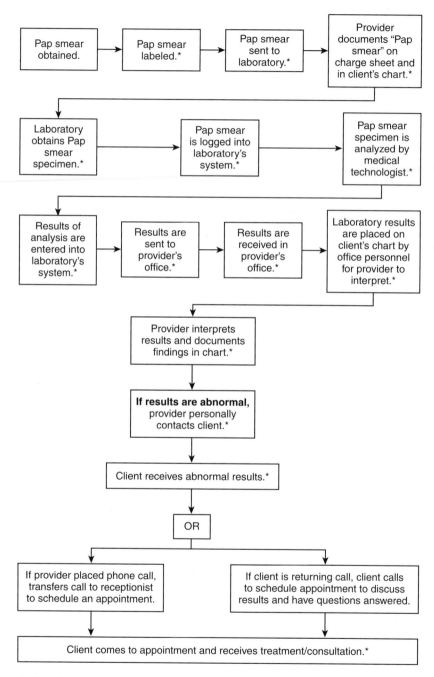

*Potential areas where errors could occur.

Figure 11-1. Flowchart of abnormal Pap smear results.

within the office, or between the office and the client:

1. Pap smear is not labeled or not labeled correctly.
2. Pap smear is not sent to lab.
3. Pap smear is not documented in client's chart.
4. Pap smear is not charged on charge slip.
5. Pap smear is not received in laboratory.
6. Pap smear is not logged into the laboratory's computer system or is logged in incorrectly.
7. Pap smear is analyzed incorrectly.
8. Pap smear results are entered incorrectly.
9. Abnormal laboratory results are not reported to the primary care provider's office.
10. Laboratory results were sent, but lost in the office.
11. Abnormal results are not attached to the correct chart.
12. The provider does not interpret abnormal results correctly.
13. Results are not documented/posted in the client's chart.
14. The primary care provider failed to notify the client.
15. The client was notified of the abnormal results, but no follow-up was conducted because the client did not schedule an appointment.
16. The client missed the scheduled appointment and did not reschedule a visit.
17. The client decided not to follow up with the provider after being notified of abnormal results.

There are many reasons why clients do not follow up on treatment. Reasons may include issues such as denial that there may be some abnormality or simply that the client forgot to make an appointment. Perhaps the client did not receive the message that an appointment was needed or did not understand the severity of the results. Miscommunication between the staff and the client is another possibility for failure to establish an appointment. Stress can play a significant role in the client's failure to make an appointment. The client may be concerned about the possible gravity of the situation and is unable to focus her attention in order to hear what the provider is saying (even though she may appear to be listening). Finally, other overriding commitments such as work or family caregiving activities may also interfere with follow-up.

As outlined, errors could occur in any of many areas. In the flowchart depicting the abnormal Pap smear process (Figure 11-1), *there are no safety checks.*

Tracking Systems

Before applying safety checks to this process, it would be beneficial to review some process improvement techniques. Edward Deming, a statistician who developed quality improvement methodologies in the 1950s, enhanced many business processes using his process improvement ideas. Some of Deming's most notable works include Toyota's process improvement to enhance quality.

Toyota was struggling with exporting goods after World War II. Deming believed that by developing better ways to work together, that is, by creating better systems, industries could produce higher quality goods for less cost (Unlimited Learning Resources, 2004). Deming believed that everyone should be involved in evaluating the system, including the customer. All people involved in the system have valuable input to share. He believed that at least 94% of errors occurred as a result of system problems rather than individual fault (Unlimited Learning Resources, 2004). His theories used statistics to look at facts, which took the "blame" away from individuals by examining processes. Deming's theories also included psychology, learning theories, and system strategies to help leaders visualize ever-changing systems differently, predict the performance of the system, and continue to improve the way in which an industry functions (Unlimited Learning Resources, 2004).

The health care industry in the United States has been using process improvement techniques for more than a decade. Some consulting firms have refined and enhanced Deming's work to develop process improvement methodologies, which are being used in health care across the United States today. Key steps include the following:

- Define the mission/vision/goal of the improvement process (Mead, 1996).
- Decision making should be based on data. Examine the existing process by collecting information about the process (Executive Learning Inc., 1994). For instance, how many abnormal Pap smear results are missed in a month?
- Examine and chart data over time to look for trends (Executive Learning Inc., 1994). For instance, how many abnormal Pap smear results are missed each month over 1 to 2 years?
- Processes need to be examined collaboratively by all members of the team, that is, "the people doing the work" (Executive Learning Inc., 1994). Managers can't possibly know all of the minor problems that may occur within each step of the process.
- Strive for using the fewest steps to do the task (Executive Learning Inc., 1994). Fewer steps within the process decrease risk for error.
- Strive for steps that promote the highest level of quality (Executive Learning Inc., 1994). Increasing the quality may enhance the cost effectiveness.
- Include steps to provide the highest customer satisfaction (Executive Learning Inc., 1994).
- Continue to evaluate: "Plan, Do, Check, Act." (Executive Learning Inc., 1994; Unlimited Learning Resources, 2004).

How does Deming's work fit into a tracking system?

Health care professionals want to provide the best care possible to clients. Assume that the goal is to have 100% follow-up on abnormal Pap smear results. Data must be collected to examine past trends in abnormal Pap smear follow-up. In the fictitious NP's primary care office created for this case scenario, retroactive abnormal Pap smear data have been collected. Out of 400 Pap smears that were collected by this NP, 18 Pap smear results were abnormal. Five out of 18 clients did not have the appropriate follow-up. Using process improvement techniques, the team decides to institute a tracking system to assist in the follow-up process for abnormal Pap smears.

What is a tracking system?

A tracking system is a process in which one can monitor a piece of datum from one encounter point to the next throughout the entire process. A tracking system can assist in collecting data for process improvement. It can also provide a safety check to ensure quality care in various steps of the process, such as the abnormal Pap smear process outlined earlier. Several systems can be utilized such as a paper system, an electronic system, or a combination of both. A paper tracking, or tickler, system is discussed next.

Paper Tracking Tickler System

A "tickler" system helps remind the provider to follow up on tests that were ordered or to evaluate clients who have been started on new medications or have been recently diagnosed with a life-changing disease. Here is an example of how a provider might follow up on Pap smear results.

The provider conducts a Pap smear. The Pap smear is sent out to the lab. In the tickler system, the provider creates an index filing system with a tab for each week. The provider documents that a Pap smear was conducted on this client and files this index card under the week during which the laboratory report is expected to be back in the office. For example, if the Pap smear was conducted on May 23, 2005, it is expected back in the office by the week of June 6 (Monday). Lab reports are delivered on Tuesdays (June 7 in this case). This reminds the provider to check for the Pap smear results and to notify the client of those results. It is imperative that a copy of all correspondence be posted in the client's chart whether the correspondence is a letter, a postcard, or documentation of a phone call. Figure 11-2 illustrates what the index card may include.

This tickler system can also be created in a notebook with divider tabs that outline the weeks that labs/follow-up calls are due. The index card can also be created on a computer, printed, and filed inside a notebook.

Note that the client, "Alec Everett," is listed on this tickler system to remind the provider to follow up on the effects the Paxil is having on the client's anxiety/depression. It is important to determine in the NP's own practice which clients are considered to be "at-risk" clients. A client with a history of depression who may be at risk for suicidal tendencies may require follow-up after medication administration, whereas a client with diabetes who is euglycemic and has no medication changes may not require a follow-up call. In the paper tracking

Client Name	Client ID	Test or Medication and Date Ordered	Test Received Back in Office or Date to Check on Client's Status	Date and Method of Client Notification	Referral and Date	Follow-up Appointment
Rosa Martinez	040259	Pap smear 5/23/05	6/08/05	Postcard 6/08/05	None; normal Pap	1 Year
Joe McGrady	064469	PSA 5/24/05	6/08/05	Telephone call 6/08/05	Urology Associates 6/08/05	Call—2 weeks Check on emotional status
Alisha Washington	123249	Hbg A1C 5/24/05	6/08/05	Telephone call—no answer Postcard sent 6/08/05	None	3 Months
Alec Everett	345378	Paxil (anxiety/ depression) 5/25/05	6/08/05	Telephone call 6/08/05	None	2 Weeks

Figure 11-2. Index card appearance of a tickler system.

tickler system, it is not cost effective to follow up on every client who is prescribed medication or who has a routine laboratory report.

Registered nurses (RNs), licensed practical nurses (LPNs), or medical assistants (MAs) responsible for drawing blood for laboratory tests in the primary care setting should also be responsible for documenting when a test has been drawn. In the tickler system noted, the RN, LPN, or MA can document when the laboratory test was drawn. The RN, LPN, or MA should also document when the specimen was sent to the lab unless there is some type of standardization such as the laboratory courier picks up all specimens daily at 5 p.m. In these cases, charting by exemption, that is documenting when the laboratory courier didn't pick up the specimens as scheduled, should be documented in the tickler system. The tickler system filing card or notebook page might appear as illustrated in Figure 11-3.

The format shown in Figure 11-3 provides a tickler system that the entire team can use to improve quality. Once again, it is important to determine what is necessary to track within the NP's practice. Rather than asking the RN, LPN, or MA to document when the test was obtained, it is feasible to simply initial next to the date that it was ordered as noted in Figure 11-4.

Client Name	Client ID	Test or Medi-cation and Date Ordered	Date Test Was Obtained and by Whom	Test Received Back in Office or Date to Check on Client's Status	Date and Method of Client Notifi-cation	Referral and Date	Follow-up Appoint-ment
Joe McGrady	064469	PSA 5/24/05	5/24/05 *RME MA*	6/08/05	Telephone call 6/08/05	Urology Associates 6/08/05	Call— 2 weeks Check on treatment and emotional status
Alisha Washing-ton	123249	Hbg A1C 5/24/05	5/25/05 *PCR LPN*	6/08/05	Telephone call—no answer Postcard sent 6/08/05	None	3 Months
Note: Lab courier picked up 5/25 labs on 5/26 at 9 a.m. due to traffic accident.							
Alec Everett	345378	Paxil (anxiety) 5/25/05	Samples given on 5/25/05— 1st dose in office *MRP RN*	6/08/05	Telephone call 6/08/05	None	2 Weeks

Figure 11-3. The index card tickler system includes documentation about clients who need tests, as well as exceptions to courier pickups.

Another option in this type of system is the use of preprinted stickers that contain the client's name and ID number. In this system, every time a client is seen in the provider's office, several stickers are generated with the client's name and medical record number, which are attached to the face sheet of the chart. These stickers can be applied to laboratory tubes and can also be placed in the tickler system. This is a time-saving device for both the provider and the support staff. Figure 11-5 shows an example of the sticker system (without bar codes).

What are some other variations of the paper tracking system?

The preprinted client bar coding stickers encode the client's ID number to be read electronically and downloaded into a computer. The bar coding can also be used to identify labs that have been ordered for the client. The process begins with the provider ordering the lab, and the order being entered into the computer. The computer generates a bar code label. This bar code sticker

Client Name	Client ID	Test or Medication and Date Ordered	Test Received Back in Office or Date to Check on Client's Status	Date and Method of Client Notification	Referral and Date	Follow-up Appointment
Joe McGrady	064469	PSA 5/24/05 *RME MA*	6/08/05	Telephone call 6/08/05	Urology Associates 6/08/05	Call—2 weeks Check on emotional status

Figure 11-4. The index card tickler system includes documentation about clients who need tests that consists of initials placed next to the test that was ordered.

identifies the client, the medical record number, and the lab test that was ordered. A duplicate of this sticker can be added to the paper tickler system or it can be read by a bar code scanner and entered into a database. A printout lists the dates, clients, and tests that were ordered. Once the lab is drawn and sent to the laboratory, the bar code is scanned into the laboratory computer, which provides a tracking mechanism for each lab test. Of course, it is important that the provider's office and the laboratory have compatible bar code and scanning systems.

The "hoarding the chart" system is the final paper tracking system that will be presented in this chapter. The "hoarding the chart" system is a paper tracking system in which the provider keeps all client charts that have pending lab tests

	Client Name	Client ID	Test or Medication and Date Ordered	Date Test Was Obtained and by Whom	Test Received Back in Office or Date to Check on Client's Status	Date and Method of Client Notification	Referral and Date	Follow-up Appointment
Stickers	Rosa Martinez 040259		Pap smear 5/23/05	5/23/05 *JD NP*	6/08/05	Postcard 6/08/05	None; normal Pap	1 Year
	Joe McGrady 064469		PSA 5/24/05	5/24/05 *RME MA*	6/08/05	Telephone call 6/08/05	Urology Associates 6/08/05	Call— 2 weeks Check on emotional status

Figure 11-5. Paper tracking system that makes use of stickers with the client name and medical record number on them.

or that require follow-up in her or his private office until the client's needs are addressed. Another "hoarding the chart" system is when the support staff keeps all client charts with pending lab tests or those requiring follow-up on a designated shelf in the medical records section of the main office.

What are some of the benefits of the paper tickler systems?

The paper tickler systems provide a method to monitor and follow up on various tests, medications, or client status. If providers and support staff are committed to this type of system, it will work. It is also beneficial for those offices that have providers who work part time. A provider can look at the tickler system, whether it is an index card version or the notebook version, to determine which clients require follow-up. It also provides a safety check. Bruder, a member of the Committee on Quality Improvement and Patient Safety, suggests the following client safety tips to include in the primary care office that uses a paper system. These steps have been adapted from Bruder (2001) "Patient Safety Tip: Tracking Cytology and Lab Test Results" to include examples of roles that may be appropriate for different responsibilities and to include other testing modalities such as radiology and special procedures.

1. All specimens, tests, or scheduling of procedures should be documented on a tracking sheet.
2. One role (RN, LPN, MA) should be responsible for keeping the log of all scheduling and specimens or tests that are sent out of the office.
3. Client instructions should include contacting the office if testing results have not been reported within a designated time frame. (Many providers suggest 2 weeks as an absolute maximum time frame).
4. One role (RN, LPN, MA) should be responsible for receiving all testing reports.
5. The provider should see and initial all testing reports before they are filed in the client's record.
6. Testing reports should be attached to the chart prior to the provider viewing the report so that the client's history, medications, and/or previous test results are readily available for comparison. This also helps prevent other testing reports being filed in the wrong chart.
7. All testing reports should be reviewed by the provider, not just abnormal reports.
8. If only abnormal testing reports are viewed by the provider, guidelines should be developed for the office staff to assist in determining what labs may be filed without the provider's review.
9. Assign the triage of abnormal labs to the appropriate level of education (RN or LPN).
10. Develop a policy for clients who fail to keep appointments to be rescheduled or follow up with a phone call within a designated time frame (recommended time same day or next day as a maximum time frame).

11. Clients who have not kept an appointment for the day should have the chart reviewed by the provider.
12. Designate a role (RN, provider, and possibly the scheduler of testing/procedures) to follow up with clients with abnormal test results. Keep a log to ensure that the client was seen and that the abnormal results were addressed.
13. Develop a method of contact for those clients without telephones.
14. Contact laboratory, radiology, and other departments to learn about the policies developed to contact the provider in the event of an abnormal testing result.
15. Learn the best method to discuss test results directly with the pathologist or radiologist or other specialist.

It is optimal that all tests be tracked to ensure quality, however it may not be cost effective to track all laboratory results for all clients. At a minimum, it is imperative that the NP track the tests of, and carefully follow up with, high-risk clients. It is also extremely important to follow up with those clients who are having tests such as MRIs or X-rays or are undergoing procedures, not only to ensure "technical" quality, but to provide emotional support as well.

A further explanation of item 12 of Bruder's adapted list can be illustrated best by using a radiology example. MRI testing is in "high demand" in many areas with some clients waiting for several weeks for an ASAP appointment even though the MRI center is open 24 hours a day/seven days per week. Many centers have "on-call" waiting lists, so that as a client cancels, another client on the waiting list can be quickly scheduled. It would be imperative for the office scheduler to track the scheduling and the obtaining of a MRI, especially for those clients whose prognosis may depend on the timeliness of an accurate diagnosis. The follow-up appointment with the provider or the consulting provider such as a surgeon should also be tracked, again to ensure timeliness of treatment especially for those clients with serious health care concerns.

Item 8 in the list adapted from Bruder may have some interesting ramifications. Here is an example: A client received a letter from the local mammography center sent according to written guidelines stating that her recent mammogram was normal. A few days later, a nurse from the client's NP's office called to set up an appointment for the client to see a surgeon. See Figure 11-6 for the diagnostic mammogram report.

The report triggered the office staff at the mammography center to send a "normal finding" letter based on the "benign" terminology found at the bottom of the report. It was fortunate that the NP's office had a tickler system in place for abnormal test results. The NP reviewed the report and notified the office nurse to contact the client to set up an appointment with a surgeon ASAP for further evaluation. If this had been missed by the NP, the client would assume that the mammogram was normal based on the letter that she received, and she would thus not have received the care that she needed.

Perhaps an additional item should be added to Bruder's list. NPs who are practicing in states that require a collaborating physician may find that insurance

---

Examination: Diagnostic Mammogram, 6/23/2005.

History: Red and painful right breast.

Findings: Bilateral film-screen mammograms were performed in the oblique-lateral and craniocaudal projections. Computer-Aided Detection was performed and used in the interpretation. There is fatty replacement of the majority of parenchyma bilaterally. There is no evidence of a breast lesion, per se. There is, however, considerable thickening of the anterior and inferior aspects of the skin surface of the right breast. This is a change from a prior 2001 study. The most plausible etiology for the skin thickening is an inflammatory process such as mastitis. Inflammatory carcinoma would be a possibility, although less likely. Clinical correlation and follow-up will be important.

Impression: BIRADS Category 2: Benign finding. Close clinical follow-up will be necessary.

Figure 11-6. Mammogram report "benign finding" triggered "normal mammogram" letter.

companies will not recognize the NP's name for billing purposes. Therefore, the lab results may be routed to the physician rather than the NP, creating a delay in notifying the client of abnormal testing results. It may be prudent to work with local laboratories and testing centers to add the ordering provider's name to the test results slip. It would also be wise to develop a method within the office in which the client's test results are delivered directly to the NP.

What are some of the drawbacks of the paper tickler systems?

Paper systems can be time intensive. Someone needs to document that the test was ordered, obtained, received back in the office, and acknowledge that it was received and interpreted and that client follow-up was provided. Errors can occur if the provider or the support staff forgets to document the client's information altogether or forgets to document any individual aspects vital to the paper tickler system such as the client's name, date, and follow-up information on the tracking sheet. It is possible for labs/tests or follow-up to be missed, especially on those busy clinic days!

The "hoarding the chart" system can become overwhelming; charts may be piled higher and higher in the provider's office waiting for results to come back. If the client does not obtain a particular lab as ordered, his or her chart might become lost in a provider's office in the "stack of many charts" until the client seeks care once again. Heaven forbid if the client's regular provider can't see the client, because the unfortunate support staff trying to find the chart of the provider's colleague will be searching for hours for this chart! A tickler system will be needed just to keep track of whose office the chart is in!

What safety checks are added to the abnormal Pap smear process when using a tickler system?

A tickler system can help eliminate potential system errors. In Figure 11-7, 14 steps were identified for potential errors. Figure 11-7 shows the use of a paper tickler system that has a safety check added. Steps with safety checks are denoted by a dagger (†).

Although the flowchart in Figure 11-7 has additional steps, some are actually time-saving steps such as "Sticker applied to the tracking sheet," rather than taking time to write out the client's name, medical record number, lab test that was ordered, and so forth. One might ask, "Is this extra documentation worth the additional time?" If there is a potential for error that impacts the client's psychological or physical health, it is absolutely worth the time! It may also be beneficial for the provider and office staff's psychological health by decreasing the ever present worry of "Was this done?" Again, note that the NP will need to decide what clients should be considered "high risk" or what tests are crucial for follow-up because using a paper tracking tickler system is time consuming.

Electronic Health Records

Is there a less time intense method to track follow-up than a paper system?

There is a less time intense method to track follow-up than the paper tickler system, which leads to a discussion of the electronic health record (EHR), also known as the electronic medical record (EMR). The EHR has been available for almost three decades. Only in the past 10 years or so has user-friendly EHR software been available to the primary care office. EHRs now have the capability to provide the following:

1. Viewing of demographic information, clinician reports, testing results, and appointment information.
2. Ordering capabilities, formatting care delivery and documentation to reflect clinical guidelines and protocols, medication prescribing including correct dosage, medication interactions, and client education.
3. Documenting clinical history, physical, and progress notes, as well as diagnoses and nursing diagnoses.
4. Providing multiple, simultaneous access by a variety of health care professionals while maintaining confidentiality concerns as well as e-mail functioning.
5. Coding and billing functions.
6. Flagging or reminders regarding abnormal testing results, follow-up, drug information, and treatment guidelines.
7. Tracking diagnosis, testing, or treatment modalities.

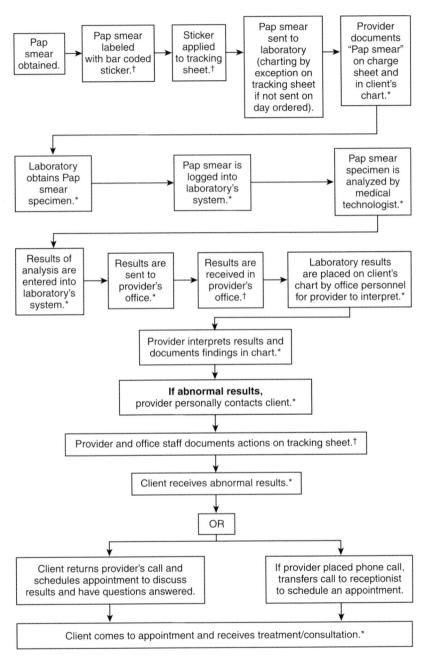

*Potential areas where errors could occur.
†Potential areas where errors might be prevented using a tickler system.

Figure 11-7. Flowchart that demonstrates the use of a tickler system.

8. Coding and insurance requirements.
9. Obtaining reports, quality projects, and research.
10. Serving as an information resource for provider and client education (adapted from Hesse & Siebens, 2002; Hodges, 2002).

Electronic health records have advanced into the Windows-compatible era. Rather than clicking on each individual word-processed page of the chart as one might think about it in a paper format, it can be somewhat interactive. For instance, when ordering a medication for a primary care client, the provider clicks on the medication that is recommended by clinical guidelines for that disease process. The provider clicks on the correct dosage. The computer correlates that particular medication with the client's allergies, and with the other listed medications that the client is currently taking in order to ensure safety. The provider then clicks to send the prescription via the computer's fax to the client's pharmacy. The computer's neatly typed prescription decreases chances for error when interpreting a busy clinician's handwriting. A medication education handout may also be printed out for the client.

How are tracking systems enhanced using an electronic health record?

The newer electronic health record also enhances tracking systems and improves efficiency in the primary care office. (*Note:* Many EHRs have the same or similar capabilities. Only a few are referenced in this section. The author does not promote any one particular EHR software company).

- Team members should be able to work simultaneously on any individual client record in the office (Brown, 2004; Physician Micro Systems, Inc., 2001).
- The system should have the ability to modify screens such as formatting a history, physical, and medical and nursing orders for specific populations of clients according to clinical guidelines (Brown, 2004; Physician Micro Systems, Inc., 2001).
- The EHR should link to the laboratory system in which the lab is ordered via computer within the client's chart. The primary care office's EHR should link with the laboratory's computer system, sending the order to lab. The client has the labs drawn. The results are entered into the system and return via computer to the client's chart. The provider needs to review and sign off on each lab result (Brown, 2004; GE Medical Systems, 2002; Physician Micro Systems, Inc., 2001).
- The system should allow for ordering and receiving of radiology digital pictures and reports such as X-rays and MRIs.
- CT scans and mammogram reports would be beneficial as well.
- The EHR should link to the client's pharmacy via fax. The provider clicks on the appropriate medication dosage and amount. The order is faxed via the EHR to the pharmacy. A screen offers current selections in correct

medication dosages. The system also reviews all current medications for drug interactions prior to allowing the provider to automatically fax the prescription to the pharmacy (Brown, 2004; GE Medical Systems, 2002; Physician Micro Systems, Inc., 2001).

- History and physical templates are available or can be created or customized to meet the provider's assessment needs (Brown, 2004; Physician Micro Systems, Inc., 2001).
- A "flagging" system notifies the provider that laboratory results are complete, abnormal, or that a diabetic's HbgA1C is due (Brown, 2004; GE Medical Systems, 2002; Physician Micro Systems, Inc., 2001).
- The flagging system can also be used to send messages or instructions to other health care team members to address client issues. For example, e-mailing Ms. Barrett, RN, within the client's EHR that the client requires further home care follow-up for dressing changes (Brown, 2004; GE Medical Systems, 2002; Physician Micro Systems, Inc., 2001).
- Nursing diagnoses and interventions should be able to be added to the EHR's software as choices for client care documentation.
- Client educational handouts regarding care, and medications or prep for lab tests should be available through the computer system (Brown, 2004; GE Medical Systems, 2002; Physician Micro Systems, Inc., 2001).
- Access to a medical/nursing library via the computer system within the electronic health record should also be available to providers (Brown, 2004).
- The ability to conduct database searches within the facility's client population for continuous quality improvement data collection should also be available (Beebe, 2004; Brown, 2004; Fischer and Blonde, 1999; GE Medical Systems, 2002; Litvin, Ornstein, Anthony, & Tanner, 2001; Physician Micro Systems, Inc., 2001; Wood, 2003).

Litvin and colleagues (2001) note that in light of all of the marvelous functions of the new electronic health record, a commitment to continuous quality improvement to provide optimal outcomes for all clients is essential to provide care according to clinical practice guidelines. The EHR should include the latest clinical practice guidelines in the development of practice standards for clients and continue to conduct outcome measurements to ensure optimal care for all clients. This also affirms Deming's continuous quality improvement philosophy discussed earlier in this chapter.

How does the electronic health record appear in a flowchart format for the abnormal Pap smear scenario?

The electronic health record flowchart has many steps, but the steps are part of the program. That is, the tracking is completed automatically, saving the provider and staff a great deal of time in manually documenting tracking information. The time-saving steps provided by the EHR are noted by the asterisk at each corresponding step in Figure 11-8.

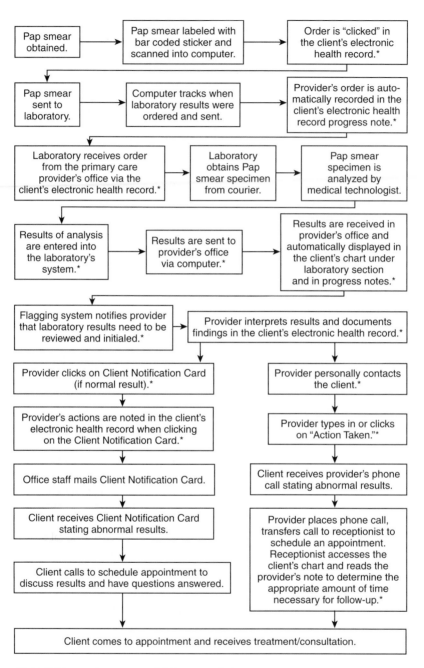

Pap smear obtained. → Pap smear labeled with bar coded sticker and scanned into computer. → Order is "clicked" in the client's electronic health record.*

Pap smear sent to laboratory. → Computer tracks when laboratory results were ordered and sent. → Provider's order is automatically recorded in the client's electronic health record progress note.*

Laboratory receives order from the primary care provider's office via the client's electronic health record.* → Laboratory obtains Pap smear specimen from courier. → Pap smear specimen is analyzed by medical technologist.

Results of analysis are entered into the laboratory's system.* → Results are sent to provider's office via computer.* → Results are received in provider's office and automatically displayed in the client's chart under laboratory section and in progress notes.*

Flagging system notifies provider that laboratory results need to be reviewed and initialed.* → Provider interprets results and documents findings in the client's electronic health record.*

Provider clicks on Client Notification Card (if normal result).*

Provider personally contacts the client.*

Provider's actions are noted in the client's electronic health record when clicking on the Client Notification Card.*

Provider types in or clicks on "Action Taken."*

Office staff mails Client Notification Card.

Client receives provider's phone call stating abnormal results.

Client receives Client Notification Card stating abnormal results.

Provider places phone call, transfers call to receptionist to schedule an appointment. Receptionist accesses the client's chart and reads the provider's note to determine the appropriate amount of time necessary for follow-up.*

Client calls to schedule appointment to discuss results and have questions answered.

Client comes to appointment and receives treatment/consultation.

*Potential areas where errors might be prevented.

Figure 11-8. Abnormal Pap flowchart that demonstrates the use of an EHR system.

An EHR system can be costly to initiate, but once the staff and the provider are comfortable with the program, it can be a cost-savings system in both client safety as well as time efficiency for staff and providers (Physician Micro Systems, Inc., 2001). See Appendix 11-1 for lists of EHR software and a comparison reference.

SUMMARY

Tracking systems are important to use in the provider's practice to ensure proper follow-up for abnormal testing results or changes in medications or to assess the emotional/physical status of a client. Whether the provider decides to use a paper or electronic medical record tracking system, continuous quality improvement should be employed to ensure optimal outcomes for our clients.

References

Bates, D., Ebell, M., Gotlieb, E., Zapp, J., & Mullins, H.C. (2003). A proposal for electronic medical records in U.S. primary care. *Journal of the American Medical Informatics Association, 10*(1), 1-10.

Beebe, K. (2004, March 8). Personal communication.

Brown, K. (2004, March 31). Personal communication.

Bruder, K. (2001). Patient safety tips: Tracking cytology and lab test results. *American College of Obstetricians and Gynecologists.* Retrieved January 6, 2004, from *www.acog. org/from_home/departments/printerFriendly.dfm?recno=28&bulletin=1968*

Committee on Quality Health Care in America. (2001). *Crossing the quality chasm. A new health system for the 21st century.* Washington, DC: Institute of Medicine/ National Academy Press. Retrieved October 7, 2004, from *http://print.nap.edu/pdf/ 0309072808/pdf_image/62.pdf*

Dovey, S., Meyers, D., Phillips Jr., R., Green, L., Fryer, G., et al. (2002). A preliminary taxonomy of medical errors in family practice. *Quality and Safety in Health Care, 11*(3), 233. Retrieved July 5, 2005, from *http://ezproxy.gvsu.edu:2144/itw/infomark/ 566/300/68785731w5/purl=rc1_HRCA_0_A91972895&dyn=3!xrn_1_0_A91972895? sw_aep=lom_gvalleysu*

Elder, N., Vonder Meulen, M., & Cassedy, A. (2004). The identification of medical errors by family physicians during outpatient visits. *Annals of Family Medicine, 2*(2), 125-129.

Executive Learning Inc. (1994). Seminar. Personal communication.

Fischer, J., & Blonde, L. (1999). Impact of an electronic medical record on diabetes practice workflow. *Clinical Diabetes, 17*(2), 89-90.

GE Medical Systems. (2002). Logician. Retrieved October 7, 2004, from *www. medicalogic. com/products/logician/features.html*

Hesse, K., & Siebens, H. (2002). Clinical information systems for primary care: More than just an electronic medical record. *Topics in Stroke Rehabilitation, 9*(3), 39-59.

Hodges, R. (2002). Myths and realities of electronic medical records. Nine vital functions combine to create comprehensive EMR. *Physician Executive, 28,* 8-13.

Institute of Medicine. (1999, November). *To err is human: Building a safer health system.* Retrieved July 14, 2004, from *www.ion.edu/Object.File/Master/4/117/0.pdf*

Litvin, C., Ornstein, S., Anthony Jr., W.E., & Tanner, D. (2001). Quality improvement using electronic medical records: A case study of a high-performing practice. *Topics in Health Information Management, 22*(2), 59-64.

Mead, A. (1996). Deming's principles of total quality management (TQM). In *Deming Distilled: Essential Principles of TQM.* Retrieved June 23, 2004, from *www.well.com/user/vamead/demingdist.html*

Phillips, R., Bartholomew, L., Dovey, S., Fryer Jr., G., Miyoshi, T., & Green, L. (2004). Learning from malpractice claims about negligent, adverse events in primary care in the United States. *Quality and Safety in Health Care 13,* 121-126.

Physician Micro Systems, Inc. (2001). *Reducing medical errors with an electronic medical records system.* Practice Partner Forum. Seattle, WA: Author.

Robeznieks, A. (2004). Error study focuses on primary care. *American Medical News, 47*(17), 1.

Unlimited Learning Resources. (2004). Retrieved June 23, 2004, from *www.4ulr.com/products/productquality/aboutdeming.html*

Wood, R. (2003). Doctors' group tries out paperless office system. *Business Review, 30*(17), 4.

12

Health Care Quality: Evaluating Clinical Practice

Jean Nagelkerk

Quality Health Care

The publication of landmark quality health care reports has prompted major discussions and widespread information dissemination. The reports have highlighted significant gaps in the quality of care and the delivery systems in the United States that have placed—and in some instances continue to place—clients at risk for adverse outcomes (Institute of Medicine [IOM], 2001; Kohn, Corrigan, & Donaldson, 1999; President's Advisory Commission on Consumer Protection and Quality in the Health Care Industry, 1998). Published reports have estimated that a significant number of errors are being made in both acute and primary care settings (Elder, Vonder Meulen, & Cassedy, 2004; Kohn, L., Corrigan, J., & Donaldson, M., 1999). Nurse practitioners (NPs), as providers of care, play a significant role in delivering quality care in many health care settings (Lamb, Jennings, Mitchell, & Lang, 2004). Their involvement in quality improvement and quality assurance activities is critical in maintaining and improving health care services and delivery systems.

What is quality care?

Quality health care is the delivery or provision of services to individuals, groups, or communities using professional knowledge and evidenced-based practice with the goal of improving health care outcomes (Mowinski-Jennings & McClure, 2004). As such, members of professional disciplines have a social and professional responsibility to educate competent practitioners. Professional standards are published through disciplinary organizations and certification and/or licensure sets minimal competency levels for practitioners. (Other definitions of terms used in this chapter are listed in Box 12-1.)

What is the NP's role in quality care?

NPs provide care within their scope of practice and adhere to the standards of care established by professional nursing organizations. They keep abreast of changing health care trends and practices and provide care based on evidence. NPs as providers of care have a responsibility to evaluate the care they provide to clients. They are often pivotal in establishing quality measures and improving the care delivered to clients in their clinical agency by assisting in the development of clinical evaluation programs or participating in existing ones. Examples of opportunities for NPs to become involved with clinical evaluation activities include:
- Serving as a member of a quality evaluation committee
- Being a peer reviewer
- Assisting with projects to improve client care in clinical agencies
- Volunteering and serving as an accreditation visitor.

What is clinical evaluation?

An essential component of clinical practice is evaluating the care provided to clients. Most health care agencies have some form of clinical evaluation that is

Box 12-1 Definitions

- *Performance measurement* is assessing to what extent the health care provider, clinic, or health plan meets a specific measure.
- *Quality assessment* is the process of evaluating whether the process of care achieved positive outcomes.
- *Quality assurance* is the process of assessing, identifying problems, applying improvements, and evaluating the outcomes to see if the corrective action resulted in improvements in care or outcomes.
- *Quality health care* is the delivery of services to patients using professional knowledge with the goal of improving health care outcomes.
- *Peer review* is the assessment by professionals reviewing the quality of care provided by their peers.

routinely conducted (McInerny, Meurer, & Lannon, 2003). Clinical evaluation, in an agency, can range from the selection of a few clinical indicators to capture data and evaluate quality to a comprehensive clinical evaluation program. No matter what quality system is in place, common clinical evaluation measures often include measuring the quality of care, the level of client satisfaction, and the outcomes achieved.

What are clinical indicators?

Clinical indicators are defined as measurable variables addressing the structure, process, or outcomes of client care (Campbell, Braspenning, Hutchinson, & Marshall, 2003). Clinical indicators include those variables that pertain to client care management and includes demographic information, diagnoses (nursing and medical), services and interventions, and outcomes. Providers can select from numerous potential clinical indicators that can be used to measure and track data to ensure and improve quality care. Examples of clinical indicators include client satisfaction, quality of life, functional capability, health promotion activities (immunizations, mammograms, digital rectal exams), knowledge, laboratory values, social support, vital signs, and recidivism rates.

Providers in collaboration with their group and employing organization must assess their practice area (specialty) and determine what clinical data they will collect to maintain and improve quality care. One method used to determine what clinical indicators to monitor is that of evaluating high-volume diagnoses or procedures. If the most common diagnosis is type 2 diabetes mellitus, clinical indicators related to this diagnosis such as HgbA1c levels, foot care, and referrals for eye exams to an ophthalmologist would potentially have a significant and positive impact on clinical outcomes. Each clinic will need to determine those clinical indicators to monitor that have a significant impact on improved client outcomes.

What is a clinical evaluation program?

Clinical evaluation programs are designed and implemented in acute, primary, and tertiary settings to maintain and improve quality client care. The purpose of a clinical evaluation program is to develop a continuous, comprehensive evaluation program that involves key internal and external stakeholders to improve and ensure quality. Within the design of a clinical evaluation program, the purpose, objective, and clinical measures are clearly defined, and routine data collection points are established with the designation of individuals responsible for specific evaluation activities. The development and implementation of a clinical evaluation program help institutionalize or establish an environment of continuous quality care improvement in an agency.

How is a clinical evaluation program developed?

The clinical evaluation program described in this section is modified from the Centers for Disease Control and Prevention's (2004) Evaluation Workgroup Steps in Program Evaluation. The steps in designing a clinical evaluation program are as follows:

1. Obtaining input from individuals involved in the clinical evaluation process
2. Describing the evaluation program
3. Determining the evaluation methods
4. Gathering data
5. Sharing the data
6. Improving clinical care.

The first step in designing a clinical evaluation system is *obtaining input* from individuals involved in the evaluation process. This includes providers, administrators, and support staff, but should also include community members and consumers or clients as well. By including those who will be involved in the process, there is a greater chance of active participation and valuing of the program and results. If individuals are not involved in the process, they may ignore, criticize or obstruct it (CDC, 2004).

There are many ways to gather feedback from stakeholders. Ways to encourage participation and feedback include scheduling a meeting or series of meetings to obtain input, developing and sending out a survey to determine the areas of strength and areas for growth in the provision of care, encouraging informal discussions about the type of evaluation system and measures that will be developed, scheduling an inservice on evaluation programs, and establishing a task force or committee of individuals who have expertise in evaluation or who are interested in learning more and guiding the agency in this process.

The second step is *describing the clinical evaluation program* by setting goals and objectives, and determining the strategies for implementation. The need to design a clinical evaluation program provides a wonderful opportunity to bring together the entire clinical staff to focus on the provision of client care services. After discussing and brainstorming the reasons why the evaluation program is being designed and implemented and the importance of continuous quality improvement, the agency team is ready to determine the program structure.

To begin, establish the goal(s) of your clinical evaluation program. A *goal* is a broad statement of the purpose of your agency. It is a global statement that includes both who will be affected and what will change as a result of your clinical evaluation program (McKenzie, Neiger, & Smeltzer, 2004). To determine a goal, the group should determine its main purpose. For many clinical agencies, maintaining and improving the quality of care and services offered and delivered are central. An example of an evaluation program goal for this case is "To provide quality care to clients." Once the goal has been set, determine the objective(s) to accomplish this goal. An *objective* is more specific and action oriented than the goal. An objective is one of the steps required to meet or accomplish the goal (McKenzie et al., 2004). An example of an objective for the goal to provide quality care to clients is "To maintain a 100% up-to-date immunization rate for all pediatric clients."

The third step is to *determine the evaluation method*. Will the evaluation design be observational, experimental, survey, or quasi-experimental? How will data be collected? Once the objectives are agreed on and the evaluation design determined, specific data collection strategies are set. A data collection strategy to assist in meeting the pediatric immunization objective is "To review immunization records of pediatric clients." A data collection point for this strategy is "To randomly select 10 pediatric charts per provider." The measure for each provider could be the percentage of clients with up-to-date immunizations. The frequency of data collection is then determined and a schedule developed. Report dates are set and an improvement plan is designed. The result is a written clinical evaluation program.

The use of charts or other documents can provide a visual representation of the program. Table 12-1 provides an example of a responsibility chart that depicts the goals, objectives, strategies, evaluation measures, frequency of data collection, individual(s) responsible for collecting and reporting the data, and the improvement plan.

The fourth step is to *gather data* specified in the evaluation program. The responsibility chart clearly reflects whose responsibility it is to collect data and how it shall be collected. It is also important that a systematic method be in place to collect the data and that the data collected are accurate. The tools that are used for data collection should be reliable and valid. The individuals responsible for collecting data should be trained, have an opportunity to ask questions, and inter-rater reliability should be established.

Common Methods for Collecting Evaluation Data. Common methods for collecting data and measuring the quality of care provided include developing a system of peer review, conducting chart audits, and using clinical tools (i.e., client satisfaction tools), to evaluate clinical measures.

Peer review. In clinical practice, providers (NPs, physicians, physician assistants) often engage in peer review (quarterly, semiannual, or annual) to assess the quality of care they provide to their clients. Peer review is typically conducted by random chart review on clinical measures or indicators and is kept private, that is, shared only with the provider who is being evaluated.

However, various consumer advocacy groups are urging openness and transparency in the peer review process so that these data are readily available to consumers and purchasers. Some providers oppose a more open and public

Table 12-1 Example of a Responsibility Chart Goal: Quality Patient Care

Objective	Strategy	Measure	Frequency	Individual Responsible	Report Dates	Improvement Plan
Pediatric immunization rate = 100%	Review 10 charts per provider (random sample)	Percentage of charts with up-to-date immunizations	Collect data quarterly	Office manager	1/1 4/1 7/1 10/1	Document in quarterly provider meeting minutes

review process. These providers have legitimate concerns regarding an open process that include (1) providers may be less inclined to critically evaluate the client's care outcomes of their peers, (2) potential legal issues may be related to this activity, and (3) it defeats the essence of a peer review process. Conversely, consumer groups feel that quality data related to client outcomes needs to be open so individuals can choose providers based on that data. The possibility of opening peer review results to the public is being debated by consumer and government groups as well as the court system and will have major implications for providers if peer review data and documents become public. Peer review is not a mandatory activity and opening the process could result in providers refusing to participate or may require regulations mandating nonvolunteer peer review. Chapter 17 provides a detailed discussion of peer review.

Chart audits. Chart audits are commonly used to collect clinical data for comparison purposes. The advantages of chart audits are that records are easily accessible, staff can be trained to pull and collect data, and there is access by the reviewer and provider to the original source. Other advantages include having the opportunity to review the audited chart to determine how best to meet the established standard, to address any questions about data accuracy, and to display data trends by using simple descriptive statistics. Disadvantages of chart audits include missing data, illegible handwriting, incomplete entries, and misfiled forms.

Tools. Measurement tools can be purchased, permission obtained to use existing ones without charge, or developed by the health care agency. The use of valid and reliable measurement tools to collect clinical data is essential. Data from implementing tools can be routinely used to identify data trends. Graphic displays of trends can be very powerful for providers in maintaining and improving care. Examples of measurement tools include client satisfaction tools, chronic illness flow sheets, and health promotion tools.

Client satisfaction is an important component of clinical evaluation. Administration of client satisfaction surveys at regular intervals allows current data to be reviewed, strengths to be confirmed, and problematic areas to be addressed and improved. The Michigan Academic Consortium (MAC) developed and tested a 19-item client satisfaction survey (Benkart et al., 2002). This survey included items on the client's experience with initial contact at the clinic, quality of treatment received, ability to understand the education provided, the overall rating of the provider visit, and likelihood of their referring a friend or family member for future care. The questionnaire was developed in English, but has been translated into Spanish, Korean, and Chinese. Box 12-2 lists some of the sample items on the MAC client satisfaction tool. The entire English version as well as translated versions of the client satisfaction tools can be accessed at *www.nnnmhc.org.*

The fifth step of the clinical evaluation program is to *share the data.* After the data is collected and summarized, the results should be presented.

Box 12-2 Sample Items on the MAC Patient Satisfaction Survey

1. It is easy to make contact with the clinic by phone.
2. The clinician answered my questions in a way I could understand.
3. The clinician explained problems and treatments clearly.
4. The clinician listened carefully to what I had to say.
5. The clinician was careful and thoughtful.
6. The clinician showed me respect and courtesy.
7. I am satisfied with the amount of time the clinician spent with me during my visit.
8. The overall quality of care I received at the clinic was good.

The presentation can be individual and private if it is reflecting only a single provider's performance, or it may be to a group of providers in the agency to compare their performance against a specific preset standard or with each other. Adequate time should be scheduled when the data is shared for questions and for development of an action plan to improve clinical care.

The sixth step is to *improve clinical care.* Clinical evaluation programs are developed to improve care in agencies. They are designed to evaluate clinical and delivery system indicators in order to enhance care and services. Part of the scheduled time for presentation should include a discussion period where data is critically analyzed and potential improvement strategies are identified, agreed on, and implemented. Additional meetings should be scheduled to review the implementation strategies and to note progress or improvement in care provided.

Are there different levels of evaluation in an organization?

Clinical care evaluation occurs at many different levels in an organization including the individual or provider level, group or clinic-based level, and system level and can be compared or benchmarked at the local, regional, and national levels. Often, not only is clinical evaluation conducted, but monitoring and evaluation of financial and business data occurs. The financial and business data include revenue (funding) and expense information. These data are critically important to evaluating the financial health of the organization.

What is benchmarking?

Benchmarking is a tool that can be used to compare and measure the performance of a specific process or indicator from a national, regional, or local data set to an organization, group, or provider (Tran, 2003). This tool assists in setting targets for improvement to attain the best possible outcomes. Pioneers of benchmarking believed that this tool had four major functions: (1) analyzing operations, (2) being knowledgeable about the competition and industry leaders, (3) incorporating best practices, and (4) establishing excellence (Tran, 2003). When benchmarking is used to examine a problem area, it is called *problem-based benchmarking.* The focus of this activity is continuous quality improvement and to provide resources and external assistance to achieve goals.

The benchmarking process entails selecting goals, allocating resources, defining processes, identifying benchmarks, collecting and analyzing data, reporting findings, and creating an action plan. Many physician practices use financial data compiled by the Medical Group Management Association (MGMA) to establish their benchmarks (*www.mgma.com*). This association conducts annual surveys to develop a large national data set that provides financial, clinical, and administrative data for varying sizes of health care practices. For example, they have data on the number of clients per provider, the cost of a client encounter, average salaries and benefits for providers, the number of administrative personnel per practice, attributes of electronic health records desirable for practices, and outcome measures for primary care and specialty practices.

Very few national data sets exist that NPs or nurse-managed center administrators can use to benchmark their clinical performance (Anderko & Kinion, 2001). A new nursing organization, the National Network of Nurse Managed Health Centers (NNNMHC), was created in September 2003 with funding from the W. K. Kellogg Foundation (*www.nnnmhc.org*). NNNMHC was created to develop partnerships that will enhance the sustainability of nurse-managed health centers and to create a data warehouse to inform policy and develop benchmarks for best practices. Network organizational members are in the process of identifying a nursing minimum data set for nurse-managed centers, influencing policy to assist nurse-managed health centers with sustainability through adequate reimbursement and transparent credentialing practices, and promoting NPs as a visible and viable provider option for clients.

NPs have the option of benchmarking their clinical, financial, and business data against large data sets such as the MGMA data or the Nursing Minimum Data Set, or they may benchmark against providers in their practice. Benchmarking can be applied to clinical, financial and business data at the individual provider, clinic, or organizational level, and may be compared to data sets at local, regional, or national levels.

Are there external clinical evaluations of providers and agencies?

In addition to internal clinical data collection, external parties may conduct or request clinical evaluation. Examples of external bodies that may request clinical data include third-party payers, health departments (if you participate in their programs, for example, immunization programs, WIC), and grant sponsors.

Each external agency is interested in specific data that relates to their members or mission. Depending on the agencies' missions, they may request or collect information on prevention measures, chronic illness management, hospitalizations, and recidivism rates for their clients. When external agencies collect clinical data, this is generally shared with the providers in order to maintain and improve quality care for their members.

Third-Party Payer Role in Quality Care. Third-party payers are interested in ensuring that quality care is provided to their members. In addition to the credentialing process that most third-party payers have established in order to verify that a provider has the appropriate education and experience, certification, and licensure, they may also establish and collect data on quality measures. They may conduct quarterly random chart audits on select clinical indicators. Examples of clinical indicators that may be selected include immunization rate, annual Pap smears, routine mammography, or a laboratory measure such as HgbA1C on clients with diabetes. The third-party payer shares this data with providers and may even provide financial incentives for meeting or exceeding their quality standards on select clinical indicators.

Are there accrediting bodies for primary care centers?

National organizations do exist that accredit ambulatory care organizations and provide a mechanism for assessment and evaluation. These assessment and evaluation mechanisms incorporate administrators, health care providers, and staff into the continuous improvement process for their organization. The Joint Commission on the Accreditation of Healthcare Organizations (JCAHO; *www.jcaho.org*), the National Committee for Quality Assurance (NCQA; *www.ncqa.org*), Accreditation Association for Ambulatory Health Care (AAAHC), and the Community Health Accreditation Program (CHAP) (Kedrowski & Weiner, 2003) are all agencies that accredit ambulatory care practices.

Accreditation Agencies. Some clinical agencies choose to apply for accreditation by an outside agency. The accreditation process is designed to assist clinical agencies in implementing quality improvement and quality assurance activities. Each accreditation agency either defines, sets parameters for clinical agencies to define, or assists clinical agencies in defining clinical and other types of indicators. As part of the accreditation process, the clinical agency establishes a clinical evaluation program to collect data on quality measures. This program establishes a continuous quality improvement process in the organization. Administrators, staff, and providers are all involved in the quality process. The awarding of accreditation to an agency signifies the commitment to quality improvement and excellence in providing health care services.

Are there national measures of quality?

A variety of national measures of quality health care exist. These measures were designed for varying purposes based on the governmental agency or professional organization that designed the indicators. The clinical indicators were defined in order to collect data for comparative purposes. Quality indicators have been designed for ambulatory care centers, acute care settings, nursing homes, home health care agencies, and residential treatment centers.

An example of a quality indicator data set for *ambulatory care settings* is the Health Plan Employer Data and Information Set (HEDIS). See the National Committee on Quality Assurance website (*www.ncqa.org*). HEDIS was developed by the federal government. It is a group of standardized performance measures that include information on services and their availability, provider qualifications, and health plans (Brooten, Youngblut, Kutcher, & Bobo, 2004). The HEDIS measures are widely collected in primary care centers disseminated via the National Committee for Quality Assistance (NCQA) web site. Examples of the HEDIS measures are in Box 12-3.

Examples of quality indicator data sets for *acute care settings* include the Nursing Report Card, ORYX, and Prevention and Inclient Quality Indicators. An example of a quality indicator data set for *nursing homes* is the Minimum Data Set (MDS) developed by the Centers for Medicare and Medicaid Services to document resident physical, mental, and functional functioning. An example of a quality indicator data set for *home health agencies* includes the Outcome and Assessment Information Set (OASIS) developed by the Centers for Medicare and Medicaid Services to document client health and functional status (Rantz & Connolly, 2004). Box 12-4 lists other measures of quality that are available.

SUMMARY

A national nursing data warehouse is important for clinical evaluation and benchmarking to capture NP client encounters because current national surveys often capture only data on physician providers because the sampling frames are based on physician practices (Jenkins, 2003). National nurse leaders

---

Box 12-3 Examples of HEDIS Measures

- Childhood immunization status
- Colorectal cancer screening
- Breast cancer screening
- Controlling high blood pressure
- Comprehensive diabetes care
- Flu shots for adults ages 50-64
- Pneumonia vaccination status for older adults
- Medical assistance with smoking cessation

Box 12-4 Measures of Quality

- Consumer Assessment Health Plan Survey
- Child and Adolescent Health Measurement Initiative of the Foundation for Accountability
- Dividend calculators developed by the National Committee on Quality Assurance
- Quality initiatives and outcome measures developed by the Foundation for Accountability
- Standards established for administration and nursing care practice in ambulatory care centers by the American Academy of Ambulatory Care Nursing

---

like Mary Mundinger, RN, PhD, are strong advocates for NP practice. By publishing research findings that define and demonstrate positive outcomes for NP care, Dr. Mundinger and others have placed NPs in the national spotlight and made them more visible to the public, legislators, employers, and insurers (Mundinger et al., 2000).

The evaluation of clinical practice is critical in health care organizations. Selecting clinical indicators is important to maintain and improve quality client care. Developing a systematic, comprehensive clinical evaluation program that identifies goals and objectives to improve processes and outcomes based on data is key to determining strengths and making quality improvement changes.

References

Anderko, L., & Kinion, E. (2001). Speaking with a unified voice: Recommendations for the collection of aggregated outcome data in nurse managed centers. *Policy, Politics & Nursing Practice, 2*(4), 295-303.

Benkart, R., Barkauskas, V., Pohl, J., Corser, W., Tanner, C., et al. (2002). Patient satisfaction outcomes in nurse managed centers. *Outcomes Management, 6*(4), 174-181.

Brooten, D., Youngblut, J.M., Klutcher, J., & Bobo, C. (2004). Quality and the nursing workforce: APNs, patient outcomes and health care costs. *Nursing Outlook, 52*, 45-52.

Campbell, S.M., Braspenning, J., Hutchinson, A., & Marshall, M.N. (2003). Improving the quality of health care: Research methods used in developing and applying quality indicators in primary care. *British Medical Journal, 326*, 816-819.

Centers for Disease Control and Prevention. (2004). CDC Evaluation Workgroup Steps in Program Evaluation. Retrieved January 31, 2005, from *www.cdc.gov/eval/framework.htm*

Elder, N.C., Vonder Muelen, M., & Cassedy, A. (2004). The identification of medical errors by family physicians during outpatient visits. *Annals of Family Medicine, 2*(2), 125-129.

Institute of Medicine. (2001). *Crossing the quality chasm: A new health system for the 21st century. Committee on Quality of Health Care in America.* Washington, DC: National Academy Press.

Internet Resources

Agency for Healthcare Research and Quality
www.ahrq.gov

Centers for Disease Control and Prevention
www.cdc.gov

The Joint Commission on Accreditation of Healthcare Organizations
www.jcaho.org

The National Committee on Quality Assurance
http://www.ncqa.org

The Foundation for Accountability
www.facct.org

The American Academy of Ambulatory Care Nursing
www.aaacn.org

Medical Group Management Association
www.mgma.org

National Network for Nurse Managed Health Centers
www.nnnmhc.org

Jenkins, M. (2003). Toward national comparable nurse practitioner data: Proposed data elements, rational and methods. *Journal of Biomedical Informatics, 36,* 342-350.

Kedrowski, S.M., & Weiner, C. (2003). Performance measures in ambulatory care. *Nursing Economics, 21,* 188-198.

Kohn, L., Corrigan, J., & Donaldson, M. (Eds.). (1999). *To err is human: Building a safer health system. Committee on Quality of Health Care in America. Institute of Medicine.* Washington DC: National Academy Press. Retrieved January 31, 2005, from *www.nap.edu/html/to_err_is_human*

Lamb, G.S., Jennings, B.M., Mitchell, P.H. & Lang, N.M. (2004). Quality agenda: Priorities for action recommendations of the American Academy of Nursing Conference on Health Care Quality. *Nursing Outlook, 52*(1), 60-65.

McInerny, T.K., Meurer, J.R., & Lannon, C. (2003). Incorporating quality improvement into pediatric practice management. *Pediatrics, 112*(5), 1163-1164.

McKenzie, J.F., Neiger, B.L., & Smeltzer, J.L. (2004). *Planning, implanting, and evaluating health promotion programs* (4th ed.). San Francisco: Pearson/Benjamin Cummings.

Mowinski-Jennings, B.M., & McClure, M.L. (2004). Strategies to advance health care quality. *Nursing Outlook, 52*(1), 17-22.

Mundinger, M.O., Kane, R.L., Lenz, E.R., Totten, A.M., Tsai, W., et al. (2000). Primary care outcomes in patients treated by nurse practitioners or physicians. *Journal of the American Medical Association, 283*(1), 59-68.

President's Advisory Commission on Consumer Protection and Quality in the Health Care Industry (1998). *Quality first: Better health care for all Americans. Final report.* Washington, DC: Author.

Rantz, M.J., & Connolly, R.P. (2004). Measuring nursing care quality and using large data sets in nonacute care settings: State of the science. *Nursing Outlook, 52,* 23-37.

Tran, M.N. (2003). Take benchmarking to the next level. *Nursing Management, 34*(1), 18-24.

13

Using Technology to Enhance Practice

Leona B. Meengs

Technology and the Nurse Practitioner

The use of technology is pervasive and continues to expand into all areas of our lives. Those professionals who take advantage of technological advancements at work will be more likely to meet the challenges of practice demands. The areas of technology explored in this chapter include the use of the Internet as a communication tool, an instrument for continued education, a reference for clinical guidelines, and a marketing tool for business. In addition, Internet e-mail can be utilized for client communication and education (Appendix 13-1), as well as for streamlining business tasks (for instance, by using e-mail to notify clients of appointments).

Likewise the personal digital assistant (PDA) enhances practice by improving the nurse practitioner's (NP's) ability to access accurate information quickly. PDA functions include basic applications that assist the NP with organization, scheduling, use of clinical reference software programs, Internet access, and client tracking. NPs who utilize the Internet, e-mail, and the PDA are more likely to remain competitive in a rapidly changing health care environment.

Using the Internet

The use of Internet technology is common in the business sector. Yet, Internet use by health care professions has traditionally been limited (Estabrooks, O'Leary, Ricker, & Humphrey, 2003). A 2000 Harris Interactive poll of 769 medical professionals revealed that 61% of the respondents' use of the Internet was for personal use and only 23% was for clinical practice. Since 2000 the impact of the Internet on practice has increased dramatically and medical professionals report that they are using the Internet more frequently and for longer durations (American Medical Association [AMA], 2002a).

How can the Internet enhance practice?

NPs who are Internet and technology savvy use a variety of sites to quickly and conveniently find clinical information. Many NPs use the Internet for clinical consultation and for obtaining updates, new protocols, and evidenced-based guidelines. The more useful and up-to-date Internet sites are often developed and updated by expert practitioners, faculty at universities, or government employees to provide information on the management of acute, chronic, and emerging diseases and current health care practices.

Enhancement of NP practice can also occur through Internet tutorials, skills modules, online workshops, and e-journal publications. Travel time can be saved by completing continuing education Internet programs from the comfort of home or earning a certificate, graduate, or doctoral degree online (Brusman Zaidel, 2003).

What types of clinical websites are useful for NPs?

Many clinically based Internet websites are useful to NPs. Listed here are a few examples of helpful websites:

- Government sites like the National Institutes of Health (*www.nih.gov*), the Agency for Healthcare Research and Quality (*www.ahcpr.gov*), and the Centers for Disease Control and Prevention (CDC; *www.cdc.gov*) are good sites for clinical research reports, evidence-based guidelines, application materials, national government research priorities, and infectious disease and bioterrorism information.
- Medical universities and nursing programs often have useful, clinically relevant websites. For example, the University of Virginia (*www.hsc.virginia.edu*) has information on making referrals, continuing education, clinical trials, and telemedicine, along with provider newsletters and a health sciences library.
- Nurse practitioner sites such as NP Central (*www.nurse.net*) have information on pertinent legislative action. This site also provides legal tips and clinical pearls along with Medicare/Medicaid coding and billing information.

- Most professional organizations have a website to provide quick access to services for their members. Member services often include access to literature databases, health and industry news, conference information and registration, discounts to journals and services, and continuing education opportunities. Many offer Internet-based career development opportunities including marketing advice, résumé development, and job postings. Professional organizations also host Internet discussion groups designed to share clinical cases, promote professional issues, and encourage political activism.
- Salary.com (*www.salary.com*) is a site that offers benefit comparisons and salary averages, résumé assistance, employment search, mortgage and moving information, and cost-of-living and salary compensation tools that compute relocation expenses. For example, an NP earning $60,000 in Grand Rapids, Michigan, may decide to accept an offer for a similar position in Bakersfield, California. Salary.com's tool indicates that a move to Bakersfield would probably mean a 7.1% increase in cost of living and a 3% decrease in salary. This represents a $4406 decrease in disposable income. To maintain the current standard of living, the NP would have to earn $64,233 at her new position. With this information the NP can negotiate a salary that takes into consideration moving cost, standard of living, and salary disparity. Salary.com has relocation aids such as home search tools, loan search tools, credit analyzers, and reports on the quality of school districts. A city comparisons and matchmaker tool matches your personal living values/preferences to U.S. city characteristics.

See Appendix 13-2 for a more complete listing of Internet resources.

How do I find Internet resources?

To find resources, perform an Internet search using a search engine. Any search engine will go directly to that specific web page if the URL address begins with *www* or *http://*. However, if the search is made with key words, phrases, or titles the choice of search engine is more critical. Google (*www.google.com*) is an outstanding search engine due to its comprehensive coverage of the web (Sullivan, 2003) and is popular because even if the key search words are misspelled, Google will respond with "Did you mean...?" and it will offer alternatives. Google also performs an image search. Choose *Images* from the Google toolbar. Type *Nurse,* select *search,* and Google will search more than 400 million image files for nurse images. Searches are also available from the *Groups, News,* and *Directories* categories.

Dogpile (*www.dogpile.com*) is another outstanding search engine and often provides more finds than Google. Besides Google and Dogpile other good search engines include AllTheWeb, HotBot, Yahoo, MSN Search, Ask Jeeves, and AOL Search (Sullivan, 2003). A medical-specific search engine, The Medical Dictionary Meta-Search search engine site, specializes in AIDS, cancer, diabetes, and stroke searches. It searches websites of the CDC, the Joslin

Diabetes Center, the National Federation of the Blind (NFB), the National Institute of Diabetes & Digestive & Kidney Disease (NIDDK), and The United Kingdom Advisory Council.

For more information on search engines and search engine tutorials visit the Boston University Medical Center: Search Engine Guide and Tutorial Site at *http://med-libwww.bu.edu/library/engines.html*. See Appendix 13-2 for more search engine URLs.

How do I know if the information is reliable?

The Internet has numerous medical information sites. The challenge for the provider as well as the client is to choose sites that consistently offer reliable evidence-based information. Universities, professional associations, and government sites are usually reliable sources. The URLs of these sites end with *.edu, .gov,* or *.org*. A reliable site should also list the author's credentials and the time the site was last updated. Another method of evaluating site reliability is to access either the McGraw Hill Healthcare and Medicine Companion (*http://web10.eppg.com/medical/lange/cmdt/index.html*) or the Health on the Net (HON) foundation (*www.hon.ch*). Both of these sites monitor and rate the reliability and usefulness of medical sites.

What types of Internet sites are clients using?

Medical information is disseminated continuously through the media. The consumer is bombarded with research reports, information on new medications, and alternative treatment modalities. Client exposure to the Internet, TV, and radio advertisements influences their health choices. The most common Internet sites that clients access for medical news are *my.webmd.com, drkoop.com,* and America Online's health channel (Grandinetti, 2000). Although providers cannot view all of the therapeutic approaches and purported cures and advances in health care, they can access news sites, forums, and discussion groups to tap into the most newsworthy information. Two popular sites specifically designed to alert health care providers about the information clients are accessing include MDConsult and Medscape (Grandinetti, 2000).

How can I help clients find good Internet resources?

Many clients are already using the Internet to access medical information. According to a Harris Poll, 110 million U.S. adults have looked on the Internet for medical information either for themselves, family, or friends and 26% of these individuals are looking for specific medical information (Taylor & Leitman, 2002b). These individuals further reported that the Internet improved their relationships with their provider (40%) and helped them understand (34%) and manage their health problems (16%), while motivating them to comply with their treatment regimen (17%) (Taylor & Leitman, 2002c).

The popularity of the Internet makes it a valuable tool for motivating, educating, and supporting clients. On the flip side, the Internet remains a source of reliable as well as unreliable information. Providers are concerned that clients may not only initiate costly treatments that lack research support but may also rely on treatments that have a deleterious effect on their health. Taylor and Leitman (2002c) found that 38% of the U.S. survey respondents judged the accuracy of Internet information without physician consultation, almost a quarter (23%) started an over-the-counter medication, and 44% obtained their medical information from commercial health pages (Taylor & Leitman, 2002b).

Clients who initiate treatment regimens without medical consultation and those who rely on commercial pages may be placing their health in jeopardy or purchasing unnecessary supplements at very high costs. Therefore, it is important for practitioners to be aware of cyber information and discuss Internet resources with their clients. Grandinetti (2000) suggests asking clients about their Internet use or incorporating the question on the client history form. By adopting this practice, practitioners will be able to initiate conversations regarding client Internet use, evaluate site reliability, thoughtfully offer reliable alternatives, and inform clients that even sites that do not advertise products or services may be misguided by well-intentioned individuals who may not have the necessary health care expertise to provide information to the public (Grandinetti, 2000).

The practitioner can also choose to be proactive and list reliable sites on their own web page or issue a letter that encourages Internet surfing, gives points on evaluating websites, lists sites that are reliable, and offers to be a partner in the process (Grandinetti, 2000). For a sample client Internet information letter to encourage appropriate use of reliable sites see Appendix 13-1.

How can I use the Internet to enhance business?

The Internet is a billboard to the world and an ideal medium for marketing your services to potential clients. In addition to marketing, websites can be used to manage accounts receivable, obtain demographic and preadmission information, disseminate client educational materials, list Internet links, post appointment reminders, collect research data, and assess client satisfaction via online surveys. According to the AMA (2002a), 3 out of 10 physicians who access the Internet have a clinical website for marketing their services and providing client education. This trend is predicted to continue (Harris Interactive, 2000; Taylor & Leitman, 2001; Vibar, 2003).

Web pages that are used only for advertising, marketing, and listing general information or services can be built and managed by the NP. Dreamweaver MX is a user-friendly authoring software program used to develop websites. However, when sites are interactive they must ensure client confidentiality according to the Health Insurance Portability and Accountability Act (HIPAA). For help with creating a HIPAA-compliant site, enlist the services of an Internet service provider who specializes in HIPAA compliance. The AMA's ConsultingLink (2002b) provides a free referral service for reliable HIPAA consultants. For more information visit *www.ama-assn.org/go/hipaa*. Besides HIPAA compliance and security issues, all websites that offer general health information should include a disclaimer that encourages users to seek advice from their personal health care provider.

How do I use e-mail to enhance my practice?

Electronic communication is fast and reliable. Communiqués can be filed, categorized, forwarded, printed, or sent to multiple parties all with the click of a mouse. E-mail has changed both our methods and expectations of communication and augmented productivity in a fast paced world. In addition, e-mail does not require computer ownership. Around the world, computers can be accessed in malls, libraries, and universities. They are often complementary amenities in hotel business or conference centers, neighborhood cafes, music stores, and other commercial establishments. E-mail also can be accessed from fee-based computer hubs or freestanding computer booths that are similar to telephone booths. Even so, e-mail retrieval is not even dependent on traditional computer availability; it can be accessed from handheld devices and mobile phones.

Can I use e-mail for client communications?

Not surprisingly, online adults want the convenience of e-mail communications with their providers. Respondents to a Harris Interactive poll report that they are willing to pay for e-mail communications (37%) and that the service would positively influence their choice of health plans (55%) and health care providers (56%) (Taylor & Leitman, 2002a). About 70% of the respondents want to use e-mail to make appointments, refill prescriptions, receive test results, or avoid unnecessary office visits (Taylor & Leitman, 2002a). Other current uses of e-mail correspondence with clients include receiving copies of medical records, reviewing educational instruction, and submitting physiological measures such as blood pressure and blood glucose readings (*The Magnet,* 2002).

Client demand for e-mail communications with their provider is growing and health care providers are responding to the allure of this new market. A 2000 online survey of physician and medical student users of Epocrates, a PDA drug reference program, found that 25.7% of the respondents used e-mail to communicate with clients (Rothschild, Lee, Bae, & Bates, 2002). Although this survey is not representative of the entire provider population, it does indicate that client/provider e-mail communications are becoming more available, especially with the younger Epocrates users who may be more adept with the use of technology.

The benefits of e-mail are appealing. They include cost effectiveness related to improved client management, a communication method that can be easily accessed and documented, and improved provider/client relationships that result in increased client satisfaction (SCPIE Indemnity Company, 2002). However, along with the benefits, health care providers have found corresponding liability risks and confidentiality issues (eRisk Working Group for Healthcare, 2002). The eRisk Working Group for Healthcare, a coalition of provider associations and liability carriers, has developed guidelines for online communications that respond to the HIPAA compliance issues of security, authentication, confidentiality, unauthorized access, and informed consent. See Appendix 13-3 for a complete list of the group's recommendations.

As with the provider/client use of e-mail, there are some considerations regarding the use of e-mail between peers, friends, relatives, and family. The ease of tapping the *Send* command accentuates the loss of one-on-one interaction and the opportunity to clarify in person. What is written, as in a letter, is translated according to the receiver's perception. However unlike e-mail, letters are usually considered formal communiqués. They begin with a greeting and end with a salutation. With e-mail there is a loss of formality and the loss of body language, voice tone, volume, laughter, or facial expression. Therein lies the opportunity for misunderstanding, potentially hurt feelings, or damaged relationships. For some personalities, a quick to the point message is acceptable, but to another it may seem brash. To avoid making e-mail "faux pas" it is good practice to follow some basic e-mail etiquette guidelines (Bliss & Sandra, 2002; Email Replies, 2003).

- Be sure you have the correct address; your acquaintances deserve to have their privacy protected. Not everyone wants their e-mail address to be common knowledge or sent to everyone else on your list of recipients. To that end, use the blind carbon copy function when sending messages to multiple parties. This function allows you to hide the addresses of separate individuals who are receiving the same e-mail.
- Maintain e-mail confidentially by avoiding the practice of forwarding messages without the sender's permission. It is safest to assume that e-mail communications are confidential communications unless stated otherwise.
- Begin your e-message with a greeting and end with a thank-you. This practice adds an air of professionalism and thoughtfulness to your communications.
- Maintain a professional profile by using spell-check functions.
- Avoid excessive verbiage. Many professionals have hundreds of e-mails to peruse.
- Use of the subject line helps the recipient to prioritize e-mail replies and makes your e-mail more likely to be addressed.

- Review your e-mail before you send it. A telephone call would be a better choice if what you have written could be misconstrued in any way.
- Avoid the use of CAPITAL LETTERS, which may be interpreted as SHOUTING.
- Avoid the use of abbreviations and symbols unless you are sure the recipient will understand their meaning.
- Avoid chain letters or advertisements; they are often considered unwanted solicitations.
- If e-mail use is for business purposes, add a confidentiality statement that addresses returning and destroying the e-mail if it was incorrectly received. For example: "This e-mail message is for the sole use of the intended recipient and may contain confidential and privileged information. Unauthorized review, use, disclosure or distribution is prohibited. If you are not the intended recipient, please contact the sender by reply e-mail and destroy all copies of the original message."

For a more exhaustive list of e-mail recommendations, visit *www.emailreplies.com*.

How can I prevent Internet and e-mail abuses?

Effective Internet and e-mail use has the potential to save money and enhance the practitioners' market and practice; however, Internet and e-mail abuses threaten employee productivity. According to the ePolicy Institute (2003a), 90% of workers admitted to web surfing at work and in 1999 the estimated cost to business owners was $500 million. Game playing, accessing inappropriate websites, and answering personal e-mail are a few of the time-consuming Internet activities that lower staff productivity (ePolicy Institute, 2003a).

To avoid potential problems, practices should develop Internet and e-mail policies that address e-mail etiquette and security measures. Examples of Internet and e-mail policy guidelines include the following: (1) Develop a policy stating that management has access to all information sent or received from the office, (2) ban games and any downloads from the Internet such as instant messaging, (3) prohibit Internet surfing that is not specifically required for work, and (4) limit use of e-mail to messaging related to work or that enables employees to work, such as notifying family if working late (Lowes, 2003). For additional guidelines, visit the ePolicy Institute's (2003b) website at *www.epolicyinstitute.com* for a comprehensive list of do's and don'ts along with a free 13-page guide for e-mail management.

Personal Digital Assistants

The PDA is a small, palm-sized, wireless personal computing device that practitioners can program to meet their individual practice needs. Basic programs include an address and date book, memo or note page, to-do list, calculator, and beam capability, which is a method of communication that allows PDAs to share information. Additional features are e-mail access, expandable memory, and all-in-one electronic devices that include PDA, mobile phone, dictation capabilities, and digital camera.

Why should I use a PDA?

Managing information for the health care provider can be a daunting and challenging task. Scheduling, networking, and mastering health care information all seem to become increasingly complex and time consuming. New drugs, drug interactions, contraindications, and new evidence-based guidelines need to be integrated into the clinician's practice. One of the greatest benefits for the practitioner is the ability to quickly download from the Internet medical software that supports clinical practice. Once downloaded to a handheld device, medical information can be easily accessed or managed within seconds from any site. These capabilities are fueling the PDA's popularity as a tool that is improving practitioner productivity while enhancing quality care (Parker, 1999).

Who uses PDAs?

According to Taylor and Leitman (2001), provider use of the PDA in 1999 was 15% and in 2001 26% with the prediction of continued growth. A recent study substantiates that prediction, reporting that 72% of respondents in family practice reported using the PDA in clinical care (Schuerenberg, 2003).

Increasingly, PDAs are used by residents, interns, students, teachers, physician assistants, NPs, physicians, and researchers to organize their schedules, enhance learning experiences, and promote interdisciplinary collaboration by coordinating client information among team members (Fischer, Stewart, Mehta, Wax, & Lapinsky, 2003; Rosenbloom, 2003). Like the growing number of health professionals who use PDAs, NPs must utilize the PDA as a resource and learning tool that will enhance and ease their transition into practice and support them in their professional growth. In that arena the PDA has become a necessity rather than a luxury.

How do universities and students use PDAs?

Universities may hire companies that have expertise in mobile learning to help in the creation of coordinated mobile environments that enhance the educational process. For example, AvantGo© (2002) provides services for universities such as Harvard Medical School, UCLA, Stanford, Ohio State, Duke, and Cornell universities. Within a comprehensive and coordinated mobile environment, students are able to access class information either wirelessly or after data synchronization. Accessible information and functions include access to directories, class schedules and calendars, guidelines, policies, lecture notes, reference materials, handbooks and animated anatomy illustrations; functions include the ability to log clinical tasks and case notes, monitor forms (i.e., charts/reports), compute medical formulas, and submit class evaluations via online surveys (AvantGo, 2002).

Student use of the PDA has become more common than not. In a recent survey, 73% of resident respondents reported that they used a PDA daily to collect data and log procedural experience (88%) (Otto & McRae, n.d.).

After student synchronization of their PDAs, faculty can review student logs, assess clinical progression, and provide feedback (AvantGo, 2002). Using PDAs for coordination of the clinical experience has also proven to be cost effective. According to AvantGo (2002), Harvard Medical School has saved $150,000 in supplies and time and they project a full return on investment within the first year.

How do I know which PDA to buy?

The most popular operating systems are the Palm operating system (Palm OS) and the Pocket PC. The choice of operating systems will depend on personal handheld computing needs and system compatibility with the practitioner's colleagues and health care institution (Fischer et al., 2003). Minimally the PDA should be able to organize and retrieve information quickly and accurately at home, office, or the client's bedside. Maximally, institutions may require the wireless advantage of Bluetooth software, which can be used to wirelessly synchronize data with a remote computer, access client records at the office/hospital, and automatically incorporate field charting into the office/hospital database (PalmGear, 2003).

When purchasing a PDA for use as a personal organizer and for storing a few references, look for a minimal processor speed of 66 MHz and internal memory of 16 MB, high resolution (320×320 pixels), expansion capability, and virus protection software. A PDA intended to utilize several large medical software references and client management programs along with Bluetooth technology will requires a minimum of 64 MB of memory and 400 MHz of processor speed. The expansion slot is a necessity for the medical professional. It can accommodate a portable keyboard, digital camera, or can expand memory up to 128 MB and provide disk space for backing up PDA programs. Memory cards slide in and out of a PDA like a desktop computer's floppy disk drive. Akin to disks, several cards can be used to hold different programs; however, most users will find a 128-MB card more than adequate. Like computers, PDA capabilities will improve annually and current programs may become obsolete or newer programs may require more memory. Upgrading to a newer PDA model will depend on the user's expectations and needs.

The Palms OS platform was first introduced in 1996 and currently runs two out of three handhelds, which translates to more than 80% of the U.S. market and 57% of the worldwide market (Palmsource, 2003). There are approximately

19,000 software titles for the Palm OS including about 400 medical software options (PalmGear, 2003). The Pocket PC operating system has almost as many software options and it is considered the ultimate handheld entertainment center with nearly 1300 entertainment options and more than 300 medical software programs (PocketGear, 2003). Software programs may be designed specifically for the Palm OS or the Pocket PC; however, many software developers offer program formats for both systems. Most hardware upgrades are available in both formats, although to accommodate them, you may need additional memory and processor speed.

Although the Pocket PC is closing ranks, the Palm OS remains the system used most often by medical professionals (Adatia & Bedard, 2002; American College of Physicians [ACP], 2001). In comparing the two systems, the Palm OS is generally less expensive and has more software program options; it is user friendly and has a longer battery life than the Pocket PC (Khoo, 2002). The Palm is considered easier to use, whereas the Pocket PC is slower and requires more memory (Franklin, 2003).

Then again, Pocket PC accepts more expansion card versions than the Palm OS (*Consumer Reports,* 2003) and offers more multimedia and games. It has Pocket Word and Excel preinstalled, works well with Outlook, and has built-in programs for network and server connection with handwriting recognition and beam options that are compatible with the Palm OS (Khoo, 2002). Additional and updated information comparing the Pocket PC and Palm OS can be found at *www.pdabuyersguide.com/tips/palm_vs_pocketpc.htm.*

Newer and more expensive models in either system may have mobile phone or digital camera/handheld combinations, and entertainment features that include gaming, audio, global positioning systems, MP3 music files, video/movie capability, dictation and recording, and voice-over-Internet protocol. An example of a newer Palm OS model is the Treo 650 smart phone (*www.palmone.com*). It has 320 × 320 pixel resolution, 32 MB of internal memory, 312 MHz processor speed, Bluetooth, phone, digital camera, email, web browser, picture and text messaging, and MP3 and video playback software. The Pocket PC HP; PAZ *(www.hpshopping.com)* boats integrated WLAN and Bluetooth, 192 MB memory, 624 MHz processor speed, MP3 software and Biometrics Security.

PDAs can be purchased from computer stores, online, or from professional organizations. The American Association of Critical Care Nurses (AACN) sells PDAs with packages that include some of the best medical software programs (AACN, 2003). The price range for a PDA is approximately $100 to $800 (*Consumer Reports,* 2003).

How do PDAs communicate?

Most PDAs communicate by using synchronization with a PC via a serial or USB port, beaming via an infrared (IR) port, or Bluetooth technology. The standard method of communication is data synchronization, which is used to share information between the PDA and PC. Synchronization eliminates the need to duplicate entries between the PDA and computer, backs up information on the PC hard drive, and is used to download software from the Internet.

Beaming is a method of wireless communication used to share information between PDAs. Items to beam include displayed records or categories from the address book, date book, memo pad, and to-do list and also notes, records, reports, documents, and presentations. The user can also use the beam function as a networking tool by designating their address and business information as a business card and beaming the card to other handheld users.

Bluetooth is a wireless personal-area network (PAN) method of communication used to link different electronic devices that are up to 30 feet apart (MediClicks, 2003; PalmOne, 2003). Bluetooth technology can be purchased; however, it may be preinstalled in some of the newer PDA models. Health care providers can use Bluetooth for communication and to eliminate duplicate devices. For example, there is now a combination cell phone/PDA on the market. Developers are working toward an ultimate device that would combine cell phone, PDA, and pager (MediClicks, 2003), and have dictation capabilities. Ideally health care providers could use Bluetooth technology to ease the workload burden, improve communications, and track or transfer client information. "Progress notes and orders could be written on a handheld device and instantly entered into the hospital's electronic medical record system" (MediClicks, 2003). Likewise SOAP notes could be dictated on the device and automatically transferred to office medical records. Although Bluetooth technology is considered a secure system it is not yet HIPAA certified (MediClicks, 2003). WiFi, a wireless local-area network (WLAN) goes a step further than Bluetooth technology. WLAN's extends linking capabilities to up to 300 feet away from a WLAN access point and thereby supports greater user mobility (PalmOne, 2003).

The PDA versatility in function is further expanded with the voice-over-Internet Protocol (VoIP) technology. For example, the Tungsten C PDA uses the Gphone program to utilize VoIP. VoIP then allows PDA owners to communicate with other handhelds over corporate networks (Palm Company, 2003). With this technology, "users will be able to pick up calls forwarded from their desk phone to their Tungsten C handheld and make calls to colleagues on the company network" (Palm Company, 2003).

How can the basic applications work for me?

Basic programs applications include date and address books, to-do lists, memo or note pages, accessory programs, and a calculator. Date book, memo/note page, or address book changes are easily made either on a computer or directly onto the PDA via the graffiti or type modes. Changes are updated each time the PDA is synchronized with the computer. Addresses can be categorized, sorted, edited, deleted, renamed, accessed, notated, hidden, and copied to paste to another program with the touch of a stylus. Addresses can also be beamed to another handheld either individually as a business card or as the entire selected category.

Schedules can be viewed in the date book by the day, week, or month. Date book calendar years may extend as far as the year 2030 while past calendar years are remembered unless purged. The alarm mode can be set to alert the user minutes, hours, or days before an event occurs. The repeat option allows one-time entry for reoccurring dates. With the Palm OS, annual events such as a birthday or anniversary can be displayed at the top of the screen. If a reminder is needed to send a card, set the alarm 3 days before. This is a great option when keeping up with birthdays and anniversaries is difficult for the busy practitioner. As with the other programs, events can be deleted, beamed, hidden to maintain confidentiality, notated for clarification, or purged from the PDA to save memory space.

The memo or note accessory is used to create brief memos that can also be categorized, edited, customized, and beamed. I use mine for clinical pearls and file them under the "medical" category I created on the launcher pad. The clinical pearls are individually filed under body systems, functional health pattern, or diseases. The memo or note accessory is a handy tool for accessing personal information such as password hints; however, if passwords are entered into the PDA, users should mask or hide them from view. Operation of the to-do list is similar to other applications and to-do lists also can be delegated by beaming them to another handheld.

An advanced option is the image software with a digital camera attachment. This option can help the provider build a consultation catalog that includes pictures of colleagues that can be pasted into the address book. Image software can also be used to follow wound healing or progression and wound pictures can be downloaded into the medical record. For additional information on both the Palm OS and the Pocket PC visit Dr. Gadget at *www.doctorsgadgets.com.*

What other programs are helpful?

Most PDAs have a basic calculator; however, you will most likely want a medical calculator. Three excellent freeware medical calculators are MedCalc, MedMath, and MedRules. MedCalc has more than 70 formulas and scores including Apgar score, body mass index, dose calculator, glomerular filtration rate, Glasgow coma scale, and pregnancy calculator. MedMath has more than 30 formulas related to internal medicine including mean arterial pressure, osmolarity, reticulocyte index, Winter's formula, and creatinine clearance. MedRules is more like a probability predictor or risk calculator than a traditional calculator. There are more than 20 formulas including the APACHE II, appendicitis, bleeding, stroke, and MI risk prediction scores. Calculators and other medical software programs are available from many online companies such as PalmGear and Medical Pocket PC. See Appendix 13-2 for additional resources.

Purchase a backup program if your PDA does not come with one. Palm has a program called MS Backup. MS Backup will back up programs in the PDA to the memory stick. When programs and data are lost, they can be restored to the handheld without synchronization or individually redownloading of each program from the PC or Internet. Another excellent backup program that is both popular and inexpensive is BackupBuddy (Hunter, n.d.).

A document reader is also a useful tool. Document readers allow users to transfer and view their text, database, spreadsheet, and presentation documents on their PDA (Adatia & Bedard, 2003). Common name document readers include Documents-to-Go, iSilo, and Installbuddy (Fischer et al., 2003). Another program, Presenter-To-Go, is used to deliver presentations from the PDA (Margi, 2003).

What can I do with PDA Internet access?

PDA Internet access puts breaking-news medical information, journal articles, medication updates, and clinical guidelines wirelessly in your palm and at the point of care. One health care provider reported that he was able to find the answer to a 3 a.m. consult question within minutes via a PDA Internet search (Vibar, 2003). PDA use for remote web access is becoming more popular with practitioners, pharmaceutical representatives, university faculty, and researchers because of easy web access to clinical information. However, to utilize a remote web access, the PDA must have a remote Internet browser installed.

The largest remote Internet server, with more than 8 million customers, is AvantGo. AvantGo is a free service that downloads selected AvantGo channels during data synchronization (Hunter, n.d.). In a user survey of 2584 practitioners, AvantGo (2003) found that the top medical PDA uses included access of clinical information (70%) and medical news (58%), medical calculator use (57%), formulary checks (50%), and access to journal articles (49%). Respondents also reported regular use of CNN. The highest reported specialty users identified were internal medicine (21%) and family practice (16%).

What health care software should I invest in?

Drug errors are one of the greatest burdens to the health care community. Drug errors are the leading cause of preventable death in the United States and cost the nation about $29 billion (Kohn, Corrigan, & Donaldson, 1999). Recent research indicates that consistent electronic guidelines have been shown to reduce medication errors in institutions and hospitals (Rosenbloom, 2003). To expand the solution to the bedside, the health care and technological communities have developed software programs that utilize the capabilities of the PDA.

PDAs are reliable, cost-effective, point-of-care tools used for referencing information and managing client care even as they contribute toward improved client satisfaction while decreasing the incidence of medical error (Adatia & Bedard, 2002; Fischer et al., 2003; Rosenbloom, 2003; Rothschild et al., 2002; Schuerenberg, 2003). Another benefit according to Grasso and Genest (2001) is fewer telephone calls to the pharmacy for drug information because of improved pharmaceutical referencing at the bedside by providers who are accessing medication information on their PDAs.

Several drug referencing programs enable the practitioner to expand electronic scrutiny at the bedside. One of the most widely used drug references is Epocrates. A study by the ACP (2001) found that 80% of the survey respondents used Epocrates to access drug information, and PalmGear (2003) reports more than 650,000 sales to health care professionals. Users report improved drug knowledge, client care, client satisfaction, reduced potential adverse drug events, and improved practice efficiency (Rothschild et al., 2002).

Epocrates is available in several versions including Epocrates RX Free, which is the basic drug and formulary reference. Drugs can be viewed alphabetically by drug or drug class. The pull-down menu option includes indications, adult dosing, pediatric dosing, drug interactions, adverse reactions, and cost information. The *Other* category includes the pregnancy and lactation rating, method of metabolism and excretion, mechanism of action, drug class, and U.S. Drug Enforcement Administration/Food and Drug Administration schedule. Other Epocrates products include Epocrates Rx Pro (drug reference plus infectious disease guidelines), Epocrates Dx (diagnosis and treatment reference), Epocrates Lab (diagnostic reference), and Epocrates Essentials, which combines the preceding programs into one program (Epocrates Ink, 2004). The Pro and Essentials versions also include alternative medicine monographs with noted drug interactions, clinical tables and guidelines, Medtools clinical calculator, and free telephone support. All the programs except MedTools are available for either the Palm OS or Pocket PC operating systems (Epocrates Ink, 2004). When downloading either Epocrates version, there is the option to download formularies. There are several choices including Care Choices HMO, Priority Health, Steelcase, and Blue Cross Blue Shield. Both versions allow you to add or edit categories. I added a "frequently used" category to find frequently used drugs with fewer stylus stokes and the notation option to insert clinical pearls or updates. Automatic updates are free and are downloaded to the PDA each time it is synchronized.

Another excellent drug database is Lexi-Drugs Platinum (AACN, 2003). There are three views: the essential, comprehensive, and comprehensive plus specialty view. All views include most of the options offered by Epocrates Rx except the formulary option, which can be purchased separately. The essential view includes elderly dosing and P450 effect. Among the additions to the comprehensive view are ethanol, nutritional, and herbal interactions, dietary considerations, client education, and nursing implications. Additions to the comprehensive plus view include specialty considerations of mental and cardio-vascular health, emetic potential, vesicant, and physical assessment monitoring and pregnancy issues. It is available for both the Palm and Pocket PC systems as an annual subscription (Lexi-Drugs, 2003).

Griffith's 5-Minute Clinical Consult is well worth the investment. The user can search by diagnosis or term and view the differential diagnosis, treatment, medications, follow-up, miscellaneous considerations, laboratory values, ICD9-CM codes and more (Skyscape, 2003). Griffith also publishes 5-minute emergency, orthopedic, and pediatric consult software.

The *Washington Manual of Medical Therapeutics* is a well-known and reputable medical reference. It covers disease management, evidenced-based guidelines, inpatient therapeutics, and drug information and dosages. The Washington manual as well as Griffith's 5-minute consults and the Taber's Cyclopedia employ smARTlink technology developed by Skyscape for integrated cross-index capabilities (Skyscape, 2003).

PEPID(2003) Portable Healthcare and Expertise is another company that sells health care software. Software suites include Emergency Medicine, Physicians' Clinical and MD/Family Physician's Suite, Clinical Nursing, Medical Student, Pre-Hospital, and Pharmacology Suites. Medical calculators and drug interaction references are available as are free demos, trials, and group sales. For more information, visit *www.pepid.com*.

Software programs that help the clinician manage client care and eliminate charging errors are becoming more popular. The PatientKeeper is an excellent program for client tracking and management (Rosenbloom, 2003). It is especially effective for the hospitalist or practitioners who make house calls. The PatientKeeper application allows the provider to access client information at the point of care. The Clinical Applications Suite includes a client list and clients' allergies, problem list, medications, vitals, clinical notes, and lab and test results (PatientKeeper, 2003).

Besides client management your practice needs to appropriately manage accounts receivable. Refused claims are often associated with inaccurate billing and coding that can be avoided with an application such as the ChargeKeeper. This program is used to improve revenue processing by automating the billing process, allowing point-of-care charges that interact with the existing billing system, and eliminating coding errors, thus, reducing claim rejections (PatientKeeper, 2003). See Appendix 13-2 for a list of software programs.

Where can I find health care software?

Several reliable sources of health care software are available. If you are looking for inexpensive guidelines, calculators, and other programs, consider the freeware or shareware offered by many of the online software companies. Other inexpensive sources are government sites. The National Heart Lung Blood

Institute (*www.nhlbi.nih.gov*) offers free evidence-based guidelines from the Obesity Education Initiative and the Seventh Joint National Committee on Prevention, Detection, Evaluation, and Treatment of High Blood Pressure (JNC-7) among others. The National Guideline Clearinghouse has a PDA/Palm guidelines index available at *www.guideline.gov* under PDA/Palm.

More comprehensive health care software can be found at health care professional sites. Many of these sites have an electronic or PDA section. The AACN and ACP both have comprehensive PDA centers. AACN offers handhelds, accessories, software, and tutorials for both Palm OS and Pocket PC systems. Both associations offer software categories that include medical, calculators, coding/billing, databases, document readers, drug guides, enhancements, handheld applets, multimedia, client tracking, references, study aids, and utilities (AACN, 2003; ACP, 2001). ACP also operates an online PDA Portal page. Use this page to access free demos of disease modules, books for PDAs, and free Palm documents and resources.

Skyscape.com offers health software expertise and is well known for its medical references. The top five software programs sold by Skyscape (2003) are Griffith's 5-Minute Clinical Consult, Physicians' Desk Reference, Nurse's Manual of Laboratory and Diagnostic Tests, Taber's Cyclopedic Medical Dictionary, and the Washington Manual of Medical Therapeutics. The advantage of Skyscape products is that they are linked and therefore information can be cross-matched or searched with minimal user effort. The Skyscape software programs are available in both the Palm OS and Pocket PC formats. The Skyscape website is a user-friendly site and can be searched by medical specialty or category; it includes online software support, promotional discounts for group purchasers, and trial versions. Other software sellers include PalmGear, Handheldmed, Pocketgear, and many more. See Appendix 13-2 for a listing of PDA software and hardware companies.

How do I protect my data?

PDA use within a wireless network can be wrought with risk from "unauthorized rogue access to malicious hackers" (Sims, 2003). Securing client information from unauthorized access is everyone's concern. The HIPAA compliance guidelines and potential penalties for noncompliance raise the anxiety threshold for all shareholders in the medical process. The three main issues that must be addressed regarding the use of PDAs in a medical setting are software protection, privacy, and confidentiality (Felkey & Fox, 2003).

To protect PDA software, purchase virus protection software if it is not already preinstalled, download software only from reliable sources, and back up data on a memory stick or PC with daily synchronization. The potential for introducing a virus into a hospital computer system via one of hundreds of PDAs is a significant concern (Felkey & Fox, 2003) and, if not already a requirement, virus protection will become a prerequisite to institutional network access.

The first step in securing information in the PDA is to utilize the preinstalled automatic lockdown option. If entering confidential client information, select an automatic lock with each Power Off option. To view information, the PDA must be unlocked with a password. If the password is forgotten, the PDA can be opened with a hard reset. This reset deletes all records; however, previously saved records can be restored with computer synchronization.

Even though the PDA is unlocked, specific events, items, or records can still be hidden or masked from view and viewed only after a password is entered. Masked records are grayed out and identified with a padlock icon; hidden records will not be visible. The preceding instructions may vary with newer Palm OS and the Pocket PC PDAs. Consult the operating manual or access online help for PDA-specific instructions at *www.microsoft.com/windows2000/support/ default.asp* and search the site with the key words *PDA tips*. Neither use of a password or lock nor hiding or masking entries in the PDA ensures HIPAA compliance when accessing a public network. HIPAA requires data encryption with 128-bit encryption algorithms when roaming a public network containing client information (Felkey & Fox, 2003; Sims, 2003). Encryption software for the PDA is inexpensive; prices range from about $10 to $50 (Morrison, 2002).

The Virtual Private Network (VPN) feature provides additional security but even with this technology in place do not assume HIPAA compliance. Before entering sensitive data into a PDA, consult with your institution's security officer or policy guidelines regarding PDA use.

SUMMARY

The Internet, e-mail, and PDA can enhance health care providers' practice by providing technical support that brings medical information to the provider, facilitates improved client outcomes and satisfaction, engages clients as partners in care, reduces medical errors, and supports faculty and students in the learning process. Technology tools can be implemented in augmenting marketing services, capturing charges, and improving client management. Nurse practitioners who take advantage of technology will find it easier to meet the growing demands of practice.

References

Adatia, F.A., & Bedard, P.L. (2002, October). "Palm reading": 1. Handheld hardware and operating systems. *Canadian Medical Association Journal, 167,* 775-780.

Adatia, F.A., & Bedard, P.L. (2003, March). "Palm reading": 2. Handheld software for physicians. *Canadian Medical Association Journal, 168,* 727-734.

American Association of Critical Care Nurses. (2003). Retrieved July 28, 2003, from *www.aacn.org*

American College of Physicians. (2001). ACP-ASIM survey finds nearly half of U.S. members use handheld computers. Retrieved July 28, 2003 from *www.acponline.org/ college/pressroom/handheld_survey.htm*

American Medical Association. (2002a). AMA study: Physicians' use of Internet steadily rising. Retrieved August 9, 2003, from *www.ama-assn.org/ama/pub/print/article/1616-6473.html*

American Medical Association. (2002b). How to "HIPPA—top 10 tips. Retrieved August 10, 2003, from *www.ama-assn.org/go/hipaa*

AvantGo. (2002). Harvard medical students learn and work through mobile solutions. Retrieved August 4, 2003, from *www.avantgo.com*

AvantGo. (2003). 2003 Physician survey. Retrieved August 4, 2003, from *www.avantgo.com*

Bliss, J.B., & Sandra, S. (2002). *Working the web: A guide for nurses.* Upper Saddle River, NJ: Prentice Hall.

Brusman Zaidel, L. (2003, January). Advance your career on-line. *Nurse Practitioner: The American Journal of Primary Health Care. Source Book for Advanced Practice Nurses,* s28, 6-11. Retrieved July 8, 2003, from *www.tnpj.com*

Center for Disease Control. (2003). Clinical guidelines available at http://www.cdc.gov

Consumer Reports. (2003). Best handheld computers – PDA: (out of 16). (2004). Retrieved August 13, 2004 from www.consumersearch.com/www/electronics/hand-held-computers-pda

Email Replies. (2003). Email etiquette rules for effective email replies. Retrieved July 23, 2003, from *www.emailreplies.com*

Epocrates Ink. (2004). Information on epocrates. Retrieved August 6, 2002, from *www.Epocrates.com*

ePolicy Institute. (2003a). Beware cyberslackers, spammers, and saboteurs. Retrieved August 10, 2003, from *www.epolicyinstitute.com*

ePolicy Institute. (2003b). E-mail do's and don'ts. Retrieved August 10, 2003, from *www.epolicyinstitute.com*

eRisk Working Group for Healthcare (2002, November). Guidelines for online communication. Retrieved August 3, 2003, from *www.medem.com/phy/phy_eriskguidelines.cfm*

Estabrooks, C.A., O'Leary, K.A., Ricker, K.L., & Humphrey, C.K. (2003). The Internet and access to evidence: How are nurses positioned? [Abstract]. *Journal of Advanced Nursing, 42*(1), 73-81. Retrieved July 23, 2003, from CINAHL database.

Felkey, B.G., & Fox, B.I. (2003). Privacy, confidentiality, and security for PDAs. *Hospital Pharmacy, 38*(4), 387-388.

Fischer, S., Stewart, T.E., Mehta, S., Wax, R., & Lapinsky, S.E. (2003). Handheld computing in medicine. *Journal of the American Medical Informatics Association, 10*(2), 139-149.

Franklin, C. (2003). How stuff works. Retrieved July 7, 2002, from *http://electronics.howstuffworks.com/pda.htm*

Grandinetti, D.A. (2000). Doctors and the web help your patients surf the net safely. *Medical Economics, 77*(5). Retrieved August 10, 2003, from *www.memag.com*

Grasso, B.C., & Genest, R. (2001). Use of a personal digital assistant in reducing medication error rates. *Psychiatric Services, 52,* 883-886.

Harris Interactive. (2000). Harris Interactive study reveals a lack of information technology use in medicine. Increased use of computers by physicians could revolutionize the medical practice—but hasn't yet. Retrieved July 7, 2003, from *www.harrisinteractive.com/news/printerfriend/index.asp?NewsID=78*

Hunter, K. (n.d.). Handheld computers in family medicine. Retrieved July 19, 2003, from *www.fammed.wisc.edu/education/res/Essentials.htm*

Khoo, E. (2002). Pocket PC or Palm OS. Retrieved July 11, 2003, from *http://asia.cnet.com/reviews/handhelds*

Kohn, L., Corrigan, J., & Donaldson, M. (Eds.). (1999). *To err is human: Building a safer health system. Committee on Quality of Health Care in America. Institute of Medicine.* Washington DC: National Academy Press. Retrieved July 29, 2003, from *www.nap.edu/html/to_err_is_human*

Lexi-Drugs. (2003). Comparison of platinum views. Retrieved July 21, 2003, from *www.lexi.com*

Lowes, R. (2003, February). Don't play solitaire, and other office computer rules. *Medical Economics.* Retrieved August 10, 2003, from *www.memag.com*

Margi. (2003). Delivering powerful mobile presentation solutions. Retrieved July 28, 2003, from *www.margi.com*

MediClicks. (2003, June). 21st Century medicine: Bluetooth: Wireless medical applications. *MediClicks,* Issue 1.49. Retrieved July 30, 2003, from *www.mediclicks.net*

Morrison, K.M. (2002). Security software for handheld computers. Protecting patient information stored in your PDA isn't just a good idea; It could be required under HIPAA. *Family Practice Management.* Retrieved August 14, 2003, from *www.aafp.org/fmp/20020600/59secu.html*

Otto, G.R., & McRae, D. (n.d.). Using hand-held computers to document family practice resident procedure experience [Abstract]. Retrieved August 7, 2003, from PubMed database.

Palm Company. (2003). Palm announces alliances invoice over IP, Wi-Fi and security for Palm Tungsten C handheld users. Retrieved August 5, 2003, from *http://pressroom.palm.com*

PalmGear. (2003). Information on PDA. Retrieved July 10, 2003, from *www.palmgear.com*

PalmOne. (2003). Pick a wireless solution to match the way you work. Retrieved August 25, 2003, from *www.palm.net*

Palmsource. (2003). Information on PDA. Retrieved July 11, 2003, from *http://Palmsource.com/palmos*

Parker, G.M. (1999). Easing workflow in the palm of physicians' hands. *Health Management Technology, 20*(10), 48-49.

PatientKeeper. (2003). Information on patient keep. Retrieved August 11, 2003, from *www.patientkeeper.com*

Pepid. (2003). Pepid products portable healthcare expertise. Retrieved August 10, 2003, from *www.pepid.com*

Pocketgear. (2003). Pocket PC software. Retrieved July 11, 2003, from *www.pocketgear.com/software.asp*

Rosenbloom, M. (2003). Medical error reduction and PDAs. *International Pediatrics, 18,* 69-77.

Rothschild, J.M., Lee, T.H., Bae, T., & Bates, D.W. (2002, May/June). Clinician use of a palmtop drug reference guide. *Journal of the American Medical Informatics Association, 9,* 223-229.

Schuerenberg, B.K. (2003, February). When Goliath can't help, David does the job. *Health Data Management,* pp. 72-80.

SCPIE Indemnity Company/American Healthcare Indemnity Company. (2002, May). Guidelines for e-mail communication with patients. *Safe Practice, 8*(2). Retrieved August 2, 2003, from *www.scpie.com/general/publications/safe_practice/200212.pdf*

Sims, B. (2003, April). Deploying secure, reliable wireless LANs in the healthcare environment. *Health Management Technology.* Retrieved August 10, 2003, from *www.healthmgttech.com*

Skyscape. (2003). The best medical and nursing reference for your handheld. Retrieved July 28, 2003, from *www.skyscape.com*

Sony, (2003). Retrieved August 8. PDA information available at *www.sony.com*

Sullivan, D. (Ed.). (2003). The major search engines and directories. Retrieved August 10, 2003, from *www.searchenginewatch.com*

Taylor, H., & Leitman, R. (Eds.). (2001, August). Physicians' use of handheld personal computing devices increases from 15% in 1999 to 26% in 2001. *Healthcare News, 1*(25). Retrieved July 8, 2003, from *www.harrisinteractive.com*

Taylor, H., & Leitman, R. (Eds.). (2002a, April). Patient/physician online communication: Many patients want it, would pay for it, and it would influence their choice of doctors and health plans. *Health Care News, 2*(8). Retrieved August 3, 2003, from *www.harrisinteractive.com*

Taylor, H., & Leitman, R. (Eds.). (2002b, May). Four-nation survey shows widespread but different levels of Internet use for health purposes. *Healthcare News, 1*(25). Retrieved July 8, 2003, from *www.harrisinteractive.com*

Taylor, H., & Leitman, R. (Eds.). (2002c, June). Four-country survey finds most cyberchondriacs believe online healthcare information is trustworthy, easy to find and understand. *Healthcare News, 1*(25). Retrieved July 8, 2003, from *www.harrisinteractive.com*

The Magnet. (2002, February 7). *Online medical liability risks increase as patients communicate via the Internet.* Retrieved August 2, 2003, from *www.medem.com/ phy/phy_magnet.pdf*

Vibar, L.A. (2003). PDA use growing in medical and other fields. *New York Times Network.* Retrieved August 5, 2003, from *www.nynewsnetwork.com*

UNIT **IV**

Your Place
in the
Community

14

Community Involvement

Patricia W. Underwood

Benefits and Strategies for Community Involvement

Community involvement is often seen as an endeavor for the established practitioner, a way to "give back" to the community. For nurses, however, it is an expected part of professional practice. The International Council of Nursing (2003) definition is quite explicit on this point:

> Nursing encompasses autonomous and collaborative care of individuals of all ages, families, groups and communities, sick or well in all settings.... Advocacy, promotion of a safe environment, research, participation in shaping health policy and in client and health system management, and education are also key nursing roles.

This chapter will examine the benefits of and strategies for community involvement that fulfills the practitioner's social contract and enhances the success of independent practice.

Why should I be involved in the community?

There are three primary reasons for community involvement: marketing your practice, building political capital, and creating change in the delivery of health care. Although the majority of your time spent in community involvement will not be compensated, it can have big returns in getting known and being seen

259

as a valued resource. Community involvement can be viewed as an important strategy for *marketing your practice*. If your name is recognized and your abilities respected, it is likely that increased numbers of clients will seek your services. There is a significant amount of "word of mouth" advertising that enhances the practices of nurse practitioners (NPs). Community involvement is your investment in this form of advertising.

Similarly, community involvement can not only establish you as a future resource, it can enable you to build *political capital*. Becoming known among community leaders and special groups within the community and making a contribution to those issues that community groups have identified as most significant to them can increase the likelihood that your ideas will be given credence. Thus your spheres of influence will be increased and your opportunities to *create health care system change* enhanced. For example, a women's health nurse practitioner (WHNP) volunteered her services providing programs on health promotion at a local shelter and also spoke on women's issues to some hospital auxiliary groups. Women in leadership positions within the community became acquainted with this nurse and recognized her expertise. The NP was invited to be part of a new community planning group that was constituted to develop strategies for increasing access to care among the underserved and minority populations. Through this forum, the NP was able to increase breast cancer screening among migrant women.

What forms can community involvement take?

Your choice of involvement will depend both on the circumstances that present themselves as well as the outcomes that are desired. The most common forms of involvement include sharing health information, volunteering service, and establishing, leading, or participating in community coalitions to address health issues.

Sharing Information. Sharing health information is often the initial form of community involvement and one that can produce substantial marketing effects. If your intent is to combine public service with marketing your practice, you need to approach it systematically. Box 14-1 suggests a step-by-step approach for sharing information.

Box 14-1 Step-by-Step Considerations in Marketing through Sharing Information

1. Assess areas of expertise.
2. Match with topics of current interest in the media.
3. Identify community groups that might desire the information.
4. Consider the cohort characteristics of your targeted audience in choosing a method for information sharing.

Develop a plan that includes a realistic appraisal of your areas of expertise. When identifying an area where you have special knowledge, do not hesitate because your experience may not be extensive. If you are comfortable with an area of knowledge for which the public has expressed a need, opportunities can be found where you can present it.

Find the match between your expertise and the community needs or local media interest. Listening to the local radio station or reading newspapers can give you cues to the "hot" topics. *Healthy People 2010* goals (see *www.healthypeople. gov*) can point the way to topics that are of interest within your local community. You may want to check with the county health department to identify the organizations that are actively focusing on particular goals. Common issues that emerge as topics for short presentations and seminars are often focused on the needs of women, children, and the elderly. An area that is frequently neglected is that of men's health. Getting information to this group is a challenge because they are less inclined to attend public presentations of health topics than are their female counterparts. A viable alternative is to encourage women to consider their contributions to the health of the significant men in their lives. It is often the women who provide the support, encouragement, or just plain nagging that is needed to push men toward healthier pathways.

The match between your expertise and topics of community interest will often reveal an obvious target/audience for that information.

Find the community groups that might desire your information on timely topics. Women's or men's organizations; church, health care, or professional groups; and community centers or residential complexes may be ideal for public presentations. Some women's shelters have a requirement of attendance at programs that are designed to improve women's health and life management skills. A piece in a newsletter or newspaper is also a good avenue, particularly for those who are more reticent about talking to sizable groups. There is an emerging market for health presentations via local radio, and in some cases television, that might be investigated. A short, regularly aired health program is not only good from an individual marketing perspective, but can do much to advance nurses as primary sources of health information in the eyes of the public. You should not be dissuaded by a concern that you have to assume total responsibility for the content. Partnering with a local school of nursing is often a very beneficial option.

Market through presentations that involve consideration of the cohort characteristics of the target group. These considerations are critical to a final decision about where and by what means information is ideally delivered. People born before 1946 and Baby Boomers (1946-1959) will be impressed by expertise conveyed in a personable manner. You may find them in organizations, churches, and clubs. By contrast, Generation Xers (born 1963-1977) are not joiners and prefer to go it alone. They are very literate when it comes to technology and tend to be lifelong learners. Generation Y (born 1980-2002) is similarly technologically competent. They have never lived without cell phones, chat rooms, faxes, and voice mail. They embrace a fast paced life and rapid change. They question everything, are impatient, and Google for information. If you are interested in reaching members of Generations X or Y, you will have to use a less traditional route than oral presentations. A website, list serve, or health chat room may be effective in connecting with these cohorts. Although developing a website or Internet newsletter among your clients may take time and technological expertise, it can provide a significant degree of control and afford an opportunity to be creative in delivering your information.

Futurist Lowell Catlett predicts that cell phones will rapidly change the way we deliver health care. They provide immediate connections, will soon replace personal digital assistants (PDAs) for handling data, and with picture capability will make distance assessment possible (Catlett, 2004). It is possible that in the near future, the cell phone may provide a new route for connecting with the community. Thus, community involvement through the sharing of information is only limited by your own creativity and inclination.

Volunteering Service. Donating services is another means of community involvement. It may range from periodic services such as providing screening examinations and camp or school annual physicals to a more regular commitment. Volunteering usually requires less preparation time than information sharing but may require a more long-range commitment if services are provided at a free clinic. This route may be less effective as a marketing technique because people who attend a free clinic are unlikely to attend your fee-for-service clinic. On the other hand, if your service is significant, it may be acknowledged in the news media.

Do not be shy or unduly modest. If you are making major contributions, notify the health editor of your newspaper to see if that person might be interested in doing a story. Such an article would not only be good for your practice by making people aware of your services, but it would give nurses increased visibility. Nurses are traditionally reluctant to seek publicity and this serves no one.

Involvement in Community Coalitions. A third means of community involvement is through the route of joining or building a community coalition. This avenue of involvement may take the greatest skill and the longest time commitment. It is not the best marketing tool, nor is it the preferred route when your time needs to be concentrated in building your practice. It does, however, provide a very comprehensive opportunity for making a difference and may be of significant value in building political capital.

Care must be taken to see that this involvement does not reflect the paternalism that is often typical of forays by professionals into the community. The paternalistic attitude that the professional knows best does little to facilitate the empowerment of community members and limits the partnerships that are necessary to producing lasting community change. If you want to become involved in community coalitions, make sure you bring with you the philosophy and skills that will maximize your success, as discussed in the next section.

Community Coalitions

What is a community coalition?

Coalitions have been defined variously according to their purposes, composition, and duration. They may serve a key role in the coordination or integration of services and resources, but their major purpose often goes beyond that. Some coalitions are composed of member organizations; however, it is useful to view community coalitions as potentially involving both organizations and individuals who represent key elements of the population. Practicing with community means that all stakeholder groups should be considered for membership, especially the least powerful and most vulnerable.

Coalitions were once defined as more temporary structures. Today, coalitions may be considered more durable (Butterfoss, Goodman, & Wandersman, 1993) but are usually time limited (Dluhy, 1990). It is important to recognize the lack of permanency of a community coalition and to push for expeditious action to address the needs identified by the community. If it is advantageous that the efforts of the coalition be sustained on a more permanent basis, the coalition may recommend being replaced by a more permanent type of structure.

Advocacy has been included as a component of some definitions of coalitions. Indeed, advocacy is critical in moving beyond the sharing of resources within the group to the acquisition of external resources and goal achievement. If carefully composed, the coalition may assume a role of advocacy on behalf of the community. It seems useful, therefore, to define community coalitions on the basis of all the factors discussed: "a structure of individuals, groups, and organizations coming together to acquire resources (power and materials) needed to effect a solution to a common problem within the community" (Underwood, 1997, p. 273).

What are the reasons for starting a coalition?

Box 14-2 lists many purposes/reasons for forming community coalitions. A major purpose is to create a sufficient power base to challenge the status quo and to engage the problem-solving process or changes required to address a need identified by the community. Coalitions have the ability to pool resources and achieve a power beyond that which any individual might accomplish. A community coalition is particularly useful for advanced practice nurses (APNs) because it affords a mechanism for bringing together community needs and programs that have been developed outside the community. Coalitions can tailor these programs to meet the conditions of the local situation.

Box 14-2 Reasons for Starting a Coalition

Outcome Achievement

Initiatives based on citizens' needs.
Planning and creation of shared vision.
Collaborative problem solving.
System/community change.
Resource acquisition.

Coordination and Integration

Provide an information sharing/networking platform.
Increase coordination among agencies and individuals.
Integrate the formal and informal helping systems.
Promote a holistic, comprehensive approach.

Individual Development

Provide community education.
Emphasize health promotion.
Create culturally relevant solutions.
Increase opportunities for citizen leadership development.

Source: Bandeh, J., Kaye, G., Wolff, T., Trasolini, S., & Cassidy, A. (1996). *Module one: Developing community capacity,* pp. 55-56. (Battle Creek, MI: W. K. Kellogg Foundation and the Health Care Forum.)

Coalitions can also provide the APN a base from which to achieve health care objectives over the objections of traditional sources of power.

As a new APN in women's health, I found myself practicing in a rural area of California. The community clearly had a need for an expectant parent education program, but the physicians (the traditional sources of power) were not supportive. I formed a coalition of a few individuals who represented the population of young mothers, a BSN prepared nurse, and a representative from the local chapter of the Red Cross. The latter organization was chosen because the Red Cross has a formal Mother-Baby Program and also certifies instructors and instructor-trainers. I obtained the certifications and, with the help of the coalition members, initiated a program. In retrospect, the coalition might have been constituted more broadly, but in this situation the outcome was achieved. A significant community need was addressed and the traditional negative sources of power were overcome.

Identifying a community need, creating a vision around that need, problem solving and strategizing to develop a plan for change, and acquiring the resources necessary to achieve that change are all essential. Along the way, interagency resources may be integrated or coordinated and the knowledge and advocacy skills of people in the community may be developed. It is critical that coalition building begin by agreeing on the need within the community that the coalition will address and by developing a shared vision of a future where that need is met.

What ingredients are key to a philosophy of community coalition building?

Instead of simply practicing "in" the community, a philosophy of practicing "with" the community will maximize the positive outcomes. Practicing with the community requires a high degree of collaborative leadership and an acknowledgment that the community must play a central role in defining its problems and in proposing solutions appropriate for and acceptable to the community. Practicing with the community effectively facilitates the empowerment of community members.

This philosophy has two essential ingredients. The first is that the *community must have the central role* in identifying those issues or problems that it sees as priorities and in selecting the means to address them. If communities have only a minimal say in identifying health issues and in setting the direction for their solution, the result often is that the health systems developed are insensitive to issues of diversity and are plagued with inefficiencies, including duplication of effort, fragmentation, unproductive competition, and lack of planning (Wolff, 1995). The community's ability to "have a say" is no guarantee that problems will be solved, but it increases the likelihood that solutions will be both relevant and coordinated.

The second key ingredient in practicing with community is an *emphasis on assets* as opposed to deficits. It is important that you focus on the community's capacity for solving its problems, rather than simply viewing it as a collection of problems to be solved by you the professional. Outside resources are more likely to make a difference when the capacity of the community is recognized and respected (McKnight, 1989).

How can I be a collaborative leader?

The philosophy of practicing with community must be accompanied by an understanding of collaborative leadership. This type of leadership does not depend on content expertise. Instead, it requires that the leader focus on the process by which the group comes together to solve a problem. Collaborative leaders safeguard that collective process and recognize that the more power and control are shared, the more these ingredients are available to use in problem solving. It has been suggested that five characteristics are essential to collaborative leadership:

- Trustworthiness
- An ability to see the big picture
- Flexibility and patience
- Abundant energy
- Hope (Trasolini, 1996, pp. 18-19).

These characteristics can be developed and enhanced through the process of self reflection.

Inspire Action. Additional principles of collaborative leadership are suggested by Chrislip and Larson (1994). The first of four principles is that collaborative leaders inspire commitment and action (Box 14-3). The emphasis is on inspiring and facilitating a process where people can solve their own problems, rather than simply directing action. For example, after several children had been struck by cars within a 2-year period in a single neighborhood, health professionals designed a program to educate parents and children about not running into the street. Unfortunately, the problem persisted. A community health nurse assembled the residents of the neighborhood to discuss what they believed was the cause of the problem and what might be the solution. The residents thought that the problem was due to too many trucks going through the neighborhood at too high a rate of speed. With the encouragement of the nurse acting as a collaborative leader, the citizens petitioned the city council to install two speed bumps and to lower the speed limit. No further incidents occurred. In this example, the collaborative leader facilitated the development of an effective solution.

Focus on Peer Problem Solving. The second principle involves peer problem solving. Power is de-emphasized as the leader works to facilitate a shared vision and engenders energy and involvement in the solution seeking process. This principle is very similar to the second factor in transformational leadership that calls for inspirational motivation (Northouse, 2004). Transformational leaders raise followers' levels of consciousness about the importance and value of specified and idealized goals, motivate followers to transcend their own self-interest for the sake of the group, and move followers to address higher level needs (Bass, 1985, p. 20). A critical difference between transformational and collaborative leadership rests in the commitment to partnership that is inherent in the latter.

Encourage Broad-Based Involvement. A collaborative leader may serve without titles that would distinguish the role. This is evident in Chrislip and Larson's (1994) third principle, which stresses the importance of broad-based involvement. It is essential to identify all of the potential stakeholders within the community and to actively seek people who have differing perspectives. The emphasis is on inclusiveness in bringing people together to

Box 14-3 Chrislip and Larson's Principles of Collaborative Leadership

Inspire commitment and action.
Become a peer problem solver.
Encourage broad-based involvement.
Sustain hope and participation.

address an issue of common concern identified by the community. Nurses are very good at this because we value giving voice to those whose voices are often ignored.

When a hospital made plans to expand its outpatient facilities within the community, it was the nurse practitioner on the team who insisted on conducting focus groups among the low-income residents to ascertain their views about the way services could be offered to best meet their needs. A couple of informal leaders from the community were then added to the planning committee. The actual location of the clinic, the hours of operation, and the particular services offered were tailored to the needs of the client population and greatly enhanced its success both from a humanitarian as well as an economic perspective.

Sustain Participation. The final principle focuses on sustaining hope and participation. Collaborative leaders convince people that their opinions are valued, celebrate even small steps toward goals, and help groups sustain their effort when the work gets hard and the inclination is to quit. Most work with the community will take time and it is often tempting to just "do it yourself." Participants may feel the same way and question why they should make time to participate in meetings that involve so much talk and seem to progress so slowly. It is important to set realistic expectations of participation from the beginning (e.g., how much decision making will be involved and how long it will take to find a location, plan renovations, design services; obtain funding, staff and equipment).

It is also important not to wait until the final outcome is achieved to celebrate. Each small achievement along the way is cause for recognition within the wider community and will ensure the continued involvement of the planning group as well as the continued community support and a sense of ownership. Collaborative leaders do not simply give lip service to valuing the opinions of others but make visible how those opinions shape the work of the group and how vital they are to ensuring success.

An understanding of the skills needed by a collaborative leader will prepare you to consider coalition work as an avenue for community involvement. One word of caution is important here. If you choose the coalition route for community involvement, you may want to get your feet wet by joining an established coalition. You can still apply all the principles of collaborative leadership but will find it an easier first step than working to develop a coalition.

Should I build a coalition?

Coalition building is a challenging but very rewarding process. It will require skill of the collaborative leader, not only to initiate but to maintain. The consolation is that if you do it right, you will not be alone. Collaboration means sharing both the work and the responsibility. It is important that you have a clear understanding of what a community coalition is, the reasons for initiating one, and the processes to be employed before making a decision to undertake such an initiative. Your commitment over the length of the project is essential. If you have any doubts about your ability to sustain the commitment needed, it would be better for your reputation not to choose the coalition building route.

Not all coalition work has to be lengthy, however. Within 6 months, one WHNP used the coalition process to implement a program to enhance breast health among migrant women. Her example will be used to illustrate the steps in coalition building. Before these can be discussed, however, it is important to clearly understand what a coalition is and for what purposes you might want to establish one.

What steps are important in building a coalition?

Lay the Foundation. So how do you get started? Box 14-4 outlines five steps in coalition building. Your first efforts may be in response to learning of a need that the community has identified that fits your areas of interest and expertise or you may simply decide that you want to become involved in the community. Either way, it is advisable to begin to lay the foundation by finding a partner within the community who has established credibility and may be interested in collaborating. You may know of an individual or you may approach an organization that is working on behalf of the target community. It is important for you to be sensitive to the cultural and political dynamics with which you are operating if you are going to be successful. If you are an established member of the community you may already possess this knowledge.

Form a Steering Committee. A critical next step is to form a steering committee. It is advisable to include representatives of the key groups who are stakeholders in the issue. You will want people who have community leadership potential, but you also want individuals who can be a voice for the less powerful segments of the community. Care should be taken to ensure that in composition and operation, professional voices do not dominate those of community members. True collaborative leadership will require your use of excellent group process management skills. Attention also needs to be given to selection of meeting times and locations and the setting of ground rules that

---

Box 14-4 Steps in Coalition Building

Lay the foundation.
Form a steering committee.
Develop organization and timetables.
Research the target issue.
Develop an action plan.

will support the participation of those whose voices are essential to the success of the initiatives that will emerge from the collaboration. The biggest mistake that well-intended professionals make when trying to work with the community is to fail to involve critical stakeholders on the basis of perceived educational, social, or economic limitations. These very individuals may make the difference in the success or failure of the coalition in achieving the desired outcomes.

Do not be discouraged if the initial steps of coalition building take longer than expected. Bringing all the important players aboard is critical to ensuring success. Implementation of action plans will move more quickly once the group dynamics have been established and commitments to a shared vision are achieved. The six R's (Box 14-5) are helpful in mobilizing grassroots members (Kaye, 1996, pp. 104-106). Providing *recognition* for the efforts individuals are making should not wait until the goals are accomplished. It is essential to the maintenance of memberships that the *rewards* of participation outweigh the costs. Fostering *respect* for each member, even when there are conflicting viewpoints, and encouraging *relationships* that reflect accountability, responsibility, and mutual support are critical. Opportunities for social exchanges can facilitate relationship development. Similarly, the *role* of each member should be clarified and the value of each person's contribution made obvious. Some members may have experienced being "tokens" on a coalition, so your job is to create substantive roles with real power. Similarly, it has been said that nothing succeeds like success. You cannot wait until the end of the project to see *results*. Small wins should be structured and celebrated along the way to generate the momentum needed to keep the energy and excitement high.

Develop an Organization and Timetables. Figure 14-1 depicts the integration of the dual activities of developing the products/outcomes that will be achieved and planning the processes and strategies that will be used by the coalition. Developing some organization for your work is critical but be cautious about being too regimented. A certain amount of give and take is involved, particularly when you are dealing with community members who

Box 14-5 Six R's of Participation

Recognition
Reward
Respect
Relationship
Role clarity
Results

Source: Kaye, G. (1996). Grassroots organizations: Building capacity. In J. Bandeh, G. Kaye, T. Woff, S. Trasolini, & A. Cassidy (Eds.), *Module one: Developing community capacity* (pp. 103-147). Battle Creek, MI: W. K. Kellogg Foundation and the Health Care Forum.

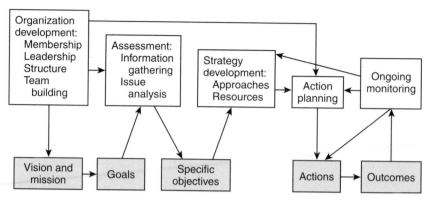

Figure 14-1. Planning processes and the products that are produced (Bandeh, J., Kaye, G., Wolff, T., Trasolini, S., & Cassidy, A. (1996). *Module one: Developing community capacity.* Battle Creek, MI: W. K. Kellogg Foundation and the Health Care Forum.)

may have different timetables. Some worksheets that might be helpful are included in Appendix 14-1. Additional materials (charts and worksheets) may be found in the workbook edited by Kaye and Wolff (1995) and are available through the W. K. Kellogg Foundation. (The W. K. Kellogg Foundation has been engaged in significant work to promote the development of community-based coalitions to promote health particularly in underserved populations. Their workbook, *Sustaining Community-based Initiatives: Developing Community Capacity,* is available online in both HTML and PDF formats at *www.wkkf.org/Programming/ResourceOverview.aspx?CID=1&ID=656.* Among their initiatives is a collaborative project by the schools of nursing at the University of Michigan, Grand Valley State University, Michigan State University, and Wayne State University to establish nurse-managed centers.)

Research the Issue. It is important that the selected issue be researched to identify what has previously been done, and what current efforts may be under way. It is also necessary to identify the political, economic, social, legislative, and unintended consequences of potential action. The latter is another area that is too often overlooked and may sabotage the successful implementation of long-term change. Community meetings, focus groups, citizen surveys, and a resource inventory may yield useful information in researching the issue. It may be helpful to include the results of these data-gathering efforts in a briefing book.

Develop an Action Plan. Action planning considerations (see Box 14-6) and strategic analysis of the issue (see Box 14-7) may occur at the same time. The *causes of the problem* may become apparent through an analysis of the community information. It is important for the coalition to then identify the

Box 14-6 Action Planning Considerations

What are the causes?
Who are the actors?
What role should actors play?
What are the barriers to the goal?
What are the strategies and programs?
What resources do we have and need?

actors and their ideal roles. *Actors* are those individuals or institutions who are most directly involved with the issue and who are in a position to help solve the problem. Their *ideal roles* include the one or two primary activities the actors could reasonably take to help solve the problem.

Barriers that are both obvious and covert must be identified so that strategies and programs can be developed to address them. *Strategies* should be creative and collaborative. It is useful to identify the full range of options that are available and to consider which strategies might influence which other strategies. The strategy that seems to influence the greatest number of other strategies can be called "the driver." Investing scarce resources in the driving strategy can be expected to yield the greatest payoff. This type of analysis replaces the usual brainstorming with subsequent plans to implement all reasonable strategies.

The final component of action planning includes an assessment of what *resources* are available and what are needed. Resources most typically come from donations by the organizations involved in the coalition. In fact, this is often the reason a particular individual, group, or agency is invited to become a member. The resources do not have to be monetary. Sometimes the most significant contributions are in the form of in-kind services. A civic or religious affiliated group may be able to donate meeting space or publicity development.

Resource development is an activity that is most effective when it is the outcome of long-standing and nurtured relationships. You never know when a contact may be helpful with a future project. One NP reported that after reading in the newspaper that there was a new director of the local senior center, she wrote a letter of congratulations. She also offered to help in any way that she could. Later, when the NP was trying to expand her practice, she was able to obtain a $28,000 grant from the senior center to be used for case management services.

Another source of resource development is local colleges and universities. Staff at these institutions may be willing to assist with grant writing to obtain

Box 14-7 Strategic Issue Analysis

Who are the allies?
Who are the opponents?
What conditions cannot be controlled?
What is the ability to mobilize?

resources in a more formal way. Local foundations are another resource that is often overlooked. Making yourself known to foundation leaders may pay off in the future when you have a project for which additional funding is needed.

As you are developing an action plan, you need to further analyze the issue. Obvious in any such analysis is a delineation of the *opponents* and *allies*. As difficult as it is, anticipating your opposition is essential if you are to develop anticipatory strategies to neutralize them. Appealing to common goals or values is often an effective approach. While identifying opponents, do not forget to fully consider potential allies and the relationships they may be able to capitalize on in promoting your issue.

The other two components of issue analysis are less obvious. Determining what *conditions cannot be controlled* is important so that precious time and resources are not wasted trying to modify them. A final thing to consider is the *ability to mobilize* support for the issue among important constituencies. The question is always one of what it will take to get people to come out in support of the goal the coalition is trying to achieve. If the issue you are trying to address is a need that has been identified by the community, it will be easier to gain the support needed.

Example of Coalition Building. A WHNP practicing in a rural area was concerned about the mortality rates from breast cancer among migrant women. She recognized the fact that migrant women were not engaging in breast self-examination (SBE) nor were they seeking routine mammograms and examination by primary care providers. As a result, the diagnosis of breast cancer was frequently made at a stage when it was less amenable to treatment. She decided to develop a coalition to see if this health behavior could be changed.

She began to *lay the foundation* by contacting the director of the local Migrant and Rural Health Association for support and to make certain that the approaches she used would be culturally sensitive. Initial *research* was conducted by going out to the migrant camps and talking to the women about the issue. She found that many of the women were amenable to health examinations but perceived considerable barriers to accessing services. The barriers included language differences for those who spoke little English, the fact that when women attended a clinic the whole family tended to come with them, and the fact that the clinics were not open during the times when the women were not picking crops. This analysis helped to *identify stakeholder groups*: migrant women, Migrant & Rural Health Association, County Health Department, the local hospital where mammography was performed, the Radiology Department, physicians, and nurses. The only other stakeholder group that might have been included was the camp/farm owners. The stakeholder groups were identified as potential members of the coalition. Individual representatives of each stakeholder group were invited to be part of a *steering committee*. Meetings were held in the evening so that the migrant women members could attend and transportation was provided. Attention was paid to the six R's as the *organization, timetables,* and *action plans* were developed. Worksheets similar to those included in Appendix 14-1 were used to facilitate the planning. The following outcomes were achieved:

- The Radiology Department agreed to be open in the evening for mammograms once a month.
- The Health Department (located across the street from the hospital) agreed to conduct health examinations on the same evening the mammograms were to be given.
- The hospital and the Health Department agreed to use a common record.
- Transportation and interpretation was facilitated by the Migrant & Rural Health Association.
- Pamphlets explaining the services and their importance were developed in English and Spanish.
- Within the migrant camps peer coaches were trained to encourage women to participate in health screening.

This project became a model for the state. It had a major impact on modifying the delivery of health care and in changing the participation of individuals from a vulnerable population in their own health practices. It also helped the nurse practitioner to gain credibility within the community and her input was solicited in future statewide planning initiatives.

This case was an example where use of a reasonable planning process involving all key stakeholders, giving attention to the six R's, obtaining needed resources, and careful issue analysis met with real success. Following these prescribed behaviors, however, does not guarantee that everything will go smoothly. All coalition efforts are met with some challenges. Anticipation of these challenges will enhance your ability to meet them.

What challenges should I anticipate?

While practicing with the community enhances the likelihood of meaningful change within that community, coalition building is not without its disadvantages as a general strategy. Being aware of these disadvantages and barriers may enable you to act to avoid them or minimize their results. Box 14-8 lists the five major disadvantages of coalition building, a major one being that they are *slow to develop.* This will be very frustrating to some members depending on their personality and preferred communication styles. Setting expectations for reasonable progress and creating small steps of measured progress may be helpful.

Three additional disadvantages occur as a direct result of the major advantage of coalitions—their inclusiveness. The presence of diverse members representing different groups and organizations may create opportunities for *policy differences* and *conflict. Power inequities* may also occur in a truly inclusive coalition, particularly if you have professionals with advanced education and community members whose education may be limited. The way to minimize

Box 14-8 Disadvantages of Coalitions

Slow to develop
Policy differences
Conflict
Inequity of power
Member turnover

some of these potential disadvantages is through setting ground rules from the beginning and reinforcing them and through paying attention to the six R's.

The final disadvantage of a coalition is *member turnover*. It is probably wise for the group to decide from the beginning whether organizations or groups need to have consistent representatives or whether anyone may be designated as a substitute. The disadvantage of disallowing substitutes is that a given group may not have representation at a particular coalition meeting. On the other hand, if there is frequent substitution in representation, the group dynamics are disrupted and the work of the coalitions is further slowed. Whatever choice the coalition makes, an excellent system to maintain ongoing communication is needed. If good communication occurs, it will help to keep even absent members informed.

Kaye and Wolff (1995) have identified a number of typical barriers to coalition success (Box 14-9). When coalition members represent different organizations, *competition and conflicts over turf* issues can occur. Appealing to the greater good and addressing potential conflicts before they emerge are key strategies to reducing these barriers. *Bad history* comes about through the "We already tried that" attitude. Knowing the history ahead of time (that is, doing your homework) can help to anticipate this dialogue. Creating a fair and open process with consistent ground rules may enable you to avoid this problem.

The *failure to act* phenomenon is perhaps the most deadly barrier. As mentioned previously, small results spur the coalition on. If the coalition spends too much time making decisions, members will be lost. The commitment to

Box 14-9 Barriers to Success

Turf and competition
Bad history
Failure to act
Dominance by professionals
Lack of common vision
Failure to provide leadership
Poor links to the greater community

Source: Wolff, T. (1995). Barriers to coalition building and strategies to overcome them. In Kaye, G., & Wolff, T. (Eds.). *From the ground up: A workbook on coalition building & community development* (pp. 40-48). Amherst, MA: AHEC/Community Partners.

action must be sustained and even small actions must be visible while planning is occurring on the larger issues.

Dominance by professionals and a *lack of a common vision* were also mentioned previously. From the onset, you must be committed to eliminating these barriers. Consistent with that admonishment, you must assume some responsibility for seeing that there is **leadership** for the projects identified. You do not always have to be the leader, but you need to make certain that this role is assumed. Similarly, there is a need to pay attention to developing new community leadership. The leadership capacity of community members may be critical to sustaining the changes achieved.

A final barrier is *poor links to the community*. Even if community representation is obtained, care must be taken to share power, avoid jargon that may not be understood, and make certain that meetings are accessible if the links are to be maintained. Again, preplanning is a major strategy for reducing the identified barriers. Consideration should also be given to the characteristics that are likely to maximize the success of the coalition.

What are the keys to success?

You may feel a little intimidated by all the challenges to successful coalition building, but nurses are well known to have skills that are likely to prove keys to successful coalitions. Nine keys to success (Wolff & Foster, 1995, pp. 31-38) are listed in Box 14-10. Many of these have already been addressed, so this may be considered a review. Successful coalitions are those that have a *strong community base* and *include all the important stakeholders*—even the least powerful. Nursing is a highly trusted profession and this public credibility enables us to encourage and support the participation of others.

As a *collaborative leader*, you will have times when you wonder if it wouldn't be easier to just do it yourself. When these temptations come, remind yourself that you are building community capacity for tomorrow and nurturing new leaders to carry on in your stead. Levy (1996) quotes an old Chinese poem that begins:

> Go to the people
> Learn from them
> Love them
> Build on what they have.
> When their task is accomplished
> Their work is done
> The people remark,
> We have done it ourselves. (p. 2)

This is the sense that you are trying to achieve with collaborative leadership.

Other keys to coalition success include planning that achieves a *shared vision and common mission. Systematic planning* cannot only occur at the onset. Successful coalitions have developed a mechanism for ongoing planning and

Box 14-10 Characteristics of Successful Coalitions

Strong community base
Inclusion of stakeholders (including the least powerful)
Collaborative leadership
Shared mission and common vision
Systematic planning
Effective ongoing communication
Formality of structure
Doable actions
Optimism and persistence

Source: Wolff, T., & Foster, D. (1995). Principles of success in building community coalitions. In Kaye, G., & Wolff, T. (Eds.). (1995). *From the ground up: A workbook on coalition building & community development* (pp. 29-39). Amherst, MA: AHEC/Community Partners.

reevaluation. When actions are identified, it is clear who will have responsibility for which initiatives. Planning is related to two other keys: *effective ongoing communication* and *structural formality*. Effective communication within the coalition and with other organizations and the wider community including the state, for example, is critical. Minutes, newsletters, and effective media messages will help to sustain the efforts of the coalition. Some degree of structural formality is necessary to sustain the work of the coalition. Attention to the dynamics of the group process is part of the structural considerations. Even coalitions that have limited resources benefit from designated persons assuming staffing duties and from the establishment of procedures for decision making. Contributions by organizational members and small grants can enhance the success of the coalition.

Early victories that stem from the selection of *doable actions* illustrate to coalition members and the wider community that this coalition can achieve the desired outcomes. Trust is enhanced along with enthusiasm. A short-term agenda is just as critical to the success of the coalition as the long-range, ultimate goal. Paradoxically, early expectations for achievement should not be set so high that they shortchange planning. A careful, realistic balance is needed.

The final keys to coalition success are *optimism and persistence*. Optimism serves to affirm the strengths of the coalition and provides a mechanism for making the work fun. The morale of the coalition is enhanced when it celebrates its accomplishments. We live in an age of quick fixes. Unfortunately, many of the problems with which community coalitions are dealing are not amenable to the quick fix. Coalitions develop slowly and while they need to have early successes to celebrate, they require the patience to maintain the effort needed for sustainable change.

SUMMARY

Where do you go from here? The exciting thing about the answer to this question is that you are only limited by your own initiative, creativity, and personal/professional vision. If Catlett (2004) is right about some of the changes in health care with new avenues for connectedness through technology, with changes in what people value, and with the growing opportunities for women to develop their own businesses, APNs have a bright future. Nurses have the people and leadership skills, the critical thinking abilities, and the knowledge and aptitude for managing evolving and complex systems that are needed to transform the way health care is delivered.

We do not have to confine ourselves to traditional structures or modes of practice. The practice of the future is in the community and where people want to reside; it will support people's preferred ways of engaging their health and reflect their preferred modes of receiving information and making decisions. Involvement with the community at your earliest opportunity will maintain your sensitivity to these diverse perspectives and changing dynamics.

Do not let the discussion of coalition building overwhelm you. Wider community contact may begin as a marketing strategy and focus on information and resources sharing. It is to be hoped that many APNs will extend that involvement to practicing with the community and the building of coalitions to address needs that have been identified by members of those communities. This chapter could only provide an overview of the process, but rest assured that there are many resources available to assist you in maximizing your success. Effective development as professionals and leaders requires that we support each other in finding our unique best ways to contribute to the worthwhile work of optimizing people's health. The demands of the future make it imperative that we work as partners and coaches with people who seek our services, that we nurture diversity, and that we cheer each other on.

References

Bandeh, J., Kaye, G., Wolff, T., Trasolini, S., & Cassidy, A. (1996). *Module one: Developing community capacity.* Battle Creek, MI: W. K. Kellogg Foundation and the Health Care Forum.

Bass, B.M. (1985). *Leadership and performance beyond expectations.* New York: Free Press.

Butterfoss, F., Goodman, R., & Wandersman, A. (1993). Community coalitions for prevention and health promotion. *Health Education Research: Theory & Practice, 8,* 315-330.

Catlett, L. (2004, November). *The future of leadership in health care.* Paper presented at the annual meeting of the American Academy of Nursing, Washington, DC.

Chrislip, D., & Larson, C. (1994). *Collaborative leadership: How citizens and civic leaders can make a difference.* San Francisco: Jossey-Bass Publishers.

Dluhy, M. (1990). *Building coalitions in the human services.* Thousand Oaks, CA: Sage Publications.

International Council of Nursing. (2003). The ICN definitions of nursing. Available at *www.icn.ch/definitions.html*

Kaye, G. (1996). Grassroots organizations: Building capacity. In J. Bandeh, G. Kaye, T. Wolff, S. Trasolini, & A. Cassidy (Eds.), *Module one: Developing Community Capacity* (pp. 103-147). Battle Creek, MI: W.K. Kellogg Foundation and the Health Care Forum.

Kaye, G., & Wolff, T. (Eds.). (1995). *From the ground up: A workbook on coalition building & community development.* Amherst, MA: AHEC/Community Partners.

Levy, B. (1996, December). *The Nation's Health,* p. 2.

McNight, J. (1989). Do no harm: Policy options that meet human needs. *Social Policy,* pp. 5-15.

Northouse, P.G. (2004). *Leadership: Theory and practice.* Thousand Oaks, CA: Sage Publications.

Trasolini, S. (1996). Leadership: Building capacity to lead a community-based process. In J. Bandeh, G. Kaye, T. Wolff, S. Trasolini, & A. Cassidy (Eds.), *Module one: Developing community capacity* (pp. 7-28). Battle Creek, MI: W.K. Kellogg Foundation and the Health Care Forum

Underwood, P.W. (1997). Building community coalitions—A critical aspect of advanced nursing practice. In V. D. Ferguson (Ed.), *Educating the 21st century nurse* (pp. 267-285). New York: NLN Press.

Wolff, T. (1995). Barriers to coalition building and strategies to overcome them. In G. Kaye & T. Wolff (Eds.). *From the ground up: A workbook on coalition building & community development* (pp. 40-49). Amherst, MA, AHEC/Community Partners.

Wolff, T. (1995). Coalition building: One path to empowered and healthy communities. In G. Kaye & T. Wolff (Eds.), *From the ground up: A workbook on coalition building and community development* (pp. 1-12). Amherst, MA: AHEC/Community Partners.

Wolff, T., & Foster, D. (1995). Principles of success in building community coalitions. In G. Kaye & T. Wolff (Eds.), *From the ground up: A workbook on coalition building and community development* (pp. 29-39). Amhurst, MA: AHEC/Community Partners.

15

Professional Involvement

Patricia W. Underwood

Making a Difference

In an effort to meet the challenges of establishing a practice as a nurse practitioner (NP), it is natural to focus all of one's attention on issues related to the clinical practice environment. Unfortunately, failure to give attention to broader professional issues can leave you as vulnerable as practicing without malpractice insurance. Professional involvement is not only an expectation of nurses in advanced practice; it is a critical strategy to ensure the efficacy of that practice.

Professional involvement may range from becoming a member of a professional association, to critically reviewing one's practice and systematically utilizing research in order to advance the profession, to actively participating in the development and modification of policy that will change the way health care is delivered. The specific direction that professional involvement will take will depend on the resources available at any given time, but involvement is an expectation of nurses in advanced practice.

Why should I get involved in professional associations?

The health care environment is extremely dynamic. Pressure for change arises from a variety of groups including consumers, regulatory bodies, and financial entities. Consumers are increasingly interested in finding greater access to safe care at a lower cost. Regulatory bodies seek to address system errors and potential fraud. At times their proposed solutions are reactive and fail to adequately consider long-term and unintended consequences. As a result, the "solutions" may create new problems. Financial entities also create pressure for change as they seek to curtail expenditures. Alone, none of us can adequately address the issues of practice regulation, quality of care, and reimbursement. As a collective group, however, we can have a major influence on shaping policy. Participation in professional associations is crucial to achieving the power necessary to ensure our preferred future and to control our practice.

Nurses have not traditionally been the power brokers in the health care arena, but we do have more power than many realize. A critical question is do we have the will to use it? A chief source of power lies in the relationships we have with our clients. People may not understand what we do, but they trust us and view us as having their best interests at heart. During the last several years, Gallup polls have repeatedly found that people trust nurses more than any other profession (with the exception of firefighters immediately after September 11, 2001). A second source of power comes from our shear numbers. There were 2.7 million nurses (American Nurses Association [ANA], 2004) as of 2002 and this includes 102,929 practicing NPs. These numbers create a formidable presence if the voices they represent are mobilized. The fact that there is an impending nursing shortage crisis at the same time that people are calling for a major transformation in the health care delivery system potentially magnifies our power and creates a tremendous opportunity for nurses (Jennings, 2001).

How do professional organizations prevent loss of power?

Unfortunately, power, or nursing agency, is too easily lost. Mason (1999) describes two ways in which nurses can lose power. It can be taken from them when hospitals redesign care delivery to take registered nurses out of the loop of critical decision making. Loss of power can just as easily occur within primary care offices and clinics when office managers and financial controllers specify the parameters of providing care without the input of nurse practitioners.

A second way in which nurses can lose power is to "become fragmented and self-destruct" (Mason, 1999, p. 7). Fragmentation is often of our own making and can take many forms. The most common examples usually relate to fighting in public. Different groups of nurses appear to want different things. The third parties to which the entreaties are addressed are not willing to become involved in settling internal disputes and often respond by eliminating the opportunity for nurses to have any voice in the issue. As Mason so colorfully remarks, "the wolves are lying in wait for nursing to lose its power" (p. 7). If lack of public unity creates a void where the powerful voice of nursing is not heard, others will gleefully step forward to fill it to our detriment.

There is a third way that nurses lose power—we give it away. It commonly happens in the many little instances when nurses ask permission to perform some intervention that is clearly within their scope of practice. It can occur in a more major way when nurse practitioners do not appreciate all the nuances of reimbursement requirements and acquiesce to physicians' desires to impose supervisory authority. After the passage of the Omnibus Reconciliation Act of 1989 (OBRA'89), there was significant potential for nurse practitioners to give away power as guidelines for Medicaid reimbursement were developed in each state. OBRA'89 provided for the Medicaid reimbursement of pediatric nurse practitioners (PNPs) and family nurse practitioners (FNPs) to the degree that this level of practice was recognized in a given state. Guidelines for reimbursement had to be developed consistent with the scope of practice of PNPs and FNPs as covered in the state's nursing practice act (or its equivalent). In Michigan, for example, the Michigan Nurses Association negotiated guidelines that would establish a contract for collaborative practice with a physician (the physician would willingly provide backup as needed) as the only requirement for reimbursement. Unfortunately, many NPs did not fully understand this and were willing to sign contracts that gave physicians authority for delegation and supervision. Thus, individual nurses gave up some of the power for independent practice that their professional association had won for them.

While no guarantee, participation in professional organizations is the best insurance against the erosion of power. Individually, we may not have the time or the political capital to ensure our voice in policy setting and control of practice. Together, we can leverage the power that is needed to address not only general nursing issues but those that are specific to the practice of nurse practitioners.

Which organizations can maximize nurse practitioners' power?

Often the answer to the question of participation in professional organizations is reduced to a question of immediate cost and resources for informing one's practice. On this basis, specialty organizations are frequently selected because their membership fees are relatively low and because they provide information specific to a particular practice focus. They are an excellent resource for achieving a defined practice mission. In addition, several specialty organizations, such as the American College of Nurse Practitioners (ACNP), National Association of Pediatric Nurse Associates and Practitioners (NAPNAP), American Association of Nurse Anesthetists (AANA), Association of Women's Health, Obstetric, and Neonatal Nurses (AWHONN), and American College of Nurse Midwives (ACNM), have associated certifying bodies (Table 15-1). The specialty organizations, however, may vary considerably in the resources they can command, particularly at the state level, for addressing broader issues of practice control, reimbursement, and regulation.

Table 15-1 Credentialing Activities of Professional Organizations

Organization	Credentialing Entity	Areas of Certification
American Academy of Nurse Practitioners (AANP) *www.aanpcertification.org*	AANP Certification Program	NP (adult, family)
American Nurses Association (ANA) *www.nursingworld.org*	American Nurses Credentialing Center (ANCC)	NP (acute care, adult, adult psychiatric and mental health, family, family psychiatric and mental health, gerontological, pediatric) CNS (adult psychiatric and mental health, advanced diabetes management, child/adolescent psychiatric and mental health, medical-surgical, pediatric)
Association of Women's Health, Obstetric, & Neonatal Nurses (AWHONN) *www.awhonn.org*	National Certification Corporation (NCC)	NP (women's health, neonatal)
National Association of Pediatric Nurse Associates and Practitioners (NAPNAP) *www.napnap.org*	National Certification Board of Pediatric Nurse Practitioners and Nurses	NP (pediatric)
American Association of Nurse Anesthetists (AANA) *www.aana.com*	Council on Certification of Nurse Anesthetists (CCNA) *www.aana.com/council*	Nurse anesthetists
American College of Nurse Midwives (ACNM) *www.midwife.org*	ACNM Certification Council *www.accmidwife.org*	Nurse midwives

Membership in a state nurses association (SNA) brings with it broader resources for monitoring the full spectrum of statutory and regulatory initiatives that may significantly affect practice. The cost of membership is higher, but it is an excellent investment in protecting the very practice you are trying to establish. Many SNAs have been successful in achieving independent prescriptive authority for NPs and in establishing appropriate guidelines for reimbursement through Medicaid. They are frequently effective in influencing health policy at a state level by placing members on boards and committees that address health issues.

Membership in a state nurses association comes with the full resources of the ANA. This includes access to certification through the American Nurses Credentialing Center. Acting in partnership, ANA and the SNAs have been successful in achieving legislative victories at the federal level that have increased the reimbursement opportunities for NPs. Coalitions of the ANA and specialty organizations have also had much success in asserting the position that control over advanced practice should rest with the profession rather than through the mechanism of a second license at the state level. This is beneficial because the profession is able to set higher standards of practice that are measurable through national certification procedures.

The answer to the question of professional association membership seems clear. To provide maximum power and security for the future, nurse practitioners should belong both to a specialty organization and to their SNA. The cost is a critical investment in the future. This imperative should not discourage anyone with immediate expectations of significant involvement. When you are starting out, commitment to advancing the profession through membership in professional organizations is enough. Advanced practice, however, carries with it an expectation of evolving leadership. Political activism is critical to the survival of the profession as well as to the creation of change within the health care delivery system so that it more effectively addresses the needs of the people we serve.

Henry (2000) has described four levels of political involvement: awareness, involvement, participant, and leader (p. 308). The level of *awareness* requires informed membership. At this level, it may be sufficient to belong to your professional organizations and follow selected political issues as the organizations share information and strategies. Very soon, however, advanced practice nurses should move to a level of *involvement;* in fact, for clinical nurse specialists and nurse practitioners, their jobs may demand it. At this level, APNs become actively involved in influencing policy within organizations. As nurses expand their political skills, become *leaders* within their professional organizations, and *participants* in the wider political arenas, it remains important to bring the profession along. This is an important consideration in avoiding pitting one segment of the profession against another, maintaining a unified voice, and maximizing nursing's power. "Nursing must see itself as politically responsible beyond influencing the legislative process through lobbying and grassroots efforts. Nursing must view itself as engaged in all of the processes that result in public policy relating to health" (Salmon, 2001, p. 349).

Policy Development

What avenues are there for policy development?

Policy development may occur at a number of levels through the mechanisms of organizational policy, standards, practice guidelines, statutes (state and federal), and regulatory and implementation guidelines. It is critical to identify the problem for which you are seeking a solution and the potential policy that may provide that solution.

Following that identification, consideration must be given to where the policy would most effectively be developed and implemented. To make such a determination, you need to consider who has jurisdiction/responsibility for and/or control of the issue. Two important principles should be kept in mind. First, creating or modifying laws is not always the most effective nor the most efficient means of enacting policy. Second, no matter where a policy is enacted, plans have to include strategies for influencing the guidelines for implementation. If attention is not given to the latter, an outcome that is much different from the original intent of the policy may occur. A case in point was the Medicaid regulations that resulted from the OBRA'89 legislation, which was discussed earlier in this chapter. Lack of attention to the guideline development might have obviated the entire intent of the legislation to recognize the independence of nurse practitioners. Opportunities for policy development in the contexts of standards, statutes, and regulations will be discussed separately.

How is policy developed through practice standards and guidelines?

The most immediate targets for policy development on the part of nurse practitioners are practice guidelines and protocols. These can promote quality care and consistency of practice within the context of an organization/clinic. The caution here is to make certain that they are not so specific that they set up standards of care that may easily be breached in the normal course of rendering care. Nurses tend to be very idealistic and write explicit standards. Such specificity may place NPs in legal jeopardy. In the absence of any written policy, however, the prevailing practice, in fact, becomes policy.

To develop and implement policy at the organizational level, NPs are advised to employ the strategies of planned change. It is especially important to take into consideration the culture of the organization within which you work and who controls it. Additional considerations include the prevailing methods of communication, sources of power, and resources available. As a base, it would be important to look at national standards and guidelines and then make certain the standards you set are consistent with the scope of practice within your state.

Standards may also be set at the national level. The ACNP, NAPNAP, AWHONN, and the National Organization of Nurse Practitioner Faculties (NONPF) are the most frequently involved organizations in setting standards that are specific to NP practice. The ANA sets the standards for general nursing practice at the RN and advanced levels. (See Table 15-1 earlier in this chapter for a list of the organizations that set standards and credentials for advanced practice nurses.) In partnership with specialty organizations, ANA authors standards for specialty areas of practice. There is a great opportunity for NPs to become involved in setting these standards. Volunteers for standard setting panels are routinely sought. You can contact ACNP or submit your name to ANA through your state nurses association. This type of professional organization activity is time limited and may be very manageable.

How is policy developed through state and federal statutes?

Statutes are the most difficult to bring about but may produce the most enduring solutions to issues of public policy. The step to address public policy through statutes should only be taken after careful consideration of other options due to the considerable resources that are needed to bring about change in this arena. To be effective, it is absolutely essential that nurses speak with one voice. If you want to be involved in the passage of legislation at the state or national level, it is advantageous to do so within the context of your state nurses association or in consort with the ANA or ACNP at the federal level.

How have nurses organized to pass legislation at the state level?

Many nursing organizations at the state and national level have taken steps to enhance their ability to speak with one voice through the development of nursing coalitions and the adoption of policies and procedures for strategically addressing issues. Henry (2000) has described the development of the Coalition of Virginia Nurses. In Michigan, a similar coalition came into being through the guidance of the Nursing Summit. The Summit is composed of the presidents of the Michigan Nurses Association (MNA), the Michigan League for Nursing (MLN), the Michigan Organization of Nurse Executives (MONE), the Michigan Association of Colleges of Nursing (MACN), and the Michigan Coalition of Nursing Education Administrators (MCNEA). The catalyst for this development was the report of a legislator who had held hearings around the state on strategies to address the nursing shortage of that time. This report listed all the nursing organizations that were represented in these well-meaning brainstorming sessions and concluded that the legislator did not know who spoke for nursing and, therefore, could take no action. Summit members wisely recognized that this was a legislator's ploy to legitimize taking no action. Rather than responding to the legislator, they determined to bring all of nursing together to develop a process for identifying and advancing a common political agenda.

All of the nursing organizations in the state of Michigan had been meeting twice a year to informally share information and organizational goals. Summit members, as part of this informal group, brought the political issue to their attention and suggested that the group be formalized and that a process for identifying a common political agenda be developed along with a mechanism for settling disputes over strategy. It was a significant milestone that nurses established a process for choosing focal issues. It was more impressive, however, that they were able to adopt a process for resolving differences over strategy. This process focused on the expectations of member organizations in the event that planned strategies to advance the agenda had to be modified. Members made a commitment to fully voice concerns about new strategies within the group, but to keep silent in public in any instances where the individual organization did not feel they could support the revised strategy adopted by the group. The Coalition of Michigan Organizations of Nurses (COMON) came into being with elected leadership and dues. At the behest of COMON, MNA (as the organization with the most political resources) provides the bulk of staff work to advance a particular issue. COMON also conducts a yearly event (Nurses Impact Day) to educate all nurses about timely issues and develop their political expertise.

How have nurses organized to advance policy at the national level?

At the national level, the Tri Council has served as a power building group. The members of the Tri Council include the ANA, the National League for Nursing, the American Association of Colleges of Nursing, and the AONE. These major nursing organizations meet several times a year to discuss issues of mutual interest. In 2002, they adopted a process similar to COMON's to enhance their ability to strategically advance political issues. This process includes a mechanism to enhance a common voice and a means for identifying a lead organization(s) on any given issue. These strategies on the state and national levels have served to enhance nursing's ability to develop "political capital."

Why is it important to build political capital?

Organizations that have built political capital are most likely to be successful in bringing about the passage of a law. Political capital is gained through long-term relationships with legislators and other political groups, a reputation for consistently providing needed information/research on issues, and an ability to deliver support for issues. Often nurses who are neophytes in the area of policy and politics will want to respond to every issue that remotely touches health care. It is important to know when it is wise to simply take no stand on an issue and when it is beneficial to expend political capital to support or oppose an issue. Political capital is not unlimited. It is like a "free spin" card that should be saved for a time when its use may be very critical in influencing the outcome in the desired direction.

Nurse practitioners have many opportunities to become involved in legislation at the state and national levels. Participating in efforts to educate yourselves on the issues and develop your political savvy is a first step. Working with your professional organization to develop and promulgate the common messages is critical. (A list of resources is provided at the end of this chapter that may help you further develop your political expertise.)

At what points can nurse practitioners influence legislation?

Typically, groups and individuals attempt to influence legislative outcomes at two points: when committees from the chamber of origin (the House or Senate) hold hearings on a particular bill and later when it comes to the floor for debate and vote. In the former instance you can participate in giving testimony and in the latter, you can work more directly to influence the vote of your representative or senator.

The most effective means of influencing the outcome, however, is to be involved in the drafting of legislation. It is important to have relationships with legislators' staff because they are the ones who are actually involved in doing the background research on a bill and drafting the legislation. Opportunities to participate in policy making at this level depend on having established long-term relationships with your legislators. Again, your professional organization can play the most critical role in opening these doors.

One of the most difficult situations in which to influence legislative outcomes occurs following a gubernatorial or presidential veto. To override a veto takes a two-thirds majority of both the House and Senate. Although extremely difficult, it is not impossible to override such a veto. With 1 in every 44 voters being a nurse, we have incredible power, if we can speak with one voice.

During Richard Nixon's presidency, there was a significant controversy over the Labor-Health, Education and Welfare appropriation levels and the funding for nurse training. Nixon twice vetoed the appropriations bill for fiscal year 1973 ("Fate of Nursing Funds," 1972). The funding of this act was important to all nurses because it provided funds for education programs and advanced training. Nurses were organized, prepared to speak with one voice, and descended on Washington en mass to lobby Congress. Sheer determination, overwhelming numbers of committed nurses who were willing to speak out, and a clear consistent message won the day. Congress voted to support the issues important to nurses. The situation was unusual but showed what nurses can achieve when we work together regardless of our level of education or practice focus.

How do nurse practitioners decide whether to aim for state or federal legislation?

A major consideration when selecting legislation as the preferred strategy to address a particular policy issue is whether to aim for the federal or state level. If the policy you want to influence is connected to a federal program, such as Medicare, the answer is obviously federal legislation. Federal legislation can be more efficient because, if passed, it can apply throughout the country simultaneously. For a program like Medicaid, which is carried out on the state level, the process is more complex. General changes need to take place at the federal level, but state-by-state development of regulations to implement the general provisions must also occur.

For issues that affect the practice of nurse practitioners within their scope of practice, such as independent prescriptive authority, the initiatives must occur at the state level. Although there have been significant efforts by ANA and ACNP to work with the National Council of State Boards of Nursing on some common expectations of nurses in advanced practice, these remain only guidelines. Each state has its own practice act or the equivalent.

Although rare, there are occasions when it is expedient to launch state and federal initiatives simultaneously. For example, a serious problem for client safety and nurse burnout is the issue of mandatory overtime. In 2000 the ANA House of Delegates took a strong position opposing this practice (ANA, 2000). ANA made passage of a federal law that would prohibit this practice as a means of staffing a legislative priority. Because efforts to achieve federal legislation are slow, some state nurses associations have felt pressured to move more quickly. Therefore, legislation on the state level has been initiated across the country. Recent research (Rogers et al., 2004) demonstrating the links between fatigue due to overtime and client errors may provide critical support for its passage.

Sometimes, when the decision is not clear regarding state versus federal jurisdiction, the question becomes one of where the legislation can be achieved most expeditiously. To achieve state and/or federal legislation, nurses must work collaboratively—not only with each other but also with consumer and health provider groups. As an individual, you can maximize your political clout by working through your professional organizations because they have the big picture that enables them to be sensitive to issues of timing. They also have the political capital needed to maximize success in achieving legislative goals. Your greatest contributions can be in identifying the areas of concern, helping acquire the data to support the recommended change, and developing the vivid illustrations of the need to capture support for the change. These can be incorporated into the strategies that will maximize success in bringing about statutory reform.

How is policy developed through regulatory change?

In addition to practice standards and statutes, a third means of policy development is through regulatory change. This strategy is often overlooked by nurses. It is especially critical that after achieving any legislative change, attention be given to how rules and regulations are developed for implementing the new law. As mentioned previously with the OBRA'89 legislation, failure to be attentive could have cost the desired gains.

Regulations can occur through the generation of implementation guidelines/rules related to a newly passed law or through formal amendment to those rules at some future point. For example, when the Balanced Budget Act of 1997 accorded nurse practitioners direct reimbursement through Medicare Part B, the Health Care Financing Administration (HCFA) was charged with developing the rules for carrying out that reimbursement. They had to define the qualifications of NPs to be eligible for reimbursement. It was initially stipulated that reimbursement would go only to nurse practitioners who possessed three qualifications: a master's degree in nursing, authorization to practice as an NP in accordance with state law, and certification by the American Nurses Credentialing Center or other recognized national certifying bodies that have established standards for NPs. Professional organizations were immediately concerned that this rule included no provisions for recognizing nurses who were currently authorized to practice as NPs by their states and who possessed national certification that did not yet require a master's degree. Letters of protest and concern were sent to HCFA. In the winter of 1999, Dr. Virginia Trotter Betts, JD, RN, who was serving as special assistant to U.S. Department of Health and Human Services (DHHS) Secretary Shalala, became involved in working with HCFA to amend this rule. A modification in the rules around the principle of not disenfranchising currently practicing NPs was negotiated. The amended rule would allow registered nurses who were licensed in their states to practice as NPs and who had received a certificate of completion from a formal advanced practice program before January 1, 2002, to meet the qualifications for reimbursement. A meeting was arranged between HCFA representatives and representatives of the major nursing organizations involved with NP practice and certification. It was anticipated that the nursing organizations would support the proposed amendment. Interestingly, two organizations were so angry that the original rules had gone out with such a glaring omission that they aggressively asserted their concerns without listening to the compromise that HCFA was willing to provide. The frustration of HCFA ended the meeting without the anticipated support of the amended rule. Fortunately, work continued after the meeting and the amended rule was eventually adopted.

What lessons are key to regulatory change?

Three important lessons can be learned from this regulatory situation. First, as previously mentioned, professional associations must be vigilant throughout the rule-making process that succeeds the passage of a law and, to the degree possible, *work with the rule-making body as the rules are developed*. Second, it is important for nurses to obtain positions of influence throughout the policy-making world, whether as elected or appointed officials. Achieving desired policy changes is much easier from internal spheres of influence than from working on the outside. The final lesson is one that cannot be overstated. Nurses and nursing organizations have to work together and understand when the timing is appropriate for individual protest and when it is time to listen and provide collective support.

What is the role of a state board of nursing in policy change?

Another important source of policy through regulation occurs at the state level via the board of nursing (BON). Boards operate differently from state to state and it is important to understand the process in your state. Most, however, make policy through formal rules or resolutions. The state rule-making avenue occurs much as it does at the federal level.

Rules are promulgated following the passage of legislation. From time to time, rules may have to be modified even while the original legislation stands. For example, a law may give the BON authority for approving nursing education programs. A rule requiring a specific process of periodic review may be modified to substitute review by a national accrediting body where appropriate. Another example might be the need to modify a rule to recognize a newly accredited national certification body for the certification of nursing practitioners. These types of changes may arise from review within the board or may be sought by professional organizations. The BON and professional organizations can collaborate in the development of new or amended rules, but the *focus* must be *on protection of the public*. It is not difficult to make a case, however, that what is in the interest of nurses in providing safe, quality care is also in the best interest of the public. Proposed rules must go through the formal rule-making process specified by the state. Public hearings are required and this is a wonderful opportunity for nurses to make their views known. Again, it is advantageous to support or oppose with one voice but put forward a variety of arguments and illustrations.

Policy can also be made through the resolution process. Sometimes this can work simultaneously with attempts at legislative reform and is often a quicker process. An example is the situation with mandatory overtime. The charge is often client abandonment if a nurse does not work additional time. While nurses are working for legislative solutions at the state and federal levels, employers have threatened to report them to the BON with subsequent loss of license if they do not comply with mandated overtime. Nurse members of the Michigan Board of Nursing were concerned about licensure being placed in the middle of this staffing controversy and about the effect of overtime on the client safety. They passed a resolution indicating that the BON expected licensed nurses (LPNs and RNs) to exercise their clinical judgment in accepting or rejecting requests to work overtime based on their ability to give safe client care. If a nurse did not believe that he or she could provide safe care, the nurse would be well within what the BON expected in rejecting that assignment. It was acknowledged that such a rejection did not in and of itself constitute client abandonment. This resolution was upheld by the attorney general for the State of Michigan. It meant that employers could not threaten nurses with the loss of their licenses. A similar resolution was subsequently adopted by the Delegate Assembly of the National Council of State Boards of Nursing. Thus, in a relatively short span of time, nurses collaborated to bring about policy changes that meant that they could not lose their licenses for refusing to be placed in a position of providing potentially unsafe care. Unfortunately, none of these resolutions prohibit employers from firing nurses, so the need for legislative redress continues.

Again, three lessons can be gained from this discussion of regulatory avenues for policy development. First, legislative achievement does not end with the passage of a bill. Attention to the subsequent rule making is essential. Second, working with the BON provides several opportunities for policy development and some of them may be very time efficient. Last, as members of a BON, individual NPs have a real opportunity to make a difference.

How is policy developed in governmental agencies?

A final major arena for policy development may be found within the activities of governmental agencies that are charged with the development of programs to enhance health and health care. Prominent among these are the DHHS, the Agency for Healthcare Research and Quality (AHRQ), and state and community health departments. Nurses have wonderful opportunities both for employment in policy-making positions in all of these agencies as well as for membership on task forces and committees that focus on specific health concerns. Individual interest and expertise in the focal area is important, but the support of your professional association can greatly enhance your chance of being appointed to a particular committee or task force. One of the ways in which AHRQ creates policy is through the publication of research-based practice guidelines for selected health problems. *Healthy People 2010,* and *Prevention: A Blueprint for Action* (DHHS, 2004) are notable initiatives to set policy direction for health promotion. The prevention blueprint focuses on diabetes, obesity, tobacco use, and health literacy.

Summary of opportunities for policy development.

Nurse practitioners have a number of opportunities for policy development. These include but are not limited to:
- Standard setting
- Development of practice guidelines
- Legislation
- Regulatory change
- Funding initiatives

Political capital or power to achieve desired policy outcomes can be maximized by working through your state nurses association and through your specialty association. You, as an individual, can make a difference, however, especially if you gain elected or appointed office. Again, your professional associations can be of immense assistance in achieving these goals. Whatever avenues of policy change you choose, it is important to remember that we, as nurses, maximize our success when we speak with one voice.

How can nurse practitioners begin to build political power?

Power to achieve desired policy outcomes for any given issue can be enhanced through long-standing relationships that have been built over time as well as by behaviors specific to the issue. Taken together, these behaviors can be referred to as the seven C's (Box 15-1). The first three—*collegiality* among nurses, public *credibility*, and recognized *contribution*—depend on relationships most effectively built over time. *Collectivity, communication, collaboration,* and *commitment* are behaviors and skills that can be developed and then applied within the context of the situation.

Collegiality. Collegiality among nurses regardless of education or practice focus is critical to maximizing political power. If we can think beyond our most immediate practice concerns and embrace those issues that are of concern to the majority of the profession, we have a force to be reckoned with. For advanced practice nurses, collegiality within the profession means that we do not have to fight our issues of reimbursement and practice autonomy alone. If we are willing to lend our time and support to issues such as mandatory overtime, we can expect a quid pro quo when it comes to an issue such as independent prescriptive authority. In other words, if nurse practitioners lend their support to issues that are clearly of great concern to staff nurses, we can expect support from the wider nursing community for issues that may be of specific concern to nurses in advanced practice.

Credibility. Credibility within immediate spheres of influence (i.e., within your organization and community) can be built by each NP by offering needed information supported by research and facts. Participation in the development of public information materials or appearing as an authority in print and electronic media are effective strategies for developing a reputation as a knowledgeable practitioner who has the public's concern at heart. A willingness to provide needed information to health care administrators and state and federal legislators also builds credibility. It is important to remember that information

---

Box 15-1 Seven C's for Maximizing Political Power

Build relationships over time through:
    Collegiality
    Credibility
    Contribution
    Commitment to pursue the issue beyond simple adoption
Plan specific strategies to enhance:
    Collectively speaking with one voice
    Communication effectiveness
    Collaboration

must be both timely and understandable. If you gain a reputation for delivering on your promises, you are more likely to have your opinions listened to and even sought. Credibility not only enhances your power in pushing your policy agenda but increases the possibility that you will learn about proposed policy initiatives early in the process when the opportunity to shape them is maximized.

Contribution. Contribution is the third of the relationship-building strategies and is especially important in developing political power in the legislative arena. Contributions may take the form of either cash or in-kind help. It can begin with a contribution to the political action committee (PAC) of your professional organization. The PAC board evaluates candidates' positions for consistency with the values and goals of the professional organization and candidates' potentials to advance nursing and health care issues. Such contributions will be used consistent with an analysis that few of us have time to conduct ourselves and, thus, will maximize your investment. In lieu of or in addition to cash contributions, working on a candidate's campaign—even if it is simply stuffing envelopes—will pay big dividends. A minimum amount of time contributed may jump start those relationships that are critical to future success in policy development. Contributions, whether cash or in kind, are no guarantee that elected officials will vote in the way that you desire but it usually means that they will listen to your position.

The principle behind in-kind contributions—being perceived to be willing to work on another's issues—can also pay off within organizations and institutions. If you are willing to work with an institutional or community coalition addressing an issue that is important to individuals in a position to make policy, those individuals will be more inclined to listen to the positions you are advocating. Thus you are developing resources for future policy achievement.

Collectivity. The relationship-building strategies enhance our power reserves. When the need for policy development or change arises, our behaviors and skills with respect to collectivity, communication, collaboration, and commitment help us to capitalize on and expand that power. Collectivity is the ability to *speak with one voice* and can best be built on collegiality. This is one of the most essential ingredients of political power and one with which nurses seem to have considerable difficulty. Frequently the lack of collectivity is not ill intentioned but stems from a desire to see policy embrace the ideal and address everyone's issues. Unfortunately such outcomes are not often consistent with political reality. Compromise is required to reach those positions that achieve the greatest good for the most people. The choice should not be between achieving the maximum ideal or nothing. Instead, we must find ways to move toward our goals without seriously jeopardizing the position of any particular nursing group, even if it means we cannot accomplish what each group wants. The reality is that achieving policy change that advances our position—even halfway—often puts us in a position to build on that success for future goal achievement. Some may argue against NP reimbursement at 85% of the physician level, but this level of reimbursement at least afforded NPs the opportunity to gain independent provider numbers and to develop a track record of independent billing and the data to use to lobby for equal pay for equal services.

Communication. Clear, effective communication that endeavors to achieve congruent perceptions and expectations is essential. Messages provided by individual professionals and groups should be consistent in their position but may vary in both language and context to be understandable by the recipient. Too many times attempts to set new policy have not come to fruition because the parties involved have held differing expectations of what each will do and have seen the issue from varied perspectives. Different ideas about the possible solutions to a given issue are critical at the onset, but it is important for dialogue to continue until a primary solution emerges.

It is also important for communication about the prospective policy to be couched in terms that all potential stakeholders will understand. For advanced practice nurses, this means avoiding the use of jargon and including examples that make the issue visible. In fact, making our practice visible to the general public is one of the key challenges to our profession. Although the public trusts nurses (most trusted profession in CNN/Gallup polls in 2000 and 2002, 2003, and 2004), they do not understand what we do and do not fully appreciate how essential our critical judgments are to health promotion. Without clear communication and practice visibility, the public cannot support our issues and concerns.

Collaboration. Collaboration and coalition building are facilitated by clear communication. Nurses collaborate with our clients on a daily basis and frequently collaborate with other health care disciplines in the provision of holistic care. Yet, when it comes to policy development, we often isolate ourselves. Health care consumers can be among our staunchest allies for policy change because our efforts are often on their behalf. It is important to assess who the stakeholders are for a given issue and to attempt to align them with our position. A little bit of political pragmatism is healthy. This means that you can feel free to collaborate with a certain group on a specific issue even if they are not a group with which you are naturally allied. For example, the United Auto Workers may not be a natural ally of ACNP and the ACNM, but these three organizations might collaborate in encouraging an insurance company and employer to include NPs and Certified Nurse Midwives (CNMs) among their health plan providers. *Involving the widest community* in moving policy is a sophisticated political strategy.

Commitment. Policy development is rarely a quick process, so commitment to stay with the issue to its conclusion is important. It is easy to support an admirable policy when there is little cost, but too often support diminishes once significant opposition has been raised. Furthermore, effort cannot be suspended once the policy is accepted. Procedures, guidelines, or regulations for implementation are usually next steps. As previously mentioned, policy can be obviated through misguided implementation. The implementation of the Health Insurance Portability and Accountability Act of 1996 (HIPAA) makes this very clear. Although HIPAA was designed to improve access to health care by facilitating the transfer of health insurance from one employer to another, some of the regulations that were initially implemented provided impediments to communication among professionals who were called to provide care in a manner that best met the client's needs. In some instances, information necessary for care during an emergency was limited due to privacy restrictions. These regulations had to be revised to better ensure that the intent of the legislation was met. Hence, full implementation was a lengthy process. This example also aptly illustrates the necessity of *paying attention to how policy is implemented* and *considering potential unintended consequences*.

The seven Cs: collegiality, credibility, contribution, collectivity, communication, collaboration, and commitment are not easily achieved on a profession-wide basis. Maximizing our power through these strategies must begin with individual efforts in the way we relate to each other, to our clients, and to those in positions to make policy.

How do I begin to develop a plan for a specific policy change?

Once you have identified an issue you believe needs to be addressed through policy, it is helpful to use the answers to a number of questions to clarify the context and specifics of the policy proposed (Box 15-2). Clarifying the problem and its background and identifying the stakeholders are early considerations that will shed light on the context of the issue and be important in framing strategies that will maximize successful adoption. Alternative options should be evaluated for their efficacy, evidentiary support, and costs/benefits. Once a preferred solution/policy has been identified, additional factors including the requirements for implementation and administration and potential

---

Box 15-2 Critical Questions for Policy Change

What is the problem that needs to be addressed?
What are the potential solutions and their advantages and disadvantages?
What evidence is there that the proposed solution will achieve the desired outcomes?
What are the financial implications including costs versus benefits?
Who are the stakeholders and what do they have to gain or lose?
What will be needed to implement the policy and who will administer it?
What are the potential unintended consequences?

unintended consequences must be considered in order to develop an effective plan for implementation.

What Is the Problem That Needs to Be Addressed? Although this question appears obvious, it must be carefully posed to make sure that you are on the right track. Sometimes enthusiasm for a particular policy emerges early and may obscure the real issue. For example, concern about the issue of pain management has led to a change in policy to include continuing education units focused on pain as a requirement for relicensure. If the problem is simply that health care providers do not have information about research on pain management, such a policy may provide a solution. If, on the other hand, the problem is that despite the availability of information on pain management, evidence-based guidelines are not being implemented, then changing relicensure or certification requirements may not address the real problem. Clarifying the specific problem that needs to be addressed is necessary to identifying desired policy outcomes and for brainstorming potential solutions.

What Are the Potential Solutions and Their Advantages and Disadvantages? Brainstorming is an activity that does not have to be restricted by more than the question of whether a suggested solution would address the identified policy goals and outcomes. Analysis of the advantages and disadvantages of any proposed policy will initially occur at a broad level and then become more specific as choices are narrowed. Criteria are selected on the basis of situational appropriateness but may include ethical and legal considerations; ability to influence cost, access to or quality of health care; consistency with professional standards and scope of practice; resources needed; and ease of implementation. Hanley (1998) suggests that "do nothing" should always be an option considered in the initial analysis.

What Evidence Is There That the Proposed Solution Will Achieve the Desired Outcomes? As the choices are narrowed, the question of supporting evidence becomes critical. Evidence that something will not work in your situation may be sufficient to eliminate an option. However, do not be prematurely dissuaded from considering an otherwise viable solution simply on the basis of historically negative anecdotal reports: "We tried that before and it didn't work." Solid evidence of the ability to achieve desired outcomes through the enactment of a particular policy will not only influence its selection but will be important for inclusion in written and oral persuasion of stakeholders to adopt the policy.

What Are the Financial Implications Including Costs versus Benefits? The actual estimated costs of policy options are important considerations in the current climate of concern about health care cost containment. Newness is an insufficient reason for policy change. Preferred solutions must achieve decided benefits and be cost effective. Achievement of cost savings or at least maintenance of budget neutrality will be a huge advantage for policy change. Actual costs along with resources needed for implementation are very important to consider when exploring the initial advantages or disadvantages of a potential policy. When you are planning a political strategy, the *perceived* costs must be considered as well. When the costs are immediate but the outcomes/benefits are in the future, as was the case with the Nurse Reinvestment Act of 2002, the work for policy acceptance is harder. When this is the case, the merits of the issue must be compelling.

Who Are the Stakeholders and What Do They Have to Gain or Lose?
Another important consideration in both selecting the preferred option and in planning strategy is identification of the stakeholders. Information about each stakeholder, their stake, and whether they will be potentially advantaged or disadvantaged by the proposed policy is essential to strategic action. Working with your professional association on state and national issues will give you access to information that can be used strategically. Policy within an institution must be addressed in the same way and it will be an advantage to pull together a coalition of stakeholders who are likely to support the issue.

What Will Be Needed to Implement the Policy and Who Will Administer It?
Fawcett and Russell (2001) have suggested that these questions are an important part of any policy analysis study. While you may not be doing a study, there is an advantage in asking these questions. It will help you to think beyond simple acceptance/adoption of the policy and may be important in seeing that changes are sustained. Considering the resources needed to actually implement the policy affords you the opportunity to build them into the adoption plan. You don't want to get a policy accepted only to find out that the resources are not there to see that it is carried out. In the same manner, it is important to think about who will control the administration of the policy. The individuals responsible will need to have both the skill as well as the commitment to make sure that the policy does not simply sit on the shelf.

What Are the Potential Unintended Consequences?
Although it is common not to consider this question, long-term policy success often depends on it. Good intentions are not sufficient if the consequences of policy implementation actually make the situation worse. The implementation of HIPAA policy, as previously discussed, is a prime example. The implementation of the HIPAA law was delayed while modifications were made to address unintended consequences. It is much more efficient if you can consider the unintended consequences from the beginning and take them into account when developing your plan.

What Political Factors May Make a Difference in Policy Acceptance?
Once you have selected the most viable, cost-effective option and have considered the stakeholders, potential unintended consequences, and what is required for

implementation, you are ready to work for its adoption. It would be nice if policies were adopted simply on the basis of their own merits. Unfortunately, this is not always the case. A number of political factors unrelated to the policy's merits may significantly influence the outcome and have to be considered in the development of strategies to promote policy adoption (Box 15-3). These considerations are appropriate for all policy arenas. It is wise to understand *how the policy advocates are perceived* by those who can influence the policy decision. When supporters of policy are perceived as trusted professionals who also have the wider interests of the public or their health care institutions at heart, change is facilitated. Thus, it is key to be able to present arguments that go beyond self-interest. Arguments are not always sufficient if the group is perceived as having little power either to advocate on their own behalf or to mount sufficient opposition. This is why developing relationships over time is so critical to future success.

It is also important to identify *who has the power* to approve the policy change. The goals and values of the decision makers will need to be addressed along with the advantages of the targeted policy to persuade them to support your position. Consistency with held values and research data that supports more effective achievement of desired outcomes with adoption of the policy are not always enough. People often ask "What's in it for me?" You need to be prepared to articulate how the adoption of this particular solution addresses their interests to gain support for your issue.

The *timing* of the issue can also influence its outcome. If a proposed policy addresses an issue that has received significant media attention advocating the development of solutions, this may facilitate its adoption. On the other hand, if there is not sufficient time to build support before a decision must be made, if data are not available to assist in positive consideration of the proposed solution, or if considerable political capital has just been expended on another issue, the timing may not be right. If the policy is being proposed as part of legislation, its priority on the legislative calendar, the length of the legislative session, the possible term limits of sponsors, and the timing of elections may all be critical considerations. The ability to select the ideal time at which an issue is addressed is not always possible. It is useful, therefore, to remember that even if the proposed policy is not accepted, the groundwork in understanding the issue has been laid and it may be reintroduced more successfully in the future.

Box 15-3 Political Factors that Influence Policy Acceptance

How the initiating group is perceived.
Who has the power?
Perception about "What's in it for me?"
Timing.

It is important to understand that no single factor will significantly influence the outcome. It is the way these factors interact with each other that is critical. An understanding of any of these political factors that may influence a particular policy will serve as a preliminary step in planning a specific strategy to achieve your intended outcomes.

What strategies can I use to influence policy adoption?

A number of specific actions have been advocated by people in the policy arena (Box 15-4). These are appropriate for any situation where you are trying to implement a change. They are designed to maximize your support and minimize your opposition.

Bipartisan Support. If you are introducing policy in the legislative arena, it is wise to have sponsors from both parties. This makes it less likely that other legislators will initially react to the proposal strictly along party lines. Although at times it may be much easier for nurses to find sponsors among a specific party, it is wise to work to gain sponsors from the other party as well. Thus you will have champions in both courts.

This tactic may be less clear if you are talking about policy within the community or an agency. The same principle still applies, however. Try to identify the various factions that may be operating and enlist cooperation from all. People are more likely to listen to someone within their own group with whom they identify. In an institutional setting this may mean gaining support from nurses, medical staff, administrators, and so forth.

Avoid "Us versus Them" Thinking. The impetus for policy development or change often arises out of a concern over the current situation. There may be a natural tendency to criticize those responsible for the way current policy is implemented. This criticism can lead to a dichotomizing of the issue. When people become defensive, they become more resistant to change. Defensiveness also leads to a personalization of the issue. If you can present your proposed policy in a manner that avoids the "us versus them" connotation, people are more likely to be open to the new idea. One way to do this is to focus on the

---

Box 15-4 Strategies to Influence Policy Adoption

Gain bipartisan support.
Avoid "us versus them" thinking.
Focus on agreements.
Be willing to compromise.
Keep it simple.
Pick your fights carefully.

potential for improving health outcomes, particularly in light of new research or the opportunity to gain new resources. Such an approach suggests that the current less desirable/less effective way of doing things may be a function of contextual constraints rather than personal failings.

Focus on Agreements. In the course of developing strategies to revise or initiate policy, differences of opinion are likely to develop. This is certainly true among nurses, whether within a single group or across organizations. Focusing on the areas of disagreement will create barriers to presenting an essential united front and to creating effective coalitions. When you are working with a variety of groups on policy development, the best strategy is to highlight those areas where agreement exists. This enables you to move the policy agenda forward. It is not necessary that those with whom you are collaborating agree on other issues. The requirement of collaboration is to have substantial agreement on the proposed policy. Sometimes agreements can be forged by considering a different outcome that can be successfully achieved by all involved. This is consistent with a "win–win" style of negotiation.

Be Willing to Compromise. A closely related strategy calls for the analysis of the proposed policy to determine those components that are essential and those that might be sources of compromise. All or nothing thinking is a significant barrier to success in policy development. Unfortunately, nurses are too often guilty of such thinking because we identify the ideal as our desired outcome. Holding ideals is good, but the unwillingness to compromise halts progress. The situations of reimbursement or independent prescriptive authority, as previously discussed, are excellent examples. When initiating a new idea, it is often hard to be totally successful on the first try. If you can compromise and get some part implemented, it is usually easier to go back for the full program.

Keep It Simple. People can understand an idea when it is clear in concept and presentation. This is hard to achieve because we are frequently dealing with complex human beings and systems. Not all of the complexity has to be included within the policy itself. Enabling legislation or implementation guidelines are places where smaller issues can be addressed.

A prime example of the detriment of complexity was Clinton's proposal for health care reform. Much excitement was generated among nurses when President Clinton proposed the Health Security Act (HSA) because it reflected many of the key points in Nursing's Agenda for Health Care Reform (ANA, 1991) and because many nurses had been afforded the opportunity to have input into its development. The HSA reflected an interesting concept to increase the access to and quality of health care while controlling the costs through "managed competition" (Weissert & Weissert, 1996). Key components of the proposal were a national board that would set the standards for health plans and regional alliances that would negotiate the purchase of health benefits among approved plans.

Through participation in mandatory regional health or corporate alliances, each company or region would devise a list of standard benefits, to be offered at the same price to all consumers. These health alliances would negotiate the best price and service from competing health plans. Each year people would have the opportunity to compare and choose a health insurance plan (Wakefield, Gardner, & Guillett, 1998, p. 351).

Unfortunately, the proposal was so complex that the general public could not understand it and was susceptible to the strong lobbying of the insurance companies to defeat it. Thus, a potentially good policy was defeated through ineffective strategies including the attempt to manage every subissue, the length of time spent in consensus building, and failure to focus the media attention on the content rather than the politics of the issue (Blumenthal, 1995; Fallows, 1996; Yankelovich, 1995). Keeping it simple is no guarantee of success in policy adoption, but if you don't try to achieve this goal your task will be very difficult.

Pick Your Fights Carefully. In the broadest interpretation, "pick your fights carefully" means that you do not have to take a stand on every issue that comes up. This is particularly important for an organization. When you get into a fight for an issue you are spending resources to be prepared, to develop your best arguments, and to mobilize stakeholders and the media. You are also spending political capital. Remaining neutral on an issue that is not part of your political agenda can yield benefits well beyond saving resources. If the policy being proposed does not affect nursing, nurses, or the public welfare, and if it is beneficial to another profession, remaining neutral is, in fact, helpful to the other profession.

Taking a strong stand in the midst of controversy has the potential to build political credibility if you win, but it can lessen your future political power if you lose. Therefore, choose your issues carefully both from the standpoint of their importance to the policy that you are advocating and the potential for winning the fight. Preparation and couching arguments in terms of public well-being are key strategies to winning.

How can I communicate with legislators?

Once you have thought through your general strategies for promoting policy, it is time to get down to specifics. You will want to communicate with those who have the authority to propose, support, or oppose the policy you are advocating. Your ability to enlist the sponsorship of legislators is best achieved as an outcome of an established relationship and through direct (face-to-face or phone) communication. But what choices do you have if you simply want to encourage a legislator to vote in a particular way? Technology has increased our options to include e-mail and voice mail and has made it easier to send a telegram. These are certainly faster than through the postal service, but the strategies for framing the content are the same. Legislators respond more favorably to individual letters/communication than to petitions or to form letters signed by individuals. Although you want to make your communication individualized, it must be brief and to the point. (See Box 15-5 for a suggested format for a letter to a legislator and Appendix 15-1 for a sample letter.) It is advisable to mention in the opening sentence what you want the legislator to do. If the amount of communication is substantial in relation to a particular issue, staff may simply sort it according to whether it is for or against a particular issue or action. You want to make sure they correctly categorize your letter.

The second thing you want to do is state who you are and clearly convey why your opinion has merit. Again, you must be brief. The fact that you are a nurse practitioner and may have substantial experience working with people who may be significantly affected by the policy is an important point. Be sure and state that you are a constituent, if this is the case. This statement should be followed by providing what you believe is the most important piece of evidence of the potential outcome of the legislation or the most vivid illustration. Legislators and their staffs will not read lengthy communications, so choose your points wisely. You can conclude by thanking them and offering to provide additional facts or information, if you believe they may view that as helpful. There are instances in which legislators simply want to know the responses (support or oppose) of their constituents. If this is the case, you may want to limit your communication to conveying that without the supporting data or illustration. This may also be more cost effective if you are sending a speedgram. Due to the screening for anthrax, mailed letters to legislators may be delayed.

Box 15-5 Sample Letter to a Legislator

Address to:

U.S. Representative	U.S. Senator
Honorable [name]	Honorable [name]
House of Representatives	United States Senate
Washington, DC 20515	Washington, DC 20510

Dear _____

I am writing to ask you to [co-sponsor/support/oppose (name & number of the bill)].

I am [if you are a constituent mention it] and a registered nurse and *[type]* nurse practitioner who [briefly state your special experience/expertise relevant to the issue]. If this legislation [passes/does not pass], [give a vivid illustration of the positive or negative impact, depending on your position. Be careful not to overstate your case, however]. You may be interested to know that [provide a key fact that will strengthen the case you are making]. Please feel free to contact me at [contact information], if further [information/statistics/data] would be helpful.

A safe and efficient means of communication is via fax. The addresses and fax and phone numbers for federal senators and representatives may be found at the following websites *www.house.gov* or *www.senate.gov*. Whatever means of communication you choose, remember that the ability to state your case simply and directly will enhance your influence.

How can I develop effective testimony?

You may have the occasion to give testimony to a legislative committee or at a public hearing in support of the policy change you are advocating. Whatever the situation, you will usually have the opportunity to present the testimony orally and to submit it in writing. Thus, you should bring a written copy. This copy should have your contact information on it. Often it is helpful to bring additional copies (perhaps 20 copies) to distribute to committee members, media representatives, and others attendees who may concur with your position.

Another thing you should consider is that speakers are usually limited to a set number of minutes. You must adhere to this religiously. At some events there is a timer and people are cut off when their time is up. If you are cut off, it will certainly detract from the points you are making. If possible, find out ahead of time the rules that will govern the conduct of the particular hearing.

It is also possible to submit a more lengthy written testimony. However, you should limit yourself to a few key points. The worst thing you can do is to try to address every issue. The most effective strategy is for people who are supporting a particular policy to carefully plan who will address which points. This way you can make sure that everything is covered and that you maximize the effectiveness of each individual piece of testimony. See Appendix 15-2 for an example of testimony.

What Is Your Message? Crafting your message should always begin by researching the issue and reading the bill or policy statement that has been proposed. Secondly, you must ask yourself these questions: What is your message, who is your audience, and how will you deliver it? The most frequent mistake people make when preparing testimony is to try to say too much. The testimony should begin with an introduction that states who you are and on whose behalf you are speaking (Box 15-6). You should also include in the introduction what you want the listeners to do. It is advisable to make no more than three points and you can include them briefly in the introduction. The body of the testimony can address each of the three points and include vivid illustrations (one per point) and facts. The conclusion should briefly summarize what you are asking for and the main points you have made. Less is truly more. If you go on at length, people may fail to retain the central points you are making. The media is also looking for sound bites and catchy phrases to include in their stories. When the ANA and other nursing organizations were trying to defeat the development of the registered care technologist (RCT),

Box 15-6 Testimony Components

Introduction

Salutation Address the person chairing the meeting and the officials who are there to receive the testimony.

Who you are (State your name and those credentials that would speak most to your credibility.)

Who you represent Are you speaking as an individual or are you speaking on behalf of an organization. Any testimony on behalf of an organization must be authorized.

State the organization's most powerful credential. For example, "I am speaking on behalf of the American Nurses Association, the voice of the nation's 2.7 million registered nurses.

What you want (I have come here to ... State your main points (no more than three).

    Point #1
    Point #2
    Point #3

Body of Testimony

Develop each of your points:
    Point #1 with an illustration and facts as appropriate
    Point #2 with an illustration and facts as appropriate
    Point #3 with an illustration and facts as appropriate

Conclusion

State your main points again and thank the body you are addressing.

they asked the public if they would like their *loved ones to be cared for by someone who had been flipping burgers only 2 weeks before?* This phrase created a vivid picture that emphasized the lack of training these individuals would have. This picture stayed with people far longer than the facts that were presented, and it contributed to the defeat of the proposed policy. Caution must be exercised in your choice of phrases, however. You don't want to just repeat slogans or phrases that are being promulgated already.

Who Is Your Audience? It is critical to be aware of your audience and to frame what you are saying in words that are relevant to them. Avoid using jargon. This is often difficult for nurses to do since we are used to speaking with other health care professionals, but it is critical for ensuring that people are following your message. Because nurses are with people at all of the important points in their lives, we often have wonderful experiences and stories to relate that can make our points very real.

The people in your target audience are stakeholders, so you should select the messages that address their stakes most closely. Legislators like to "do good" particularly when it is cost effective or at least cost neutral. The public wants to protect what they have (for example, client safety legislation), to increase positive outcomes (for example, legislation to lower taxes), and to see that critical needs are addressed (for example, child health insurance laws). Highlight your audience's stake, speak in language they understand, and use meaningful illustrations and they will pay attention.

Although research and careful preparation of testimony has been emphasized, Lustberg (2003) has indicated that the effectiveness in achieving the desired outcome is influenced 7% by the content, 38% by voice tone, and 55% by body language. Thus, it is important to consider how you are going to deliver your message. Above all you want to convey an open, positive presence (smile at every opportunity, raise your brow, and appear welcoming). Maintain good eye contact with the primary recipients of your testimony. You want to engage them and in effect say "come, join me in this position." Stand or sit erect and use natural gestures. Speak with a confident voice, at a volume sufficient to be heard and appropriately modulated. Speak conversationally (Lustberg, 2003). You want to appear warm and likable because it will make your audience more open to the points you are making. You need to be careful, however, not to create a false bond with them because it will not ring true and may have the opposite effect.

SUMMARY

It is obvious from the discussion that the opportunities for professional involvement are only limited by time and personal choice. Hopefully, it is equally obvious that professional involvement is imperative for ensuring that

---

 Resources to Help Develop Political Expertise

American Nurses Association website, *www.nursingworld.org.* The ANA website includes information on political strategy, legislative activities, and the latest information on policy issues critical to the nursing profession.

Buresh, B., & Gordon, S. (2002). *From silence to voice: What nurses know and must communicate to the public.* Ottawa: Canadian Nurses Association.

Congressional Directory. Order through Capitol Advantage, (800)659-8708.

Mason, D.J., Leavitt, J.K., & Chaffee, M.W. (Eds.). (2002). *Policy and politics in nursing and health care* (4th ed.). Philadelphia: W.B. Saunders Company.

Milstead, J.A. (2004). *Health policy & politics: A nurse's guide.* Frederick, MD: Aspen Publishers.

Policy, Politics, & Nursing Practice. Journal published quarterly by Sage Publications, Thousand Oaks, CA.

future practice according to standards and reimbursement rates determined by nurse practitioners is in your hands. It is certainly beyond the scope of a single chapter to deal with the politics of policy development in a comprehensive way, but you now have a few tools to guide you. Involvement in a professional organization is an excellent investment in your future. Whether your involvement is simply as a member or as an active leader, you can make a difference.

References

American Nurses Association. (1991). Nursing's agenda for health care reform. Retrieved May 4, 2004, from *http://nursingworld.org/readroom/rnagenda.htm*

American Nurses Association. (2000, June 28). *ANA House of Delegates sends strong message on mandatory overtime and nurse staffing.* Retrieved May 4, 2004, from *http://nursingworld.org/pressure/2000/pr0628.htm*

American Nurses Association. (2004). *Nursing facts: Today's registered nurses—numbers and demographics.* Retrieved September 2, 2004, from *http://nursingworld.org/ readroom/fsdemogrpt.htm*

Blumenthal, D. (1995). Health care reform—Past and future. *New England Journal of Medicine, 332,* 465-468.

Department of Health and Human Services. (2000). *Healthy people 2010: Volumes I and II.* (GPO stock no. 017-001-00547-9). Retrieved April 24, 2005 from *http://www. healthypeople. gov/Publications*

Deparment of Health and Human Services. (2004). *Prevention: A blueprint for action.* Retrieved May 2, 2005 from *http://aspe.hhs.gov/health/blueprint/*

Fallows, J. (1996). *Breaking the news: How the media undermine American democracy.* New York: Vintage Press.

Fate of nursing funds uncertain as congress adjourns. (1972). *American Journal of Nursing, 72,* 2139-2140.

Fawcett, J., & Russell, G. (2001). A conceptual model of nursing and health policy. *Policy, Politics, & Nursing Practice, 2,* 108-116.

Hanley, B.E. (1998). Policy development and analysis. In D.J. Mason & J.K. Leavitt (Eds.), *Policy and politics in nursing and health care* (3rd ed., pp. 125-138). Philadelphia: W.B. Saunders Company.

Henry, J. K. (2000). Political activism: Moving the profession forward. In J.V. Hickey, R.M. Ouimette, & S.L. Venegoni (Eds.), *Advanced practice nursing* (2nd ed., pp. 306-316). Philadelphia: J.B. Lippincott.

Jennings, C. (2001). The evolution of U. S. policy and the impact of future trends on nursing practice, research, and education. *Policy, Politics and Nursing Practice, 2,* 218-227.

Lustberg, A. (2003, March). *Communication tips for the 21st century.* Presentation at the midyear meeting of the National Council of State Boards of Nursing, Savannah, GA.

Mason, D.J. (1999). Nurses dancing with wolves. *American Journal of Nursing, 99*(8), 7.

Rogers, A.E., Hwang, W., Scott, L.D., Aiken, L.H., & Dinges, D.F. (2004). The working hours of hospital staff and patient safety. *Health Affairs, 23,* 202-212.

Salmon, M.E. (2001). Nursing in a political era. In J.M. Dochterman & H.K. Grace (Eds.), *Current issues in nursing* (6th ed., pp. 346-351). St. Louis, MO: Mosby.

Wakefield, M., Gardner, D.B., & Guillett, S. (1998). Contemporary issues in government. In D.J. Mason & J.K. Leavitt (Eds.), *Policy and politics in nursing and health care* (3rd ed., pp. 125-138). Philadelphia: W.B. Saunders Company.

Weissert, C.S., & Weissert, W. G. (1996). *Governing health: The politics of health policy.* Baltimore, MD: Johns Hopkins University Press.

Yankelovich, D. (1995, Spring). The debate that wasn't: The public and the Clinton plan. *Health Affairs,* pp. 7-23.

16

Professional Collaboration

Ruth Ann Brintnall

Collaboration

Collaboration between providers is a quintessential element of effective, efficient health care. Across settings, evidence supports that when communities of health care providers collaborate, client outcomes improve (Hamric, Spross, & Hanson, 2005; Hanson, Spross, & Carr, 2000). As a growing body of health care providers, nurse practitioners (NPs) who utilize collaboration have consistently demonstrated effective health care outcomes that are cost effective and yet high in client satisfaction (Cunningham, 2004). Where collaboration exists, outcomes centered on the client occur and relationships between the client and health care team are strengthened. When collaboration is absent, or ineffectual, health care becomes fragmented and competitive.

The benefits of collaboration between providers have been recognized by multiple professional and health care organizations. The American Nurses Association (ANA), the American Association of Critical Care Nurses, the National Institutes of Health, Society of Critical Care Medicine, and the Joint Commission on Accreditation of Healthcare Organizations have all acknowledged the positive effects of collaboration on health care services (ANA, 1980; Higgins, 2003). Moreover, the vision for health care reform described in the recent Institute of Medicine's study, *Crossing the Quality Chasm: A New Health System for the 21st Century* (2001), calls for collaboration across settings in a national effort to make our health care system more equitable, more efficient, and more client centered. When used effectively, collaboration works, and the partnerships that evolve between providers (such as registered nurses, physical therapists, occupational therapists, radiation therapists, speech and language pathologists, physician assistants, and physicians) as collaboration occurs promote mutual respect, minimize traditional hierarchical relationships, and promote satisfaction for providers and patients alike.

What is collaboration?

Collaboration is defined as a group of individuals who intentionally work together for a common goal (Jansky, 2004; Kenny, 2002). Other definitions of collaboration include these:

> Collaboration is a dynamic, interpersonal process in which two or more individuals make a commitment to each other to interact authentically and constructively to solve problems and to learn from each other in order to accomplish identified goals, purposes, or outcomes. The individuals recognize and articulate the shared values that make this commitment possible. (Hanson et al., 2000, p. 232)

Collaboration is

> ... integration of the perspectives and skills of each team member, and a process of complex problem solving. Collaboration implies the generation and evaluation of new problems (and plans) which result directly from the integration of individual contributions rather than simply the coordination of individual ideas. (Lamb & Napodano, 1984, p. 26)

As such, effective collaboration begins with the individual and in turn incorporates each team member as he or she contributes to comprehensive client outcomes. Effective collaboration among health care providers is critically important as health care providers are increasingly challenged to deliver efficient and effective care, and more than ever before, providers offer health care services in multiple-specialty groups and multidisciplinary health maintenance organizations. Because nurses have historically modeled effective collaboration between disciplines, opportunities for nursing as a discipline to champion collaboration exist as changes in our health care system continue to unfold. Evidence suggests that collaboration makes a substantial difference across settings and across disciplines. At the same time, professionals who work in collaborative environments describe higher levels of work satisfaction and have stronger commitments to clients and the organization.

What are the benefits and barriers to collaboration?

Multiple benefits and barriers to effective collaboration have been documented. Benefits to collaboration include:
- Improved client outcomes
- Increased provider satisfaction
- Cost-effective care
- Efficient use of resources
- Shared accountability for outcomes

In contrast, barriers include:
- Poor communication
- Value conflicts between providers
- Role confusion and ambiguity
- Competition for services
- Inconsistencies in regulation of practice

What are successful strategies that foster collaboration?

Multiple strategies have been shown to be effective in enhancing collaboration across health care settings. Of those, role socialization and role modeling seem to be particularly important. Thus, professional nursing programs should include content on team building, communication skills, and role and value clarification, as well as practice opportunities that offer interdisciplinary and team activities. Professional nurses in the workplace should seek an environment that values interdisciplinary collaboration and provides opportunities that incorporate nursing. Several interdisciplinary strategies in clinical practice have proven innovative and successful. Examples of successful strategies for interdisciplinary collaboration include:
- Interdisciplinary team conferences
- Interdisciplinary clinical rounds
- Interdisciplinary educational programs and continuing education
- Interdisciplinary quality improvement teams
- Interdisciplinary product line teams
- Formal and informal interdisciplinary consultation
- Interdisciplinary journal clubs

Two specific examples of improving client care quality using an interdisciplinary approach are the Schwartz Center Rounds pioneered by the Kenneth B. Schwartz Center (*www.theschwartzcenter.org*) and the organization huddle process described by Cooper and Meara (2002).

Schwartz Center Rounds were created by the Kenneth B. Schwartz Center to provide a forum for improving relationships and facilitating understanding between caregivers and their providers. As such, the Schwartz Center Rounds program provides an opportunity for multidisciplinary exchange because it brings caregivers from across disciplines together to discuss their thoughts, experiences, and feelings. In addition to team building, other benefits of Schwartz Center Rounds have been improved communication, a stronger sense of connection, and a greater appreciation for the role of colleagues. Schwartz Center Rounds has been used as an effective forum by members of the multidisciplinary team to examine important ethical issues and discuss challenging cases. The format provides a comfortable and relaxed setting where members of the multidisciplinary team can dialogue and support each other as they engage in difficult and stressful roles.

The organizational huddle process described by Cooper and Meara (2002) is another example of an innovative strategy that promotes collaboration. The organizational huddle is a problem-focused model that occurs as an ongoing rather than a scheduled process. The huddle process uses the concept of the ensemble to enhance communication and minimize barriers in the organization. By blending the expertise of multiple providers, higher outcomes are achieved. Huddle participants focus on their individual contributions, yet at the same time assume accountability for the group outcome. The huddle meets for only brief periods (15 minutes) as frequently as three times a week. There is no agenda and minutes are not taken. The success of the huddle depends on open communication, respect, and accountability as participants resolve problems, share information, and seek support from each other. In an environment of mutual goal setting, huddle participants produce comprehensive, informed, and timely decisions.

Other opportunities to collaborate exist in most settings. For example, professional organizations may have an interdisciplinary focus with shared governance opportunities. Local health projects or community initiatives often also seek professional volunteers. Interdisciplinary rounds or journal clubs that meet at regular intervals are still another excellent way to facilitate team building.

Collaborative Practice

Is collaboration the same as collaborative practice?

Collaborative practice is one method that is used to collaborate with a health professional or group of professionals. Within their professional roles, all NPs are expected to effectively collaborate with other health care providers. However, in certain roles the expectation of collaboration is more formal and means that specific shared accountability for client outcomes is expected. These roles, referred to as *collaborative practice,* usually require a formal contract.

What is collaborative practice?

Several definitions of collaborative practice have been posed in the literature. Most definitions imply a synergistic relationship between providers with common components such as shared decision making, client-centered goal setting, and collegiality. The American Medical Association and the ANA have developed the following definition of collaborative practice: "Collaboration is the process whereby physicians and nurses plan and practice together as colleagues, working interdependently within their scopes of practice with shared values and mutual acknowledgment and respect for each other's contribution to care for individuals, their families and their communities" (ANA, 2004). In earlier descriptions of collaborative practice, Siegler and Whitney (1994) identified several important components of collaborative practice that continue to be appropriate today. For example, they described these requirements: Collaborative partners must be assertive and yet work together in a cooperative manner; partners must also have differing expertise and yet work in a reciprocal manner; and last, partners must provide a unique perspective, or product, as the result of their combined approach.

How collaborative practice is defined for any partnership is critically important because the agreed-on definition of collaboration often sets the tone for the practice. Before NPs enter formal collaborative roles, they must have a keen understanding of how the definition of collaboration for their practice will be translated into purpose, functions, and responsibilities.

What types of collaborative practice roles have worked?

Across settings, there are multiple examples of success stories for advanced practice nurses (APNs) who practice as clinical nurse specialists (CNSs), NPs, certified nurse midwives (CNMWs), and certified registered nurse anesthetists (CRNAs). Advance practice nurses in collaborative roles have been successful in rural and underserved areas, outpatient clinics, private office settings, home care, community practices, acute care settings, and other settings. While the awareness of collaborative advance practice roles may be most visible to the public for CNMWs and CRNAs (Conger & Craig, 1998), APNs in other roles and other settings have been highly successful. For example, APNs have established roles with other health care providers in the acute care settings (Buchanan, 1997; King & Baggs, 1998); pediatric NPs have developed roles for inpatient services (Niemes, Barnaby, & Schamberger, 1992); geriatric APNs have collaborated to impact the discharge patterns of hospitalized elderly (Naylor, 1990; Neidlinger, Scroggins, & Kennedy, 1987); CNSs have comanaged care following cardiac surgery to reduce the length of stay (Lombness, 1994); NPs have managed complex HIV clinic populations with high-quality outcomes (Aiken et al., 1993); and NPs have developed collaborative models in the oncology practice setting (Bush & Walters, 2001; Kedziera, & Levy, 1994; Kleinpell & Piano, 1998). Still other APNs have worked to developed innovative roles in perioperative care and ambulatory surgery units (Guido, 2004).

As an example, an exemplar of a novice NP's experience developing a collaborative role is provided in Appendix 16-1.

What are the skills and characteristics of NPs who are successful in a collaborative practice?

NPs are leaders in their work environments and in communities. They help shape health care policy and advocate for vulnerable populations. NPs in collaborative roles frequently share common qualities such as these:

- Confidence
- Self-direction
- Clinical competence
- Conflict resolution skills
- A vision for the potential of NPs as a health care resource
- Flexibility
- Affability
- Humor
- Ability to effectively communicate with all members of the health team

How do I develop a collaborative practice role?

NPs interested in a collaborative role should begin by reviewing the nurse practice act in their respective state. The state board of nursing is another essential contact, and often, state boards of nursing have information on collaborative practice or formats for collaborative practice that NPs are required or encouraged to use. The National Council of State Boards of Nursing is another helpful resource for state-by-state information. A listing of organizations and helpful websites for NPs to explore as they develop collaborative arrangements is given at the end of the chapter. Table 16-1 lists state NP organizations and may also be helpful in exploring state-by-state practice. The ANA and other nursing organizations in the NP's area of interest should also be explored. Many professional nursing organizations also offer helpful websites and listservs or provide access to members who have pioneered collaborative roles and may act as mentors.

In all cases, the elements of collaboration must be clear before roles are implemented, and a written, legal document is essential. The document should guide all parties with regard to role and function to minimize ambiguity and duplication. At a minimum, NPs who are considering roles in collaborative practice should review the following:

1. The state nurse practice act and the occupational regulations of the state public health codes in their state that govern NP practice within the state
2. National standards of practice, such as *American Nurses Association Standards of Advanced Practice* or the *American Academy of Nurse Practitioners Scope and Standards for the Nurse Practitioner*, or related specialty standards such as the *Oncology Nursing Society Standards for Advanced Practice*

Table 16-1	Nurse Practitioner Organizations State by State
Alabama	North Alabama Nurse Practitioner Association
Alaska	Alaska Nurse Practitioner Association
Arizona	Coalition of Arizona Nurses in Advanced Practice
	Southern Arizona Nurse Practitioners–AzNA
California	California Coalition of Nurse Practitioners
Connecticut	Connecticut Nurse Practitioner Group, Inc.
Delaware	Advanced Practice Nurse Council of the Delaware Nurses Association
District of Columbia	Nurse Practitioner Association of the District of Columbia
Florida	Florida Nurses Association
Illinois	Illinois Nurses Association Council of Advanced Practice
Indiana	Coalition of Advanced Practice Nurses of Indiana
Iowa	Iowa Society of Nurse Practitioners
Kentucky	Kentucky Coalition of Nurse Practitioners and Nurse Midwives
Louisiana	Louisiana Association of Nurse Practitioner
Maryland	Nurse Practitioner Association of Maryland
Massachusetts	Massachusetts Coalition of Nurse Practitioners
Michigan	Michigan Council of Nurse Practitioners
Mississippi	Mississippi Nurses Association, Special NP Interest Group
Montana	Montana Nurses Association, Council on Advanced Practice
Nevada	Nevada Nurses Association
New Hampshire	New Hampshire Nurse Practitioner Association
New Jersey	New Jersey State Nurses Association's Forum of Nurses in Advanced Practice
New York	Nurse Practitioner Association of Greater Rochester
	Nurse Practitioner Association of New York
	Nurse Practitioners of New York
North Carolina	North Carolina Nurses Association
Ohio	Ohio Association of Advance Practice Nurses
Oklahoma	Oklahoma Nurse Practitioner Association
Oregon	Nurse Practitioners of Oregon
South Carolina	SC NAPNAP Chapter
South Dakota	Nurse Practitioner Association of South Dakota
Tennessee	Tennessee Council of Advanced Practice Nurses
Texas	Texas Nurse Practitioners
Utah	Utah Nurse Practitioners
Vermont	Vermont Nurse Practitioner Association, Inc.
Virginia	Virginia Council of Nurse Practitioners
	NAPNAP Hampton Roads Chapter

Continued

Table 16-1 Nursing Practitioner Organizations State by State—cont'd

Washington	ARNPs United of Washington State, WA State NP Group
	ACNM WA State Chapters VI-3 and V1-10
	NAPNAP WA State Chapter
	NPGS Nurse Practitioner Group of Spokane
	PSONS Puget Sound Chapter of the Oncology Nursing Society
	PSNPA Puget Sound Nurse Practitioner Association
	WSNA Washington State Nurses Association
	WSNPA West Sound Nurse Practitioner Association
Washington, D.C.	See District of Columbia
Wisconsin	Nurse Practitioner Forum of the Wisconsin Nurses Association

Adapted from Nurse Practitioner Central Nursing Organization. Retrieved October 3, 2004, from *http://nurse.net.*

3. Prescriptive drug privileges and Drug Enforcement Agency (DEA) regulations for NPs including mechanisms for securing a DEA number for prescribing controlled substances (See Chapter 4 for a discussion of this process.)
4. Mechanisms for obtaining a Medicare/Medicaid provider number (see Chapter 6 for a discussion of this process; the June 2002 "Report to the Congress: Medicare Payment to Advanced Practice Nurses and Physicians Assistants" may also be helpful)
5. Clinical privileging information for local health care facilities and/or hospital credentialing
6. State-by-state requirements and drug-prescribing restrictions, such as the table published by the journal *Nurse Practitioner* each January

What about barriers to NP collaborative roles?

Barriers to advanced practices are real, and collaborative practice is not for everyone or every environment. Common barriers across settings include:
• Reimbursement
• Role confusion
• Prescriptive authority
• Legal recognition of NP practice (Neale, 1999; Sheehy & McCarthy, 1998; Sheer, 1996)

State regulation of NP practice, local practice milieu, and organization barriers are also obstacles for NPs in many settings. Other barriers include confusion about the NP role, sex-role stereotyping, and conflicts in the traditional hierarchy of relationships (Sheer, 1996). Efforts to develop a collaborative role can be especially frustrating if the planned collaborative partnership contrasts local practice norms. Even when state practice regulation is favorable and advanced practice nursing is recognized, all parties must anticipate that the collaborative role might face a mixed welcome.

NPs also find personal barriers as they develop their roles as well. Such tasks as leaving familiar or traditional roles, developing new relationships, establishing credibility, building networks, and meeting resistance from nurses or other health care providers have been documented by NPs in pioneering advance practice roles (Brown & Draye, 2003).

Finally, the NP must accept that even when collaborative practice is successful, the efforts of NPs may not be revered or welcomed by some. Unfortunately, barriers to collaborative and independent practice for NPs still exist in some medically dominated communities. In those settings, NPs may be perceived as the competition by physicians as dwindling paybacks and managed care continue to impact health care. Thus, the NP in a collaborative role must be willing to accept "pioneer" status as the benefits of collaboration undergo further empiric scrutiny.

Collaborative Agreement

How do I develop a collaborative agreement?

Considerable thought and preparation is imperative prior to engaging in a formal collaborative agreement. Dialogue between would-be collaborators allows all parties to articulate their scope of practice, personal goals, and describe perceived contributions to the practice so that full potentials can be reached. To a large extent, failure to define role expectations before entering a collaborative agreement invites disappointment for all parties. When complete, the written contract serves as a mechanism for discussion and evaluation of roles and function, and at the same time, provides the legal framework to protect providers.

The NP should consult others in similar roles and seek examples of collaborative contracts or agreements from several sources. Local NP groups or national professional nursing organizations, such as the ANA or the American College of Nurse Practitioners (ACNP) can be helpful sources of information and sample agreements.

Most NP contracts or agreements have spelled out responsibilities such as the terms under which the NP will manage care, specific qualifications of providers, expected obligations of the employer, mechanisms for compensation, and particular provisions for enforcement of the terms of the contract (Herman, Ziel, & Kleinpell-Nowell, 1999). Prior to signing an agreement or contract, NPs must thoroughly review and understand all components of the agreement that will impact their professional and personal goals.

What do collaborative agreements look like?

Collaborative agreements vary greatly in format and appearance. A collaborative agreement is a formal, legal written statement that defines collaborative, complementary roles and working relationships for the practice (Herman, Ziel, & Kleinpell-Nowell, 1999). The collaborative agreement delineates the rights and responsibilities of each practitioner and provides the basis for a legally sound collaborative practice (Herman, Ziel, & Kleinpell-Nowell, 1999). Negotiating an effective contract is critical to successful practice and requires an informed approach much like other business transactions in life. Unfortunately, business and negotiating skills are not always stressed in graduate nursing programs, and this may disadvantage the novice NP. Reviewing the proposed contract with an attorney with regard to your responsibilities is a solid investment. Verbal contracts are not appropriate in the health care environment of today. Specific strategies for negotiating agreements are well described in Chapter 5. Additional examples of collaborative contracts can be found in the literature (Buppert, 2005; Kamajian, Mitchell, & Fruth, 1999).

With respect to collaborative contracts, the NP should look for common components in them such as the following:

- A clear job description indicating roles and expected functions including any possible limitations on role function such as hospital admitting privileges or drug-prescribing restrictions
- Particular privileging or license required for the practice
- Fiscal compensation such as salary, bonus, continuing education, sick leave, and retirement structure including health care coverage and insurance packages (life, disability, and malpractice)
- Practice issues such as private office space and equipment needs, call schedules, billing and reimbursement structure, evaluation process, professional dues and journals, and reporting structure, if present
- Terms of employment including length of contract, criteria for contract termination, or issues such as non-compete clauses should the partnership fail

What about collaboration and agreements with professionals other than physicians?

Formal and informal collaborative relationships are common among NPs and other health care providers who share mutual client goals or a common purpose. NPs often collaborate with other APNs in research, practice, and education within their roles. With NPs and other health providers, collaboration may take the form of a referral, consultation, or informal opinion. Collaboration may be sought for advice, a specialized skill or service, or by client (or third-party) request (Goolsby, 2002). Collaborative relationships with certain health care providers are expected for optimal client outcomes but may not require formal contracts. For example, collaborating with nutritionists, occupational therapists, physical therapists, or speech-language pathologists might be accomplished quite effectively with informal relationships.

In other situations, more formal agreements may be appropriate. For example, Conger and Craig (1998) describe a collaborative model of practice for CNSs and NPs where APN roles overlap and complement each other. In this model, the traditional roles of teaching and coordination of care were incorporated in the CNS role and therapeutic treatments were managed for the NP role. Consistent with the synergistic perspective of collaborative practice, combination of services provided by two providers in complementary roles for this practice resulted in better outcomes for their clients.

At times, the specialized skills of NP faculty are sought by groups of health care providers in private practice. In that case, collaborative roles or contracts for services may also be developed between schools of nursing and private practices as partners. An example of a collaborative contract between a university and a private practice is given in Appendix 16-2.

Referrals and Consultation

How do I establish referrals and consultations with other professionals?

Although the consultation and referral process for physicians is well established, the referral and consultation pattern between NPs and other providers is not well described in the nursing literature. Nonetheless, NPs who wish to build their practice with others can impact the process by seeking out other providers who share common values and goals, and yet offer services that complement outcomes for clients.

NPs can support each other and their APN peers by establishing and using APN referral networks. When referral opportunities arise and where appropriate, APNs can easily refer clients to each other. For example, a Family Nurse Practitioner (FNP) may refer a pregnant client to a midwife, or an adult NP may refer pediatric clients to a FNP or Pediatric Nurse Practitioner (PNP), and a PNP could refer a child with a difficult rash to an NP who specializes in dermatology. To be effective and efficient in referring clients to NPs and other health care providers, it is important to establish your referral and consultation network.

There are many different ways to establish your referral and consultation database. It is important to help your receptionist, medical assistants, or registered nurses to develop a referral system so that your clients receive care from your preferred provider network. You can either use a paper or electronic system to categorize your specialty's referral network (i.e., dermatology, obstetrics, gastrointestinal, wound care, optometrist, ophthalmologists) with specific NP, physician, or other health care professional information listed on the card. Data on each card should include name of the provider, credentials, title, address, phone number (back line), fax, and if possible insurance panel participation. The development of a comprehensive referral network can save the busy

NP time, develop a strong relationship with a specialist, and offer informal opportunities for consultation with specialists to discuss care plans or new treatments. These relationships can be invaluable.

How do I inform the health care community about my practice?

Informing the health care community of your practice by means of a *notification of practice* announcement may help visibility (see Appendix 16-3). Local professional organizations such as the ANA, Sigma Theta Tau, or other professional health care groups can often provide directory lists in your area. Announcements should be sent to provider offices and institutions that may benefit from your services. For example, a gerontology nurse practitioner might send announcements to area nursing homes, gerontology networks, and local senior centers. If you are willing to make house calls for seniors, make it known. Likewise, if you are skilled in the area of adolescence care and are willing to schedule after-school appointments, weekend hours, or provide services, such as sports physicals, indicate such on your announcement. When your practice opens, send a second announcement on your letterhead to affirm that you are available and accepting clients.

Depending on the practice discipline, participating in local nursing and interdisciplinary groups may increase your visibility in the community and, at the same time, serve as a source of referrals. Opportunities in education are also increasingly available as schools of nursing seek clinical preceptors or adjunct faculty. In general, look for gaps in health care services including the care of underserved populations in your area that might benefit from your care. When referrals or consultations come your way, promptly send out your follow up letter and include a statement of appreciation.

In your correspondence, the following information is helpful whether you are requesting or responding to a referral or consultation (Goolsby, 2002).

1. Demographic data
2. Summary of the present problem including present symptoms
3. Summary of health history, family history, and social history
4. Summary of findings including laboratory or diagnostics tests
5. Perceptions of the problem and management options
6. Summary of discussions with client and client preferences.

SUMMARY

As health care needs continue to evolve for society, NPs will be well positioned to make a significant contribution to the health care needs of society. To maximize their potential, ongoing documentation of NP effectiveness will be critical and role clarity will be essential. Moreover, coordinated efforts to inform health consumers, lawmakers, and other health disciplines of the scope and potential of NPs will be critical. NPs will need to engage in deliberate efforts to

Internet Resources

American Association of Colleges of Nursing
www.aacn.nche.edu/

American Association of Critical Care Nurses
www.aacn.org/

American Association of Nurse Anesthetists
www.aana.com/

American College of Nurse-Midwives (ACNM)
www.acnm.org/

American College of Nurse Practitioners
www.acnp.org

American Nursing Association
www.nursingworld.org/

Centers for Medicare and Medicaid Services
www.HCGA.gov/medicare/mcarpti.htm

Clearinghouse to APN links
www.nurse.org/orgs.html

Healthy People 2010
www.health.gov/healthypeople

National Council of State Boards of Nursing
www.ncsbn.org

Nurse Practitioner Central
www.npcentral.net/

Practice Guidelines
www.guideline.gov

confront barriers and establish their position as effective providers of care in collaborative and independent roles.

References

Aiken, L.H., Lake, E.T., Semaan, S., Lehman, H.P., O'Hare, P.A., et al. (1993). Nurse practitioner managed care for persons with HIV infection. *Image: Journal of Nursing Scholarship, 25,* 172-177.

American Nurses Association. (1980). *Nursing: A social policy statement.* Kansas City, MO: Author.

American Nurses Association. Collaboration and independent practice: Ongoing issues for nursing. *Nursing Trends and Issues.* Retrieved January 13, 2004, from the *www.nursingworld.org/readroom/nti/9805nit.htm.*

Brown, M.A., & Draye, M.A. (2003). Experiences of pioneer practitioners in establishing advanced practice roles. *Journal of Nursing Scholarship, 35,* 391-397.

Buchanan, L. (1997). The acute care nurse in collaborative practice. *Journal of the American Academy of Nurse Practitioners, 8*(1), 13-20.

Buppert, C. (2005). *Nurse practitioner's business practice and legal guide* (3rd ed.). Boston: Jones and Bartlett Publishers.

Bush, N.J., & Watters, T. (2001). The emerging role of the oncology nurse practitioner: A collaborative model within the private practice setting. *Oncology Nursing Forum, 28,* 1425-1432.

Conger, M., & Craig, C. (1998). Advanced nurse practice: A model for collaboration. *Nursing Case Management, 3,* 120-127.

Cooper, R.L., & Meara, M.E. (2002). The organization huddle process: Optimum results through collaboration. *The Health Care Manager, 21*(2), 12-16.

Cunningham, R.S. (2004). Advance practice nursing outcomes: A review of selected empirical literature. *Oncology Nursing Forum, 31,* 219-235.

Goolsby, M.J. (2002). *Nurse practitioner secrets.* Philadelphia: Hanley & Belfus.

Guido, B. (2004). The role of a nurse practitioner in an ambulatory surgery setting. *AORN Journal, 79,* 606, 608-610.

Hamric, A.B., Spross, J.A., & Hansen, C.M. (Eds.). (2005). *Advanced practice nursing: An integrative approach.* Philadelphia: W.B. Saunders Company.

Hanson, C.M., Spross, J.A., & Carr, D.B. (2000). *Advanced practice nursing: An integrative approach.* Philadelphia: W.B. Saunders Company.

Herman, J., Ziel, S., & Kleinpell-Nowell, R., (1999). Collaborative practice agreements for advanced practice nurses: What you should know. *AACN Clinical Issues, 10,* 337-342.

Higgins, A. (2003). The developing role of the nurse consultant. *Nursing Management, 10*(1), 22-28.

Institute of Medicine. (2001). *Crossing the quality chasm: A new health system for the 21st century.* Washington, DC: National Academy Press.

Jansky, S. (2004). The nurse-physician relationship: Is collaboration the answer? *Journal of Practical Nursing, 54*(2), 28-30.

Kamajian, M., Mitchell, S.A., & Fruth, R.A. (1999). Credentialing and privileging of advanced practice nurses. *AACN Clinical Issues, 10,* 316-336.

Kedziera, P., & Levy. M. (1994). Collaborative practice in oncology. *Seminars in Oncology, 21*(6), 705-711.

Kenny, G. (2002). The importance of nursing values in interprofessional collaboration. *British Nursing Journal 11*(1), 65-68.

King, K.B., & Baggs, J. (1998). Collaboration: The essence of acute care nurse practitioner practice. In Kleinpell, R.M., & Piano, M.R. (Eds.), *Practice issues for the acute care nurse practitioner.* New York: Springer Publishing.

Kleinpell, R.M., & Piano, M.R. (Eds.). (1998). *Practice issues for the acute care nurse practitioner.* New York: Springer Publishing.

Lamb, G.S., & Napodano, R.J. (1984). Physician-nurse practitioner interaction patterns in primary care. *American Journal of Public Health, 74,* 26-29.

Lombness, P.A. (1994). Difference in length of stay with care managed by clinical nurse specialists or physicians assistants. *Clinical Nurse Specialist, 8,* 253-260.

Naylor, M. (1990). Comprehensive discharge planning for hospitalized elderly: A pilot study. *Nursing Research, 39,* 156-161.

Neale, J. (1999). Nurse practitioners and physicians: A collaborative practice. *Clinical Nurse Specialist, 13,* 252-258.

Neidlinger, S.H., Scroggins, K., & Kennedy, L.M. (1987). Cost evaluation of discharge planning for the elderly. *Nursing Economics, 5,* 225-230.

Niemes, J., Barnaby, K., & Schamberger, R.C. (1992), Experience with a nurse practitioner program in the surgical department of a children's hospital. *Journal of Pediatric Surgery, 27,* 1038-1042.

Report to the Congress: Medicare payments to advance practice nurses and physician assistants. (2002). Medicare Payment Advisory Commission.

Sheehy, C.M., & McCarthy, M.C. (1998). *Advanced practice nursing: Emphasizing common roles.* Philadelphia: F.A. Davis.

Sheer, B. (1996). Reaching collaboration through empowerment: A developmental process. *Journal of Obstetric, Gynecological, and Neonatal Nursing, 25,* 513-517.

Siegler, E.L. & Whitney, F. W. (Eds.). (1994). *Nurse-physician collaboration: Care of adults and the elderly.* New York: Springer Publishing.

Additional Reading

Hickey, J.V., Ouimette, R.M., & Venegoni, S.L. (1996). *Advance practice nursing: Changing roles and clinical applications.* Philadelphia: J.B. Lippincott.

Kuehn, A.F. (2004). The kaleidoscope of collaborative practice. In L. Joel (Ed.), *APN: Essentials for role development.* Philadelphia: F.A Davis.

McCloskey, B., Grey, M., Deshefy-Longhi, & Grey, L.J. (2003). APRN practice patterns in primary care. *The Nurse Practitioner, 28*(4), 39-44.

Richmond, T.S., Thompson, H.J., & Sullivan-Marx, E. (2000). Reimbursement for acute care nurse practitioner services. *American Journal of Critical Care, 9,* 32-38, 59-61.

Salipante, D.M. (2002). Developing a multidisciplinary weaning unit through collaboration. *Critical Care Nurse, 22*(4), 30-39.

17

Professional Responsibilities

Leona B. Meengs

The Professional Role of the Nurse Practitioner

As professionals we are obligated to exhibit behaviors that advance the integrity, practice, accountability, and community involvement of the nurse practitioner (NP) profession. As such, the NP exercises accountability in several domains: (1) providing timely, cost-effective, and quality care; (2) maintaining competencies; (3) participating in research; (4) preceptoring and mentoring; (4) advancing the nursing profession through leadership in nursing organizations, community settings, and in political arenas; and (5) nurturing personal growth. By establishing goals, setting priorities, and budgeting our time we can accomplish our work and still have the time to relax, enjoy our family, and play. However, learning to manage time effectively can be a challenging task.

Making the Most of Time

As clinicians, we are continually expected to be more productive by learning new procedures, decreasing the time per client office visit, and increasing the number of clients seen per day. At the same time we must deliver quality care while maintaining a cost-effective practice. This is often a difficult task in the clinical setting where the type of office visit, age of the clients, type of insurance, and complexity of decision making are not always in our control. Therefore, effective time management skills are essential to maximize productivity despite the unanticipated variables of clinical practice.

What are my time management goals?

Time commitments must be evaluated in relation to both professional and personal goals that reward you for working hard but also support a healthy lifestyle with a balance between work and recreation. Identifying your goals is the first step in successful time management. Do your goals include seeing more clients per day, charting after every visit, delegating more, streamlining the practice, researching and implementing evidence-based practice, mentoring, or getting home on time?

Prioritize your goals and determine which are realistic and attainable and then map out a goal achievement plan that specifies activities to accomplish the goal. Finally incorporate into your plan a method to track and measure outcomes and celebrate successes. The next step in time management is to develop an action plan that includes assessing your personal style.

What is my personal style?

An important component of time management is incorporating your personal style into your strategies and action plan. For instance, if you need an organized environment to function, keep your desk or work area free of clutter. However, if clutter ignites creativity, allow only stimulating clutter. Another element of your personal style may be your circadian rhythm. Try scheduling your most demanding tasks at your time of optimal functioning. Whether you are a morning, afternoon, or evening person, this technique will probably enhance your productivity. Incorporating personal style into your time management plans may help you to improve your clinical management skills.

An obvious option is to focus on your areas of maximal effectiveness. However, it is also valuable to identify areas in which you are less effective. Incorporate elements of your personal style to enhance areas of weakness. For instance, if you thrive on lists, you may want to post reminders and guidelines, maintain a log for client follow-up, or incorporate visual reminders such as a large musculoskeletal poster in your office. While posters may prove to be helpful references, especially if you have limited experience in this area, they also can be incorporated into client education. The same can be done with colored brochures that identify the different inhalers or birth control options. Hanging a calendar in every room also cues clients in identifying dates of symptom onset. This simple strategy may prevent the loss of valuable minutes because some clients may spend considerable time backtracking events.

Conveniently placed informational materials are not only effective for client teaching but also function as great reminders for the provider. Relying on memory alone can be a *stumbling block* to learning; anticipate busy days and implement time-saving strategies beforehand (Solberg, 2003). When you are looking for a client education handout or client assessment or survey tool, remember that drug company representatives, professional organizations, and Internet sites are great resources. Besides incorporating your personal style into practice, "know what to put first and what to put off" (Weiss, 2003, paragraph 5).

Perhaps your personal style happens to be procrastination. Procrastination is a behavior that we all exercise to some degree. It is often a conduit to lost ideas, energy, and motivation. It primarily involves tasks that do not fit into the work-flow or require more time and energy than we are willing to expend. The tasks that you dislike the most are unfortunately easily left for later; however, one can increase the palatability of a task by developing a system of management. One example may be the development of documentation, routine exam, dictation, consultation, or referral templates (Backer, 2002). These templates can be used not only to maintain standards, but also to facilitate the process of interdisciplinary collaboration.

Another method of minimizing procrastination involves a change in work habits and the commitment to develop both routine and flexible strategies. The old adage of our grandparents that Monday is laundry, Tuesday is shopping, and Saturday is lawn care helped a generation to accomplish a myriad of often repetitive and boring tasks. In reality, we cannot rigidly follow this example; however, we can choose a time slot to focus on a particular project in an environment without interruption and then commit to the plan. Another option may be to simply find someone who is skilled at and would enjoy undertaking a particular project more than you. Take into consideration the skills and gifts of colleagues and staff and form partnerships that encourage the sharing of ideas. Working in a collaborative manner not only enhances productivity and creativity but can also be a means by which you can empower others to make needed changes. Meanwhile, you can focus your energy in areas where you are maximally productive.

How do I maximize my strengths?

Identifying and maximizing your strengths is crucial to time management. Vaccaro (2000a) advocates the 80/20 rule to improve individual time management. This rule states that 20% of one's productive time utilizes personal areas of strength and therefore produces 80% of the desired results (Vaccaro, 2000a). The areas of strength for providers would most likely include those responsibilities and duties that require professional attention such as assessment, diagnosis, management, and treatment.

Vaccaro (2000a) suggests that the 80/20 rule can also be applied to relationships in that most of your support probably comes from 20% of your colleagues, family, and friends. Keeping this in mind it is important to recognize, encourage, and inspire those who are supportive (Vaccaro, 2000a).

The following outcomes measure your success at working in your personal 20% (Vaccaro, 2000a, p. 2):

- You're engaged in activities that advance your overall purpose in life.
- You're doing things you have always wanted to do or that make you feel good about yourself.
- You're working on tasks you don't like, but you're doing them knowing they relate to the bigger picture.
- You're hiring people to do the tasks you are not good at or don't like doing.
- You're smiling.

Do I multitask or focus?

The preceding ideas are achievable goals; unfortunately, a nursing background often includes conditioning to *do it all,* which is the forerunner of overcommitment and micromanagement. To succeed and survive, nurses traditionally rely on the ability to multitask to the extreme. Surprisingly, new research indicates that a major weakness may be a person's reliance or tendency to depend on one's ability to multitask (Rubinstein, Meyer, & Evans, 2001; Smith, 2001; Vaccaro, 2003). Multitasking often involves a trade-off between efficiency and effectiveness; it causes valuable time loss, especially for the novice practitioner, who must continually refocus on the previous interrupted task (Rubinstein et al., 2001). It is important to recognize that as a novice your ability to multitask, assist others, or participate in additional projects may better be limited until you are more assimilated to the NP role.

To limit the urge to multitask, try bundling your tasks by saving review of lab work or response to telephone messages for one time slot. In the long run, focusing on the current task rather than multitasking may actually be a more effective and expedient method of accomplishing your goals especially in your first year of practice. As you become more proficient at the individual components of the NP role, you will be able to focus on multiple components (Smith, 2001). Yet, multitasking still plays a role if one recognizes the trade-offs. Depending on the task, you will need to determine whether multitasking or focusing is the tool to complete the task.

How and when do I delegate?

Imagine you are paying someone to perform every task you currently take on. Is each of these tasks really worth your salary? Can you afford to answer the phone or respond to interruptions for tasks that can wait or be delegated? Acknowledge that time is one of your most valuable commodities and prioritize you tasks according to importance and level of greatest return in terms of your goals (Eade, 1998), and then commit to a plan. Compile a list of activities that must be completed, supervised, or delegated by the provider; then invest in the time to provide adequate on-the-job education for staff, which, in the long run, will result in valuable time savings (Eade, 1998).

Once a task is delegated, leave it there and do not be sidetracked by everyone else's emergencies. Allow others to be accountable for their work. Your job is to encourage, empower, and evaluate outcomes.

How can I limit interruptions?

In most health care environments, NPs are bombarded with multiple interruptions. By virtue of your presence and availability, you will be questioned on many office policies and procedures. One strategy for limiting interruptions is to limit your availability. High visibility often increases the frequency of daily interruptions; however, visibility can be limited with the procurement of office space. In negotiating a job offer, NPs, like most other professionals, should advocate for an office not as a luxury but as a necessity that facilitates productivity. A quiet space is needed for dictation, charting, chart review, and private meetings with physician, clinicians, staff, and clients. If a private office is not available, share an office with a colleague. It is important to secure a quiet place to work, think, and refocus.

Other methods for eliminating distractions include having the discipline to avoid opening every piece of junk mail or e-mail you receive. Trash the correspondence that you do not recognize and use spam-limiting technology to block unauthorized or unrecognized e-mails. Limit distribution of your personal e-mail address and fax, telephone, and cell phone numbers. Use the e-mail file system as a method of recording communications. Employ the same tactics for voice mail. Remember to be discriminating; your time is valuable.

Finally, learn to limit distractions by saying "no." Ronald L. Hofelds recommends four steps to saying no: "Step 1, open your mouth; step 2, say no; step 3, close your mouth; step 4, keep it closed" (quoted in Weiss, 2003, p. 1). One could add a fifth step: Ignore the urge to defend or qualify your response.

How can I streamline office operations to save time?

A multitude of methods are available for helping to ease office operations. One long-standing time saver is the flag system. This system uses multicoloured plastic flags mounted on the wall of each client or exam room. Colors indicate different disciplines as determined by the organization. Tip the red flag for physicians assistance, green for the nurse, and yellow for the X-ray technician. I am not sure why some offices do not use this system. It is an effective method of communicating client needs whether signaling for the X-ray technician, nurse, medical assistant, or provider. The alternative is constantly stopping your progress, searching for the wanted individual, and verbalizing your request.

Other ineffective office practices may be managed by streamlining protocols and guidelines with the use of templates for reporting office lab results, tracking high-risk clients, and charting follow-up phone calls. You may also want to trial chronic disease flow sheets to ensure that you are providing evidence-based care. An example of a diabetes care flow sheet can be found in Appendix 17-1. It is also well worth the effort to keep the chronic/acute illness and medication flow sheets up to date. When your flow sheet is up to date, trends such as exacerbations of asthma or refractory sinusitis and medication history can be easily tracked. Another important function is tracking. Chapter 11 provides a discussion on the design and implementation of tracking systems such as an abnormal laboratory or diagnostic test. While you may forgo the tracking process because you remember what happened three visits ago, your colleague will have to query the last several progress notes. Providers who are asked to see your clients in your absence will appreciate your organization.

Effective office practices include developing a plan with the scheduling staff to restructure the client schedule to ease client flow (Backer, 2002), reduce waiting times, and obtain previsit demographics via mail or e-mail. In addition, office staff can be taught to incorporate into the schedule a balance between complicated and uncomplicated, sick and routine, unplanned and planned (Secor, 2002), and family and single visits. One office technique is to schedule planned visits before lunch and leave the late afternoon fairly open for unplanned visits. This system works well if there is a level of assurance that the unplanned visits will fill in the schedule. Otherwise try to schedule unplanned visits between routine, uncomplicated visits.

Address low-priority issues such as responses to phone calls and prescriptions during breaks in the client flow. Communicate your response, order, or prescription refill on a memo and delegate the follow-up phone calls. Consider using a reminder phone call, postcard, or e-mail system to reduce missed visits, report laboratory and test results, and remind clients of periodic screening test, immunizations, and tertiary disease management appointments. Incorporate technology when possible for document management, to track client follow-up, or for automated e-mail reminders. Dictation is a quick method of documentation but requires additional staff hours for transcription. If changing to a dictation method feels overwhelming, start by using a dictation template and initially incorporating the use of dictation for office memos, reports, and referral and consultation letters. In addition, provide timely up-to-date care by following guidelines that you can download on your personal digital assistant, post in your office, or paste into your favorite pocketbook or on postcards. Besides streamlining office procedures and your approach to client visits, streamline your communication skills.

When does effective communication save time?

Effective communication always saves time, eliminates mistakes, improves relationships, and reduces frustration. The first step in improving communication is to determine the best method of communication. Sensitive issues such as those that are related to conflict or those that have an emotional component are best addressed face to face, while communication via e-mail, voice mail, or memo is effective for follow-ups and confirmation of dates. When using e-mail or memos, review your note for legibility, accuracy of spelling, and clearness and conciseness of information. Remember to clear up misunderstandings in communication as soon as possible. Take into account that e-mail can be copied, forwarded, and made public without your knowledge despite privacy and confidentiality appendixes; therefore, it is imperative that all communications remain considerate, respectful, and appropriate.

How can I create time?

Monitor how much time you spend on trivial Internet surfing, television viewing, and electronic games. Most of these activities do little for the enrichment of your professional or personal life. Consider completing a 24-hour activity log to identify time robbers both at work and at home (Table 17-1). If you find that an extraordinary amount of your downtime is spent on these activities, consider setting time limits or work toward gradually incorporating optional activities that promote personal health such as exercise and meditation.

If you do find yourself sidetracked, easily distracted, or continuously handling crises, you may want to work toward prioritizing activities. Use Table 17-2 to

Table 17-1 Managing Time and Eliminating Time Robbers

Directions: For a 24-hour period, write down in a small notebook all activities that you complete as well as the time you engaged in the activity. After you have made a 24-hour record, determine the number of minutes engaged in each activity. An example of how to set up your chart is shown here.

Time Started	Time Completed	Activity	Total Time in Minutes

This activity is useful in at least three ways. First, it identifies any time robbers such as interruptions, unproductive meetings, telephone solicitations, unorganized activities, and time wasters that may be filling your day. Second, it shows you what activities you chose to spend your time doing. That way you can compare these activities to your personal and professional goals to see if they are congruent, or if you need to reprioritize your activities. Finally it shows your style of time management. Are you managing a crisis constantly? Are you spending all of your time in professional activities? How much personal time do you have?

Source: Adapted from and reprinted with permission from Nagelkerk, J. (2005). *Study guide for Huber leadership and nursing care management* (3rd ed.). Philadelphia: W.B. Saunders Company.

Table 17-2 Prioritizing Goals

Directions: Identify those personal and professional activities that are most important to you and prioritize them. This is the easy task because you have already established your goals. Now, make a daily or weekly list of activities that you need to accomplish and check them off as they are completed. This checklist should be a tool and should not become the center of time management. An example of a checklist is shown here. You may rank your activities according to their priority or star those that are most critical to complete first. This activity will help you organize your daily and weekly workload into a manageable list.

Activities to Accomplish	Date to Be Completed	Check When Completed
1.		
2.		
3.		
4.		
5.		
6.		
7.		
8.		
9.		
10.		

Source: Reprinted with permission from Nagelkerk, J. (2005). *Study guide for Huber leadership and nursing care management* (3rd ed.). Philadelphia: W.B. Saunders Company.

help you accomplish your goals. Prioritizing your daily goals will help you to manage your time effectively. In addition, you will be highly valued by your employer because effective time management is often one of the best methods of providing cost-effective care.

Providing Cost-Effective Care

What are strategies for providing cost-effective care?

NPs are valuable partners in clinical practice groups. They provide high-quality, cost-effective care (American Academy of Nurse Practitioners [AANP], 2000) with profits that are similar to those of the physicians' groups at a fraction of the cost and with no additional risk to clients. Employers often recruit NPs because they are highly skilled at health promotion (a traditional nursing value), client screening, and client satisfaction. These outcomes ensure provider incentive perks, which are financial incentives for high participation by clients in health promotion activities, provided by payers, for the collaborating physicians in practice groups. Successful NPs also increase practice profits by streamlining office procedures, improving client flow, and developing templates and encounter forms.

Additional strategies to ensure NP value in the practice group include not only increasing the number of clients seen per day but also increasing the average charge by carefully completing the bill forms to include all the services that are provided, judiciously using resources, and by petitioning payers for reimbursement equal to the physician rate (Buppert, 2001). By increasing the number of clients seen per day from 15 to 20 or 25 the NP can increase the practice profits from about $17,000 to $63,000 or $109,000, respectively (Buppert, 2001); consequently, the funds available for a potential bonus are also increased. However, even more profit can be generated by correctly charging for services. For example, an NP can charge for ten 40-minute counseling visits and realize a profit of $170,000 with the same revenue/salary/overhead formula as the above formula (Buppert, 2001). The importance of becoming an expert in billing and coding correctly cannot be underrated because your success is directly related to your ability to generate income (Abel & Longworth, 2002; Buppert, 2001).

The final strategy involves political activism (Buppert, 2001) and requires the combined efforts and support of all nurse practitioners. Currently, NPs are reimbursed by Medicare at 85% of the physician's level when the physician is not on site. However, Medicare provides 100% reimbursement under the *incident to* clause, when the collaborating physician is on site. Nurse practitioners will become a more valuable income-producing member of the care team when billing and charging regulations become equitable. For information regarding billing and other legislative issues that affect the NP practice, access the Internet site of the American College of Nurse Practitioners (ACNP) at *www.acnpweb. org*; the American Academy of Nurse Practitioners at *www.aanp.org*; Thomas Legislative Information on the Internet at *http://thomas.loc.gov*; your state legislative site, for instance, the Michigan legislature at *www.michiganlegisla- ture.org*; or FirstGov at *www.firstgov.gov*.

Providing Quality Care

Maintaining quality of care for your clients is achieved by working within your scope and standards of practice, following national clinical practice guidelines, documenting effectively by adhering to documentation standards, tracking client outcomes, and maintaining client satisfaction. The NP scope of practice and standards of practice are established by the licensing, credentialing, certi- fying, and specialty organizations. In addition, it is imperative to know and maintain competencies in your area of practice through continued education. Nurse practitioners also adhere to the American Nurses Association (ANA) *Code of Ethics* and the *Nursing Social Policy Statement* available from the ANA (*www.nursingworld.org/ethics/code/ethicscode150.htm*). The AANP position statements and *Scope of Practice for Nurse Practitioners* are listed on their website. The *AANP Standards of Practice and a Proposal for a Code of Ethics for NPs* (Peterson & Potter, 2004, p. 123) can be found in Appendix 17-2. In addition, confidentiality must be maintained by following the Health Insurance Portability and Accountability Act (HIPAA) requirements. Tips for HIPAA compliance and a free guide to HIPAA implementation are available from the American Medical Association (AMA) and can be found at *www.ama-assn.org/go/hipaa*.

National clinical practice guidelines are available from a variety of sources including the Agency for Healthcare Research and Quality (*www.ahcpr.gov.the*); the National Heart Lung Blood Institute (*www.nlhbi.nih.gov/guidelines*); and disease-specific organizations including the American Diabetes Association (*http://www.diabetes.org*), American College of Cardiology (*www.aac.org*), and American Academy of Otolaryngology-Head and Neck surgery (*www.entnet.org*). See Appendix 13-2 for a more comprehensive list of health care websites.

How can I demonstrate that I am providing quality care?

Your knowledge of and adherence to national guidelines must be supported by your documentation. You can opt for any of several methods to monitor your own effectiveness and whether or not you are following practice and documentation guidelines. One method is to use a generic or disease-specific tracking sheet at the beginning of clients' charts. This easily accessible and complete record of client visits, diagnosis, and treatment will help you to easily recognize problem patterns and track laboratory values, treatment regimens, and client outcomes. Table 17-3 provides a sample of a generic client problem list. Another method of ensuring quality of care is the use of disease- or population-specific encounter forms. A sample hypertension encounter form (Ebell, 2004) can be found at *www.aafp.org/fpm/20040300/79atoo.html*.

Another strategy to ensure quality of care is to conduct self-audits. Self-audits provide immediate feedback and the opportunity for self-improvement without the risk of disciplinary action. You can focus your self-audit on a specific client population or your documentation and coding practices. Initially consider doing a self-audit monthly; as you improve, you can decrease the frequency to a biannual schedule. Ask office staff to randomly pull three or four charts you

Table 17-3 Client Problem List

Date	Chronic Problems	Acute Problems	Treatment/Intervention

have dealt with since your last self-audit and use practice guidelines, medical review sheets, or tracking forms to measure your effectiveness. Use these results to monitor and reassess your personal goals for improving your practice and prepare you for audits conducted by employers and insurance companies.

Two tools that employers and insurers use to monitor documentation effectiveness are medical record reviews and client satisfaction surveys. Your results are compared to not only other providers in your setting, but may also be measured against national standards. Knowing the criteria against which you are to be measured is crucial to your success. Appendix 17-3 is an example of a Client Satisfaction Survey and Appendix 17-4 is an example of a Provider Peer Review Form.

If you practice within the ethical, legal, and evidenced-based parameters for your profession, you are practicing with professional responsibility and are less likely to provide unsafe care or experience poor client outcomes. In addition, you must demonstrate that you have maintained competency in your specialty.

Maintaining Competencies

Nurse practitioners are expected to demonstrate that they have acquired and maintained professional competencies in their area of specialty. Care competencies for adult, family, gerontological, pediatric, and women's health have been developed by the National Organization of Nurse Practitioners (NONPF) and the American Association of Colleges of Nursing (AACN). Besides care competencies, NP graduates are expected to exhibit core competencies of the NP practice as identified by seven domains: (1) management of client health/illness status, (2) nurse practitioner-client relationship, (3) teaching-coaching function, (4) professional role, (5) managing and negotiating health care delivery systems, (6) monitoring and ensuring the quality of health care practice, and (7) cultural competence (NONPF & AACN, 2002). A detailed description of the core and care competencies can be found at *www.nurse.org/acnp/clinprac/np.comp.spec.areas.pdf.*

Are there requirements for maintaining competency?

One requirement for recertification (adult and family NPs) is to earn at least 75 contact hours of continuing education or 5 academic semester hours per year (American Nurses Credentialing Center [ANCC], 2003). In addition, presentations or lectures at your specialty level, publication of a book chapter or article, and earned preceptor hours can be used toward maintaining competency and recertification. NPs who accumulate 1000 to 1500 practice hours, depending on the certification specialty, are not required to take the recertification exam if they meet the other recertification criteria (ANCC, 2003). You should check specialty recertification criteria at *www.nursingworld.org/ancc/certification/recert/reqs/nprecert.html* for the most updated requirements.

"Of the 75 continuing education credits, 50% must be earned from an ANCC accredited provider or from one of the providers [shown in Box 17-1]" (ANCC, 2003).

Maintenance of practice competencies, as well as optimal job performance including effective use of time, the delivery of quality care as evidenced by client satisfaction and outcomes, and the cost effectiveness of your practice, is covered under the umbrella of professional responsibility. Your level of performance in these areas is not only evaluated by insurance payers and employers but also by peer review.

Peer Review

Peer review is a component of the quality control process. According to the ANA (1988), peer review is "an organized effort whereby practicing professionals review the quality and appropriateness of services ordered or performed by their professional peers" (p. 3). Although peer review is only one component of the review process, it plays an important role. Peer review is used to evaluate the quality of provider performance and involves the review of a provider's procedural skills, clinical performance, documentation, coding and billing practices, or scholarly work (abstracts, articles, or books) submitted for publication.

Who provides peer review?

Review criteria are often determined by the employing organization as are documentation standards. Professional organizations often issue clinical practice guidelines that guide practice and establish professional standards. Journal editors develop publishing criteria for manuscript preparation and acceptance and utilize peer review to ensure manuscript accuracy. Employing organizations and insurance companies set credentialing standards for providers who perform

---

Box 17-1　Continuing Education Providers

- American Academy of Family Physicians (AAFP)
- American Academy of Nurse Practitioners (AANP)
- American Academy of Physicians Assistants (AAPA)
- American College of Nurse Midwives (ACNM)
- American Psychiatric Nurses Association (APNA)
- Emergency Nurses Association (ENA)
- National Association of Nurse Practitioners in Women's Health (NPWH)
- National Association of Pediatric Nurse Practitioners (NAPNAP)
- Accreditation Council of Continuing Medical Education (ACCME) accredited organizations. For example, the American Academy of Pediatrics and the American Psychiatric Association. (ANCC, 2003, p. 2)

clinical procedures. Peer review of the clinician is a component of quality assurance programs and plays a major role in ensuring quality care and client safety (Gluck & Scarrow, 2003; Livingston & Harwell, 2001).

Are there different types of peer review?

Peer review of clinician performance can be conducted either anonymously by a contracted independent medical review organization or internally with disclosed peer review audits. The advantages of an internal peer review are increased awareness and education acquired by the reviewers within the group, group-specific audits to particular problem areas, team involvement, cost effectiveness of an internal versus a contracted review, and immediate feedback versus that of a protracted review process (Bradshaw, 2000). Disadvantages may include biased reviewers, ulterior competitive motives, confidentiality issues, disciplinary action, and nonstandardized methods of measurement (Livingston & Harwell, 2001).

The advantages of a contracted audit include less time commitment and responsibility to already busy providers, confidentiality and therefore increased likelihood that the reviewer will be more forthright, elimination of internal bias and competition, and comparison to national standards and guidelines. Cost is the major disadvantage. The goals of peer review are to promote quality care, ensure client safety, identify areas for growth, and establish professional accountability (Gluck & Scarrow, 2003).

What are the review criteria?

The review criteria are dependent on several factors including whether it is a review of resource utilization, clinical skills and procedures, quality of care, adverse events, practice patterns, scholarship, or annual performance evaluation.

Performance evaluation includes a review of the practitioner's job description and the extent to which performance reflects that description. Box 17-2

Box 17-2 Elements of the NP Job Description

- Job title and classification
- Job summary
- Primary responsibilities: clinical, educational, and leadership/supervisory
- Qualifications: education, experience, and skill
- Licensing requirements
- Certification requirements
- Collaborating and reporting relationships
- Compensation and benefits
- Methods of evaluation

lists the elements of an NP job description, and Appendix 17-5 lists an NP job performance evaluation tool.

Besides practitioner performance that reflects their job description, evaluation also includes practitioner cost effectiveness in ordering diagnostics, accuracy of billing, client safety and quality of care, number of client visits, and client outcomes and satisfaction.

What are the controversies related to peer review?

The most controversial area of peer review is that of medical competency in determining eligibility for hospital privileges. An unfair negative review or disciplinary action may result in not only the loss of privileges but exclusion from insurance panels and therefore a significant impingement on the ability to practice (Livingston & Harwell, 2001). Likewise, a biased review that allows a provider to continue to practice despite questions of fraudulent behavior or substandard quality could result in criminal charges against the reviewer, employers, and hospitals (Livingston & Harwell, 2001; Ryan, 2003). Hospital privileges are governed by the board of directors, which often relies on peer review; however, recent criminal prosecution cases underline the ultimate responsibility of the board and the fact that the federal government does not have to abide by state confidentiality rulings regarding peer review (Livingston & Harwell, 2001; Ryan, 2003).

Are poor reviews of health care practitioners tracked or monitored?

The National Practitioner Data Bank (NPDB) was created in 1986 to encourage health care entities to identify, discipline, and track practitioners with poor clinical outcomes or unprofessional behaviors (U.S. Department of Health and Human Resources, Health Resources and Services Administration [DHHR-HRSA], 2001). Likewise the Healthcare Integrity and Protection Data Bank (HIPDB) was created in 1996 to "combat fraud and abuse in health insurance and health care delivery" (DHHR-HRSA, 2001, paragraph 3). The HIPDB reports include statistics by state and profession and the number of medical malpractice reports along with the reporting agency. These reports are available on the NPDB site found at *www.npdb-hipdb.com.*

Health care entities that are required to report nurse practitioner HIPDB-related claims are "medical malpractice payers, HHS office of Inspector General; federal and state licensure or certification agencies, federal and state law enforcement and investigative agencies, federal and state government agencies, health plans and federal and state government agencies" (DHHR-HRSA, 2001, pp. 2-3). Although, "healthcare practitioners, providers, and suppliers are not eligible to report" they "may self-query at any time" (DHHR-HRSA, 2001, p. 2).

Are there other roles for peer review?

Peer review can be used as an educational tool. Paukert, Chumley-Jones, and Littlefield (2003) found that peer review of charts by residents is an effective method of learning and improving overall performance. Reviewing the charts of providers is a nonstressful opportunity for students to internalize clinical pearls, learn precise phraseology, and trace critical thinking patterns. Likewise, it provides students with the opportunity to experience the audit process from both the reviewer and provider perspective.

Peer review is also used in scholarship and annual performance evaluations of educators. An additional benefit of anonymous review, for those seeking publication, is that it provides an avenue of entry for the novice writer because reviewers are not influenced by title, past successes, or professional affiliation (Chan, 2003). However, it is useful to seek internal reviews of scholarly work because it may build collegial partnerships that are mutually beneficial and increase the likelihood of publication.

Do I need specialized training for peer review of manuscripts?

Research has shown that training for peer review has marginal benefits. According to Schroter et al. (2004), differences between trained peer reviewers and the control group were statistically significant; however, benefits were obscure 6 months after training and the review improvements were not of editorial importance. However, it may be helpful to attend a review session at a professional meeting or ask your mentor to describe how she or he reviews manuscripts. This may provide you with useful tips and strategies for reviewing articles.

Do I need experience?

The expectation for peer reviewing is that you be an expert in the content area of the submitted article. In addition, personal experience in submitting an article for peer review is helpful. As a student, when encouraged to publish a scholarly paper by faculty, take advantage of the opportunity. If your colleagues or mentors make the effort to encourage you, they probably will be willing to provide assistance throughout the manuscript preparation and submission process.

It is also helpful to expand your portfolio of experiences by submitting articles to different journals. For instance, a family nurse practitioner with certification in hospice and palliative care, as well as experience in diabetes research, may have the opportunity to submit articles to the *Journal of Advanced Nursing, Advanced NP, Diabetes Care, Diabetes Educator, Gerontology,* and the *Journal of Hospice and Palliative Care.* The opportunities are boundless. If you have published extensively or have published a few articles in several different journals, you are more likely to be offered an opportunity to review manuscripts based on your versatility (Hall-Johnson, 2004). Likewise, it is to your benefit to expand your scope of experience to include articles in research, education, theory, and clinical practice (Hall-Johnson, 2004). A single project can be viewed from different perspectives (i.e., theoretical, implementation, results, and clinical application); therefore, you may garner several different publishable articles from the same project.

How do I apply for scholarly peer review opportunities?

The following tips are useful for breaking into the field of peer journal review. Contact editors for whom you have had articles accepted, send your request via e-mail and include your name in the subject field, all your contact information, your experience, writing, nursing, educational, research background, and resumé (Hall-Johnson, 2004). You can also get your foot in the door by submitting letters to the editor regarding a specific article or by requesting to write reviews or abstracts; your goal is to gain name recognition (Hall-Johnson, 2004).

What makes a good review?

Your hard work has paid off; you have been asked to write a review, and you are wondering where to start. The editor will provide review guidelines. The most important guideline criteria are usually that the articles meet the objectives, standards, and guidelines of the specific journal, will be of interest to the subscribers, offer new insight or information, and address an area where information or research is lacking. In addition, determine if the article information and literature review are up to date, the methods section is strong, the tools are reliable and valid, and the limitations are discussed. Remember you were asked to review this particular item because of your background and experience. After reading the manuscript you should be able to determine if the writer is knowledgeable about the subject matter. Are you satisfied with the level of information, and is it applicable to practice? Is the writing clear, concise, and thorough or is there a need for charts, tables, or diagrams to improve clarity; are the introductions and conclusions adequate and is there a discussion regarding future research needs and clinical application?

For the review to be helpful to the writer, it must be legible, clear, concise, and follow the reviewer guidelines provided by the editor. It is helpful for the novice writer when the reviewer types out specific suggestions and references them with the manuscript page number. It is also helpful if the reviewer makes copies of the manuscript pages where there is a need for clarification or topic expansion and makes notations on that page. Besides suggestions, corrections, and critique, remember to provide encouragement as well as direction; you do not want to discourage the novice writer (Davidhizar & Bechtel, 2003).

In summary, your responsibilities as a reviewer are to present a written review to the author, determine if the material reflects the latest research, ensure that the information is appropriate for the journal and advances the profession, and maintain confidentiality (Davidhizar & Bechtel, 2003). After appraising the reviewer's recommendations, it is acceptable for the author to choose to implement, modify, or decline some of the recommendations. NPs who perform peer review, publish articles, and submit editorial reviews are not only active in role modeling professional behaviors but also are actively advancing the profession of nursing.

Advancing the Profession

Both NPs and registered nurses are professional nurses who adhere to many of the same high standards of the nursing profession. Both are expected to exhibit behaviors of professionalism; but, what is professionalism? *Professionalism* is defined as the "conduct, aims, or qualities that characterize or mark a profession or a professional person" (*Merriam-Webster On-Line Dictionary and Thesaurus,* 2004). Who or what authorities decide the characteristics of the professional? We can accept the *Merriam-Webster* definition: A *professional* is one who "engages in one of the learned professions characterized by conforming to the technical and ethical standards of a profession. . . ." Yet, regardless of technical and ethical standards, the layperson may regard a professional as one who has obtained higher education, licensure, certification, and employment.

These definitions seem rather generic. While most individuals understand the roles and expectations of the nurse, many people are unfamiliar with the role of a nurse practitioner. Neither *Merriam-Webster* nor the proletarian definitions capture the distinctive significances and multiple roles that distinguish the professional nurse practitioner. Adams and Miller (2001) identified categories of professional behaviors of nurse practitioners that extend the *Merriam-Webster* definition to include "education preparation, autonomy, theory, and adherence to the ANA Code of Ethics, as well as participation in publication, research, professional organizations, and community services, as well as maintaining competency" (pp. 204-205).

Research, an often overlooked contribution, has significant impact on the advancement of the nurse practitioner profession. The NP role in research can be multidimensional and ranges from utilizing research in providing evidence-based care or participating as a subject in completing surveys or questionnaires to functioning as a primary or co-investigator in a research project. Research findings support NP effectiveness as clinicians in areas of quality, care management, and cost effectiveness. As such, nursing research has been instrumental in advancing the role of the NP in all areas of client care. Continued participation of nurses in research will continue to have a positive impact on not only nursing opportunities but also on client outcomes.

In addition to utilizing research, nurse practitioners have the ongoing responsibility of preceptoring the NP student and mentoring the novice practitioner. Besides teaching, preceptoring, and mentoring within the nursing profession, NPs must also educate society—laypeople, other professionals, clients, employers, and insurers—about what, where, when, and how NPs perform their duties, increase health care access, and negate the inadequacies of our health care system.

How do I educate the public regarding the NP role in health care?

Health care practitioners are frequently referred to as physicians or even physician assistants. However, rarely does the nurse practitioner receive recognition in the media as a health care provider. Newspapers, news journal and magazine articles, and television shows often discuss or portray health care issues, practitioners, policies, and dilemmas without recognition or inclusion of the nurse practitioner as a health care provider. Consequently, nurse practitioners expend much of their energy describing, advocating, defending, and promoting the NP role in a predominantly medically minded society. Notwithstanding, there is still a general lack of understanding regarding what nurse practitioners contribute to the health care milieu.

Educating the public about the NP role will take a collected effort on the part of all NPs. Each nurse practitioner can promote his or her role and profession in a variety of ways, including producing scholarly work, teaching nursing courses, promoting NP-friendly legislation, serving in community programs, and joining coalitions. Nurse practitioners should respond to media editors when NPs are clearly invisible in health care discussions, news events, and editorials. In correcting these omissions, the NP also has the opportunity to publicize NPs as excellent communicators and health care practitioners. Equally important to educating the public, is passing on knowledge and experience through mentoring novice practitioners and preceptoring NP students.

The Nurse Practitioner as a Mentor. The *Merriam-Webster On-Line Dictionary and Thesaurus* (2004) defines a *mentor* as a "trusted counselor or guide, tutor, coach" and a *protégé* as "one who is protected or trained or whose career is furthered by a person of experience, prominence, or influence." Mentoring is a give-and-take relationship (Restifo & Yoder, 2004). Mentors provide guidance, encouragement, opportunity, and links to influential persons within the health care community; protégés can support their mentor's work in projects, research efforts, and publications (Restifo & Yoder, 2004). In addition protégés can acknowledge their mentors with nominations for awards and community recognition.

Mentoring has long been considered a professional responsibility and has traditionally been defined as a partnership between the novice and the expert; however, some professionals have developed mentor relationships outside of these parameters. For instance, new PhD tenure track faculty have reported that group mentoring between themselves and their peers has accelerated their professional entry into the enclave of research publication and grant awards (Jacelon, Zucker, Staccarini, & Henneman, 2003). They have found that the sharing of experiences and individual strengths creates a synergistic-like force that accelerates career advancement.

Besides the novice, other more experienced professionals continue to enjoy meaningful mentor relationships for their ability to infuse a diverse layer of experience and add a flavor of richness to their own writing, research, and professional perspectives. As such, mentoring and being mentored remain not only career-long responsibilities but also ongoing benefits. In fact, there may often be a chain of beneficiaries to the mentoring movement. An example of a chain of mentor activity is one in which an undergraduate student is mentored by a graduate student who is mentored by a faculty member who is mentored by another more experienced member of the profession. A mentoring relationship may begin as merely an informal sharing of mutual interest or a willingness to be contacted for information and guidance, but eventually develops into a relationship of shared ideas, work, encouragement, and inspiration.

The benefits of having a mentor are numerous, yet finding mentors can be a difficult task. Juliet Santos (as quoted by Tumulo, 2004, paragraph 16) states that practicing NPs commonly avoid mentorship, indicating the "lack of time and mentoring experience" as major barriers. To fill the mentor gap, Santos developed an online mentorship service, which can be found at *www.npmentorship.com* (Tumolo, 2004). Additional suggestions for finding a mentor are listed in Box 17-3. Professional groups are especially helpful in locating mentors because group members often have shared interests in promoting individuals within their organization. In addition, local group members frequently have multiple contacts with similar interest and because they are active in the local community, they can inform their protégé of job opportunities before they become public knowledge. Other potential mentors

---

Box 17-3 Strategies for Finding a Mentor

1. Position yourself in mentor-rich environments.
2. Attend journal clubs and continuing education seminars.
3. Join professional associations.
4. Become active in your local chapter of the Sigma Theta Tau International Honor Society of Nursing.
5. Participate with online NP support and network groups.
6. Offer to help a potential mentor with a project.
7. Deliver timely, professional, and comprehensive results.
8. Volunteer for committee positions, mission trips, and humanitarian efforts.

include previous preceptors, instructors, faculty, or even fellow graduates. Your nursing or graduate alumni club is also a good network source.

Besides the benefits, a mentoring relationship can involve barriers and obstacles. Conflicts can arise because of differing expectations (Ulrich, 2003). To avoid conflict, expectations and responsibilities should be made clear at the onset of the relationship (Restifo & Yoder, 2004; Ulrich, 2003). The relationship between mentor and protégé should be amicable and the communication clear. Both parties should be able to tactfully exert their opinions, which should be respectfully accepted by the other. An ideal mentor should be able to acknowledge areas of potential conflict of interest and commit to crediting the novice for her or his contribution (Ulrich, 2003). Likewise, novices should encourage, support, and work faithfully toward mutual goals while acknowledging the contributions of their mentors toward their work and professional development.

What are the characteristics of a good mentor? Restifo and Yoder (2004, pp. 7-8) list the characteristics of a good mentor:

- Positive attitude and outlook
- Caring approach toward others
- Savvy insider, seasoned veteran, and experienced practitioner
- Compatible, personal chemistry
- Model employee, exemplary professional
- Good communicator, especially listener
- Someone you trust, respect, and admire
- Likes learning, loves people
- Experience as a protégé

Having a mentor can be a momentous force in your career development, and the protégé experience will sequentially prepare you to be an excellent mentor (Restifo & Yoder, 2004). Besides mentoring, which is often within the context of a long-term relationship, NPs often serve as preceptors who *mentor* students in the short term but in a more formal clinical experience setting.

The Nurse Practitioner as a Preceptor. Preceptoring is a combination of activities that includes role modeling, teaching, mentoring, encouraging, and inspiring a student. According to the *MSN Encarta* (2003), a preceptor is a "specialized tutor: a specialist in a profession, especially medicine, who gives practical training to a student." A preceptor is more often than not a volunteer who is assigned a specific student (Restifo & Yoder, 2004). Preceptoring has long been considered a responsibility of the medical and nursing professions; however, the increasing productivity demands of practice have in some cases increased the burden and diminished the joy of preceptoring. Consequently, some nurse practitioners and physicians are less willing to function in this capacity.

Ensuring the availability of excellent preceptors while maintaining an optimal experience for the student requires effective collaborative planning by the faculty advisor, preceptor, and student (Cloutier, Shandro, & Hrycak, 2004;

Lockwood-Rayermann, 2003; Mamchur & Myrick, 2003; Myrick & Yonge, 2004; Yonge, Ferguson, Myrick, & Haase, 2003). The plan must incorporate required competencies, facilitate student learning, and provide preceptor incentive and training. Methods of ensuring successful clinical rotations include good student/preceptor matches, preceptor orientation and training modules, student orientation plans, and development of procedural, experiential, and clinical hour logs to track student progress. In addition, a comprehensive package of easily available incentives is advantageous in recruiting and retaining clinically excellent professionals for the preceptor role.

Why is student/preceptor matching important? Good matching increases the likelihood that both the student and preceptor will have a positive clinical experience (Lockwood-Rayermann, 2003). When the preceptor is a physician, an important factor in matching is the acknowledgment of cultural, educational, and philosophical differences between the traditional modes of medical and nursing education. Mamchur and Myrick (2003) reported that NP students found "shared similar beliefs about the profession" (p. 193) a significant source of student preceptor conflict. This finding underscores the importance of shared beliefs, philosophies, and models of care between the preceptor and student. However, with NPs and physician preceptors, differences in the nursing and medical care models and educational preparation may contribute toward preceptor/student conflict.

NP students enter the clinical portion of their training with very individualized experiences in comparison to most medical students and residents who often have clinical experiences and classroom preparation that are similar to those of their physician preceptors. Medical students and residents receive the bulk of their classroom education prior to their clinical rotations, which then tends to require full-time participation. Conversely, NP students may receive the didactic education simultaneously with their part-time clinical rotation experience. Consequently, there may be a disparity between the two groups in the knowledge gained from classroom learning experiences.

While NPs tend to recognize the learning needs of NP students, other provider preceptors may identify with the learning needs of the third- or fourth-year medical student in comparison to the first- to seventh-year resident. After all, those with a medical educational background have lived a very similar training experience. In comparison, there is a wide variation in the NP students' background. While one may have medical-surgical experience, another may have pediatric, occupational health, or palliative care expertise, inpatient versus ambulatory care background, or one year compared to 30 years of nursing experience. As a result, the preceptor, either NP or physician, may have a very limited understanding of the student's level of experience and knowledge. As a result student and preceptor expectations may differ. Indeed, preceptors cited NP student "lack of competency on the part of the student relating to knowledge level, skill level, and the disparities between preceptor and student expectations" (Mamchur & Myrick, 2003, p. 194) as a major source of conflict.

Research by Myrick and Yonge (2004) uncovered an additional point of potential contention: "Often [nursing] faculty require, if somewhat subliminally, that students adjust to the practice setting with minimal disruption, while at the same time expecting them to reflect their newly acquired and often disparate educational ideals" (p. 375). Faculties are strained with finding and maintaining an adequate number of preceptor sites for a growing number of NPs in an era of increased competition from other nursing schools, medical students, and residents. The risk of losing a clinical site may be considered greater than the risk of unresolved student/preceptor conflict.

In addition, preceptor/student conflict has notably been ignored and often considered a result of an individual student's "personal and idiosyncratic [behaviors]" rather than "commonplace and collective" events (Mamchur & Myrick, 2003, p. 190). Contrary to common perceptions, Mamchur and Myrick report that 24% of undergraduate nursing students report preceptor conflict. Despite the finding that graduate students tend to experience less conflict, Myrick and Yonge (2004) were alerted to certain preceptor behaviors that had a significant impact on the success or failure of the graduate's clinical experience. Because conflict is more common than previously thought, it is important to assume that the graduate student is a serious adult learner, is success oriented, has a level of expertise, and is motivated to earn excellent preceptor evaluations that could culminate in exceptional job references.

Despite student motivation, their success or failure is intricately associated with their relationship with their preceptor and their clinical experience (Mamchur & Myrick, 2003; Myrick & Yonge, 2004). Therefore, mutual expectations and positive relationships in the student preceptor union are crucial in developing the student's critical thinking and self-confidence (Mamchur & Myrick, 2003; Myrick & Yonge, 2004).

Taking into account these recent research findings, nursing faculty should strive to promote a cohesive plan for enhancing relational experiences between students and preceptors. One method used to attain this goal is the student and preceptor matching process.

How are students and preceptors matched? Matching student and preceptors is a first step toward ensuring positive experiences. Therefore, it is essential to assess students' educational and experiential backgrounds, learning styles, goals, and desired areas of specialization. Likewise, course description, objectives, and expectations should be clearly conveyed to the preceptor. In addition, to achieve an ideal match it is imperative to assess the preceptor's teaching and leadership style along with student expectations.

The preceptor's teaching and leadership style is an influential factor in student and preceptor compatibility (Lockwood-Rayermann, 2003). Lockwood-Rayermann suggests that matching the student's reaction to a task and learning needs with the preceptor's leadership style enhances the clinical experience for both parties. Box 17-4 illustrates how to match goals with rationales.

Box 17-4 Student Matching According to Leadership Style

Preceptor Style/Behaviors

Directing (high directive, low supportive)
Coaching (high directive, supportive)
Supporting (high supportive, low directive)
Delegating (low directive, low supportive)

Student Approach to Task(s): Learning Needs

Unable, unwilling, insecure: Student needs structure and direct supervision.
Unable but willing: Student needs a mentor and role model and to feel *safe* when asking questions.
Able but lacks confidence: Student needs feedback and recognition.
Able and willing: Student needs autonomy.

Source: Data from Lockwood-Rayermann, S. (2003). Preceptor leadership style and the nursing practicum. *Journal of Professional Nursing, 19*(1), 34-35.

Preceptors who tend to direct may be better suited for a student's first practicum experience, whereas those who tend to delegate may be a better choice for the student's final practicum or a student who is experienced and confident. Matching students and preceptors according to preceptor style and students' response to a task may alleviate some of the conflict that students and preceptors report (Lockwood-Rayermann, 2003). See the appendixes for examples of a preceptor letter (Appendix 17-6), preceptor matching survey and key (Appendix 17-7), preceptor and clinical site survey (Appendix 17-8), student matching survey and key (Appendix 17-9), and NP student assessment form (Appendix 17-10).

Besides leadership style, Myrick and Yonge (2004) report that certain preceptor behaviors either "cultivate or curtail" (p. 374) critical thinking (Box 17-5). Student reaction to these behaviors is either to explore and participate in the decision-making process or to simply respond in a manner that is expected (Myrick & Yonge, 2004).

Given the recent evidence of student and preceptor conflict (Mamchur & Myrick, 2003; Myrick & Yonge, 2004), the deleterious effects of mismatched partnerships (Lockwood-Rayermann, 2003), and the difficulties in finding acceptable preceptors and clinical sites (Cloutier et al., 2004; Ryan-Nicholls, 2004), preparing and supporting nurse practitioners in the preceptor role cannot be undervalued.

Preceptor orientation. Effective preceptors assess their students' needs and develop and follow teaching plans. For an excellent module on teaching, download the Preceptor Orientation Module presentation developed by the Kirksville College of Osteopathic Medicine (KCOM) found at *www.kcom.edu/academia/preceptors/orientation.htm*. The orientation module includes preceptor

Box 17-5   Cultivating or Curtailing Preceptor Behaviors

Cultivating Behaviors

Respect
Flexibility
Openness
Safety/trust
Encouragement of skepticism
Independence of thought (truly valued)

Curtailing Behaviors

Role consciousness
Constraining
Closed
Unsafe
Unquestioning
Process is really about pleasing the preceptor; critical thinking dissipates

Source: Adapted and reprinted from Myrick, F., & Yonge, O. (2004). Enhancing critical thinking in the preceptorship experience in nursing education. *Journal of Advanced Nursing, 45,* 374.

preparation exercises, and both Ground Rules and Expectations guidelines (Appendix 17-11) and an Ambulatory Care Student Self-Assessment exercise. These teaching aids help the student and preceptor develop mutual expectation while preparing the office staff for the preceptor experience (KCOM, 2003).

Besides orientation modules, NP preceptors should adopt a model or framework to guide their teaching. A common model used in the medical and ambulatory care settings is the One-Minute Preceptor. This model provides a step-by-step guide for interaction: "(1) Get a commitment, (2) probe for supporting evidence, (3) teach general rules, (4) reinforce what was done right, (5) correct mistakes, and (6) follow up with a positive comment" (Neher & Stevens, 2003, p. 391). See Table 17-4 for the goals and interventions that apply to the One-Minute Preceptor.

The goal of the One-minute Preceptor method is to assess the student's critical thinking process and thereafter fill in the knowledge gaps with bite-size pieces of information. Consequently, busy preceptors who adopt a teaching framework are both effective in producing positive student outcomes and efficient in their use of time.

Preceptor preparation is vital; however, to be maximally effective, it must coincide with student orientations. Although it is traditionally the responsibility of nursing faculty to ensure comprehensive student orientation and learning guidelines, NP students should be proactive in identifying opportunities that address their individualized learning needs.

Table 17-4 One-Minute Preceptor

Preceptor Goal	Preceptor Intervention
Commitment:	What is your assessment or plan?
Supporting evidence:	Do you want to consider any other diagnosis?
General rule:	Order a HGA1c every 3 months if blood sugar is not well controlled.
Reinforce:	Your client teaching was excellent.
Correct mistakes:	Before diagnosis, confirm elevated blood sugars with a subsequent reading
Positive follow-up:	The ACE inhibitor was an excellent choice.

Source: Data from Grover, M. (2003). Teaching general rules during ambulatory education. In W. Huang, (Ed.), For the office-based teachers of family medicine. *Family Medicine, 35,* 160-162.

What are the components of the student orientation plan?

A comprehensive orientation plan prepares the student for success. Because many preceptors are busy practitioners, they often do not have the time to provide an appropriate orientation. Therefore, students should be given guidelines and self-orientation goals and encouraged to seek additional information by asking questions of office managers and paramedical staff. Box 17-6 lists items that should be included in the orientation.

How can I assist students in transitioning into their new roles? As noted earlier, the nursing and medical cultures are products of two different professions with different philosophies, different educational backgrounds, and different approaches to health care. These differences may have an influence on the experiences of the NP student. When two cultures come together for common goals, differences in expectations often arise. To alleviate a disparity

Box 17-6 Essentials of the Orientation

1. Introduction to staff
2. Familiarization with the organization's mission statement
3. Review of emergency protocols
4. Review of office procedures
5. Overview of documentation guidelines and parameters
6. Preceptor expectations regarding student autonomy
7. Introduction to office templates, forms, and stock medications
8. Office staff responsibilities and delegation routines (Do they use the flag system? Is there another method of communication? Do physicians routinely perform paramedical tests?)
9. Location of educational materials, medical supplies, and drug samples
10. Work station, computer access, library privileges, and location of additional learning modules, case studies, and reference books
11. Information regarding lunchroom, breaks, and food service

in expectations, students should be encouraged to prepare an outline of background experiences and learning objectives with specific goals for their precepted clinical experiences. Faculty who assign clinical preceptors can ask students about their strengths and weaknesses and also ask preceptors about their leadership styles. Faculty can then match clinical sites and preceptors to student needs (Lockwood-Rayermann, 2003).

It is equally important for faculty to inform preceptors of the level of independence a student should experience in the clinical setting in order to meet course objectives. While some preceptors expect the students to take initiative and be autonomous, others expect the student to observe for a prolonged period. It is important to not only discuss expectations with the student but to also promote increasing autonomy during the clinical rotation. When preceptor and student expectations are shared, the student is more likely to flourish and the preceptor is more likely to enjoy the teaching experience. In addition, the resulting relationship is a good foundation for alternative learning strategies.

What other teaching strategies promote student success? Additional strategies for preparing students for successful clinical rotations include student-maintained procedural, experiential, and clinical hour logs. These logs are used to promote student reflection of learning activities, function as guidelines for learning goals, and provide preceptors with an outline of student experiences, skills, procedures, rotations, and learning gaps. As the faculty member and/or preceptor, you can review the logs with students and plan clinical experiences for them to gain new skills. These logs not only help students progress clinically but also help preceptor and faculty members remember student skills and the clinical rotations when they are queried for a reference. Maintained logs are a benefit for the NP student when applying for a position; it is beneficial to have documentation of supervised procedures, skills, and experiences for potential employers.

Students' procedural and experimental logs should include the date, procedure/skill performed, and the preceptor's signature. Optional log information includes the site or clinic where the procedure was performed and the client's diagnosis. Your faculty liaison should have template logs available for your use. Appendix 17-12 is an example of a procedural and experiential log. Table 17-5 is a sample of a clinical hour log.

The procedural log should include nursing and medical skills and the additional procedures learned in the student's clinical rotations. Completing a log and obtaining the appropriate signatures at the time the procedure is completed ensure that the graduating student will be one step closer to obtaining ambulatory care and hospital privileges. Besides student preparation for clinical rotations and future employment, faculty members must remember to continuously build relationships with potential preceptors in the community.

Why provide preceptor incentives? Many preceptors teach for the personal gratification of encouraging, mentoring, and preparing the novice

Table 17-5 Clinical Hour Log

Date	Site	Preceptor	Specialty	Hours
_____	_____	_____	Acute care	_____
_____	_____	_____	Dermatology	_____
_____	_____	_____	Family medicine	_____
_____	_____	_____	Internal medicine	_____
_____	_____	_____	Long-term care	_____
_____	_____	_____	Mental health	_____
_____	_____	_____	OB/GYN	_____
_____	_____	_____	Orthopedic medicine	_____
_____	_____	_____	Palliative medicine	_____
_____	_____	_____	Pediatric	_____
_____	_____	_____	Wound clinic	_____

practitioner for independent practice. However, personal gratification may be a diminishing factor in recruiting physician and NP preceptors. The demands of a busy practice and the expectations of increased productivity may force preceptors to reevaluate their ability to expand their professional responsibilities beyond those directly related to the practice. As such, it is increasingly important to acknowledge and reward those who are willing and able to engage in the additional responsibilities entailed in functioning as a preceptor.

The preceptor incentives should be easily attainable and generally acceptable to a wide range of professionals. Box 17-7 shows a few examples of incentives that preceptors may appreciate.

Preceptoring can be as beneficial and rewarding to the preceptor as it is to the student, but it requires a concerted effort on the part of all stakeholders. As a nurse professional you can work as a change agent to unite the stakeholders and promote excellent learning opportunities for the nurse practitioner student. In addition, as you develop your professional roles you will undoubtedly have increasing opportunities to function as a change agent not only in advocating for students but also in leadership opportunities by promoting change in both your professional practice and in the community.

Leadership

Leadership can be defined as the "... position of a leader, the quality displayed by a leader, the act of leading ..." (*New Webster's Dictionary and Thesaurus*, 1992). However holding a leadership position and functioning as a leader are not necessarily the determining factors in leading successfully. Successful leadership is more often dependent on one's ability to "(1) model the way, (2) inspire a shared vision, (3) challenge the process, (4) enable others to act, and (5) encourage the heart" (Kouzes & Posner, 2002, p. 13). The successful leaders

Box 17-7 Preceptor Incentives

- Continuing education credits for recertification
- Access to the university library database
- Access to professional services available to faculty
- Season pass to athletic events
- Free or discounted access to the university recreational facility
- Bookstore discounts or gift certificates
- University discount or gift certificates for technology, software programs, and person digital assistants
- Free access to university hosted seminars and conferences
- Provision of end-rotation surveys to measure preceptor satisfaction
- Sending of thank-you cards from students and faculty after every rotation
- Students bringing in cookies or snacks for the office staff at the completion of a rotation
- Student nominations of their preceptors and mentors for special recognition or awards
- A small thank-you gift for the preceptor from the student at the end of the clinical rotation

of today reflect these qualities and are also portrayed as champions, facilitators, motivators, change agents, collaborators, and pioneers.

In all areas of professional influence including maintenance of satisfied and productive workforces, creation of community coalitions, headship in professional organizations, and activism in political arenas, effective leadership requires patience, flexibility, and the willingness to continuously cultivate one's leadership skills. As such, today's leaders are more introspective and open to constructive critique and evaluation from employers, supervisors, colleagues, and staff regarding their leadership style. Kouzes and Posner (2002) have developed a survey tool used by leaders to solicit feedback from supervisors, peers, and subordinates to help them assess and strengthen their leadership skills. Survey results can be viewed as graphs and compared to a self-assessment. The tool helps leaders to assess areas of strength and weakness and provides the information needed to develop a leadership growth plan.

While cultivating leadership skills, seize prospective leadership opportunities. Box 17-8 lists some of the types of organizations that offer opportunities for NPs to experience leadership roles. Resist the urge to sidestep leadership opportunities because you feel unprepared. You will never feel totally equipped for a new leadership opportunity because every opportunity is a risk-taking event, and in every leadership experience, success or failure, you will learn from your mistakes and develop increasing expertise (Kouzes & Posner, 2002).

Besides assessing and improving your leadership style and taking advantage of leadership opportunities, there are some common do's and don'ts (Box 17-9) for aspiring leaders to remember.

Box 17-8 Leadership Opportunities

- Alumni chapters
- Committee opportunities
- Community coalitions
- Opportunities for public speaking
- Professional organizations
- Sigma Theta Tau International Honor Society for Nursing
- Teaching opportunities
- Volunteer organizations

Personal Growth

In addition to professional responsibilities of the NP role, we must remain accountable to ourselves in the maintenance of healthy and active lifestyles and relationships. Nurse practitioners invest an extraordinary amount of time into career training, advancement, and productivity often to the detriment of personal relationships, job satisfaction, and spiritual growth and contentment. Remember, a rigid focus on educational and career success can strain relationships and have an adverse effect on overall quality of life. The professional demands can become overwhelming. Without boundaries and goals, relationships with friends and family may suffer. You will need to balance professional activities and career advancement with personal relationships and activities. There will be many career opportunities, and you will need to make choices based on your priorities and the effects that your career choices will have on your personal and family life.

Vaccaro's (2000b) philosophy of "creating the time of your life" (p. 1) rather than simply trying to create more time is worth remembering. She advocates the practice of "mindfulness" (p. 1) in which one completely focuses on the present, and on occasion "breaks rank" (p. 2) from the routine. Disengaging from our run-on mental lists, pagers, and phones allows us to create the memorable moments that make practice fulfilling. Breaking the routine falls in line with what we know about teaching, the average human attention span, and the ability to retain information. Occasional breaks from routine are invigorating and are often the ingredient to a satisfying balance between work and relaxation (Vaccaro, 2000b).

SUMMARY

You have worked hard and made sacrifices to attain your goals. Now you will have to work hard as a professional to maintain your ideals, protect your practice and avoid litigation, advance the nursing profession, and maintain a healthy lifestyle. To protect your ideals take the high road of integrity, adhere to the Nursing Code of Ethics, follow professional standards of care, and your

Box 17-9 Leadership Do's and Don'ts

Do

- Build trust and promote loyalty.
- Allow everyone the right to grow intellectually.
- Make error the opportunity for growth rather than cause for punitive disciplinary action.
- Encourage others to think *outside of the box.*
- Credit those who contribute toward your successes.
- Listen.
- Build teams and team camaraderie.
- Encourage openness.
- Negotiate.
- Develop effective conflict resolution skills.
- Develop an open door policy: be available, accessible, and visible.
- Squash negativity.
- Take time to recharge.
- Forgive.

Don't

- Micromanage; this is counterproductive.
- Discourage creativity or new ideas.
- Breech confidentialities.
- Take disagreement personally.
- Show favoritism among staff.
- Lose faith, hope, and compassion.
- Exhibit territorial behavior.
- Let your career monopolize your life.

state board of nursing's nurse practitioner act, rules, and guidelines. Safeguard your practice by providing timely, evidence-based, cost-effective health care.

In addition to providing superlative health care, protect your practice by perfecting your documentation, coding, and billing skills. To advance your profession, join NP organizations and access information regarding legislation that affects NP practice. Actively promote your profession in the political arena by writing letters to legislatures, visiting your state capital, and casting your vote.

Engage in opportunities to mentor not only the novice practitioner but one another. Take advantage of leadership roles so that you can not only facilitate change for better care and healthier nursing environments, but also role model the professional behaviors of encouraging, inspiring, and promoting. The challenges of the nurse practitioner profession are many, but you have taken up the challenge and endured the academic preparation. Your new goal is not only to survive the transition into practice but to thrive in your achievement and live a fulfilling professional and personal life.

References

Abel, E., & Longworth, J.C. (2002). Developing an economic IQ in primary care. *Journal of the American Academy of Nurse Practitioners, 14*(1), 1-10.

Adams, D., & Miller, B.K. (2001). Professionalism in nursing behaviors of nurse practitioners. *Journal of Professional Nursing, 17*(4), 204.

American Academy of Nurse Practitioners. (2000). Nurse practitioners—Providers of quality primary health care documentation of cost effectiveness. Retrieved September 9, 2004, from *www.aanp.org*

American Nurses Association. (1988). *Peer review guidelines: American Nurses' Association.* Kansas City, MO: Author.

American Nurses Credentialing Center. (2003). Recertification requirements for nurse practitioners. Retrieved October 15, 2004, from *www.nursingworld.org/ancc/certification/recert/reqs/nprecert.html*

Backer, L.A. (2002, June). Strategies for better patient flow and cycle time: These tried-and-true techniques will increase revenue, reduce expenses and improve satisfaction with your practice. *Family Practice Management.* Available from *www.aafp.org/fpm*

Bradshaw, R.W. (2000, April). Using peer review for self-audits of medical record documentation. *Family Practice Management.* Retrieved September 17, 2004, from *www.aafp.org/fmp/20000400/28usin.html*

Buppert, C. (2001). How NPs can increase profits for their practices. Retrieved November 18, 2001, from, *http://nurses.medscape.com/CBuppert/GreenSheet/2001/v03.n10/green0310.01.html*

Chan, Z.C. (2003). Letter to the editor. Peer review gives voices to the novice researchers. Response to: "Peer review: Evidence-based or sacred cow?" *Nursing Research, 52*(1), 67-68.

Cloutier, A., Shandro, G., & Hrycak, N. (2004). The synergy of clinical placements. *Canadian Nurse, 100*(3), 10-14.

Davidhizar, R., & Bechtel, G.A. (2003, Summer). Tips for manuscript reviewers. *Nurse Author & Editor, 13*(3). Available from Proquest database.

Eade, D.M. (1998, January/February). Time management five keys to peak performance. *Clinician News.* Retrieved March 3, 2004, from *www.adv-leadershipgrp.com/articles/time.htm*

Ebell, M.H. (2004, March). Improving patient care: A tool for evaluating hypertension. *Family Practice Management.* Retrieved October 6, 2004, from *www.aafp.org/fmp/20040300/79atoo.html*

Gluck, P.A., & Scarrow, P.K. (2003). Peer review in obstetrics and gynecology by a national medical specialty society. *Joint Commission Journal on Quality and Safety, 29*(2), 77-84.

Grover, M. (2003). Teaching general rules during ambulatory education. In W. Huang, (Ed.), For the office based teachers of family medicine. *Family Medicine, 35,* 160-162.

Hall-Johnson, S. (2004). How can I become a journal reviewer? *Nurse Author and Editor, 12*(1), 4-5.

Jacelon, C.S., Zucker, D.M., Staccarini, J., & Henneman, E.A. (2003). Peer mentoring for tenure track faculty. *Journal of Professional Nursing, 19,* 335-338.

Kirksville College of Osteopathic Medicine. (2003). Preceptor orientation module. Retrieved October 20, 2004, from *www.kcom.edu/academia/preceptors/orientation.htm*

Kouzes, J.M., & Posner, B.Z. (2002). *Leadership the challenge* (3rd ed.). San Francisco: Jossey-Bass.

Livingston, E.H., & Harwell, J.D. (2001). Peer review [Editorial opinion]. *American Journal of Surgery, 182*(2), 103-109. Retrieved April 6, 2004, from Ovid database.

Lockwood-Rayermann, S. (2003). Preceptor leadership style and the nursing practicum. *Journal of Professional Nursing, 19*(1), 32-37.

Mamchur, C., & Myrick, F. (2003). Preceptorship and interpersonal conflict: A multidisciplinary study. *Journal of Advanced Nursing, 43,* 188-196.

Merriam-Webster On-Line Dictionary and Thesaurus. (2004). Retrieved September 6, 2004, from *www.m-w.com*

MSN Encarta. (2003). Retrieved June 17, 2004, from *http://encarta.msn.com/dictionary_/preceptor.html*

Myrick, F., & Yonge, O. (2004). Enhancing critical thinking in the preceptorship experience in nursing education. *Journal of Advanced Nursing, 45,* 371-380.

Nagelkerk, J. (2005). *Study guide for Huber leadership and nursing care management.* Philadelphia. W.B. Saunders.

National Organization of Nurse Practitioners (NONPF) & American Association of Colleges of Nursing. (2002). Nurse practitioner primary care competencies in specialty areas: Adult, family, gerontological, pediatric, and women's health. Prepared for U.S. Department of Health and Human Services, Health Resources and Services Administration, Bureau of Health Professions, Division of Nursing. Retrieved October 14, 2004, from *www.nurse.org/acnp/clinprac/np.comp.spec.areas.pdf*

Neher, J.O., & Stevens, N.G. (2003). The one-minute preceptor: Shaping the teaching conversation. In Huang, W. (Ed.)., *For the office-based teacher of family medicine. Family Medicine, 35,* 391-393.

New Webster's Dictionary and Thesaurus of the English Language. (1992). Danbury, CT: Lexicon.

Paukert, J.L., Chumley-Jones, H.S., & Littlefield, J.H. (2003, October Supplement). Do peer chart audits improve residents' performance in providing preventive care? *Academic Medicine, 78*(10), S39-S41.

Peterson, M., & Potter, R.L. (2004). A proposal for a code of ethics for nurse practitioners. *Journal of the American Academy of Nurse Practitioners, 16*(3), 116-124.

Restifo, V., & Yoder, L.H. (2004). Partnership: Making the most of mentoring. *Nursing Spectrum-Career Fitness Online.* Retrieved August 31, 2004, from *http://nsweb.nursingspectrum.com/ce/ce190.htm*

Rubinstein, J.S., Meyer, D.E., & Evans, J.E. (2001). Executive control of cognitive processes in task switching. *Journal of Experimental Psychology: Human Perception and Performance, 27,* 763-797.

Ryan, T.J. (2003, September/October). The prosecution of peer review. *Michigan Health & Hospital Magazine,* pp. 20-23.

Ryan-Nicholls, K.D. (2004). Preceptor recruitment and retention. *Canadian Nurse, 100*(6), 19-22.

Schroter, S., Black, N., Evans, S., Carpenter, J., Godlee, F., & Smith, R. (2004). Effects of training on quality of peer review: Randomized controlled trial [Abstract]. *BMJ [Clinical Research Ed.], 328,* 673. Retrieved March 24, 2004, from Proquest database.

Secor, R.W. (2002). How I get home in time for dinner. *Medical Economics.* Retrieved March 3, 2004, from *www.memag.com/be_core/search/show_article_search.jsp?searchurl=/be_core/conten...*

Smith, D. (2001). Multitasking undermines our efficiency, study suggest. *Monitor on Psychology, 32*(9), 63-66.

Solberg, L.I. (2003). The KISS principle in family practice: Keep it simple and systematic. *Family Practice Management, 10*(7), 63-76. Available from *www.aafp.org/fpm*

Tumolo, J. (2004). Bridging the great abyss. *Advance News Magazines for Nurse Practitioners.* Retrieved July 21, 2004, from *http://nursepractitioners.advanceweb.com*

Ulrich, C.M. (2003). Research mentors: An understated value? *Nursing Research, 52*(3), 139.

U.S. Department of Health and Human Services, Human Resources and Services Administration. (2001). National practitioner data bank: Healthcare integrity and protection data bank: Fact sheet for practitioners, providers, and suppliers (HRSA No. 2039001-OY1-00929.01.00). Chantly, VA: Author. Retrieved October 8, 2004, from *www.npdb-hipdb.com*

Vaccaro, P.J. (2000a, September). The 80/20 rule of time management. *Family Practice Management.* Retrieved March 3, 2004, from *www.aafp.org/fmp/20000900/76the8.html*

Vaccaro, P.J. (2000b, November/December). Creating the time of your life. *Family Practice Management.* Retrieved March 3, 2004, from *www.aafp.org/fpm/20001100/64crea.html*

Vaccaro, P.J. (2003, May). Forget about time management: Focusing your attention is the key to getting more done. *Family Practice Management.* Retrieved March 3, 2004, from *www.aafp.org/fpm/20030500/82forg.html*

Weiss, G.G. (2003, March 7). Don't have time? Read this. *Medical Economics Archive.* Retrieved March 3, 2004, from *www.memag.com/be_core/search/show_article_search.jsp?searchurl=/be_core/conten...*

Yonge, O., Ferguson, L., Myrick, F., & Haase, M. (2003). Faculty preparation for the preceptorship experience: The forgotten link. *Nurse Educator, 28*(5), 210-211.

Appendixes

Culminating Clinical Behaviors

Family Nurse Practitioners

The following list, although not all inclusive, is a compilation of family nurse practitioner student goals of clinical experiences. Please use hash marks for number of times encountered. Seek out needed experiences.

	✓
I. Medical History (Able to obtain complete history of that which is appropriate and applicable for the patient concern.)	
A. Review of pertinent information from chart	
B. Chief complaint and HPI	
C. Past medical history	
D. Family history	
E. Psychosocial history	
F. Review of systems	
G. Able to record completely, accurately, and concisely	
II. Physical Exam	
A. Able to perform physical exam appropriate to patient needs	
1. Mental status (part of neuro)	
2. Vital signs	
3. Integumentary system	
4. HEENT (to include thyroid)	
5. Respiratory system	
6. Cardiovascular system (to include lymphatic system)	
7. Abdomen	
8. Musculoskeletal system	
9. Neurological system	
10. Genitourinary	
a. breast exam	
b. pelvic exam	

	✓
c. hernia check	
d. prostate exam	
e. rectal/anoscopic exam	
11. Complete gyn exam	
12. OB exam	
13. Family planning exam	
B. Able to record completely, accurately, and concisely	
III. To provide appropriate evaluation, management/referral, follow-up, and chart documentation for the following:	
A. Integumentary	
1. Eczema	
2. Psoriasis	
3. Contact/irritant dermatitis	
4. Tinea versicolor, pedis, cruris, corpora	
5. Pityriasis rosea	
6. Scabies	
7. Pediculosis	
8. Alopecia	
9. Ingrown nails	
10. Acne	
11. Abscess	
12. Warts	
13. Skin cancer	
14. Moles/skin tages	
15. Nonspecific rash	
16. Cellulites	
17. Childhood eczema	
18. Liquid nitrogen use	
19. Lesion removal	
20. Other	
B. HEENT	
1. Eyes	
a. conjunctivitis	
b. hordeolum/chalazion	
c. iritis	

Continued

	✓
d. foreign body	
e. corneal abrasion	
f. hay fever/allergy	
g. retinal disease	
h. cataract	
i. glaucoma	
j. cover/uncover test	
k. strabismus	
l. other	
2. Nose/sinus	
a. epistaxis	
b. allergic rhinitis	
c. sinusitis	
d. polyps	
e. other	
3. Ears	
a. otitis media serous	
b. otitis media infectious	
c. otitis externa	
d. eustachian tube dysfunction	
e. ceruminosis	
f. hearing loss	
g. tinnitus	
h. other	
4. Throat-mouth	
a. stomatitis	
b. tonsillitis	
c. pharyngitis	
d. mononucleosis	
e. hoarseness	
f. buccal lesions	
g. parotitis	
h. peritonsillar abscess	
i. temporomandibular joint (TMJ) syndrome	
j. other	

	✓
5. Neck	
a. adenopathy	
b. thyroid disease	
c. carotid bruit	
d. other	
C. Respiratory	
1. URI	
2. Sinusitis	
3. Bronchitis	
a. acute	
b. chronic	
4. Asthma	
a. pediatric	
b. adult	
5. Asthma education	
6. Emphysema	
7. Pneumonia	
8. Influenza/flu vaccine	
9. Croup	
10. Differential Dx cough	
11. Risk factors/occupational/environmental hazards	
12. Other	
D. Cardiovascular	
1. Chest pain	
2. Gallop, murmur, bruits, pulses	
3. Atrial fibrillation	
4. Heart failure	
5. Aortic stenosis	
6. Mitral valve prolapse	
7. Hypertension	
8. Chronic stable angina	
9. Hypercholesterolemia/lipid management	
10. Heart disease risk factors	
11. CAD	

Continued

	✓
12. Arterial insufficiency	
13. Venous stasis	
14. Other	
E. Abdomen	
1. Gastroenteritis-viral, bacterial, parasitic	
2. Differential Dx abdominal pain pediatrics and adults	
3. GERD	
4. Peptic ulcer disease	
5. Irritable bowel syndrome	
6. Inflammatory bowel disease	
7. Differential Dx-vomiting, diarrhea, constipation	
8. Hepatitis/cirrhosis	
9. Gall bladder disease	
10. Hemorrhoids	
11. GI bleeding-referral/follow-up	
12. Acute appendicitis-referral/follow-up	
13. Pancreatitis	
14. Other	
F. Musculoskeletal/Rheumatologic	
1. Arthritis-OA, RA	
2. Sprain/strain	
3. Cervical/neck strain	
4. Back pain	
5. Plantar fascitis	
6. Tendonitis	
7. Arthralgia	
8. Fibromyalgia	
9. Rotator cuff/shoulder	
10. Knee pain	
11. Lupus	
12. Ankylosing spondylitits	
13. Sjogren's syndrome	
14. Dermatomyosites	
15. Polymyalgia Rheumatica	
16. Temporal Arteritis	

	✓
17. Sclerode	
18. Osteoporosis	
19. Sports Physical	
20. Hip fracture	
21. Other	
G. Neuro	
1. Headache	
2. Dizziness/vertigo	
3. Fatigue/weakness	
4. Fainting/syncope	
5. Radicular pain	
6. Carpal tunnel syndrome	
7. Parkinson's disease	
8. MS/ALS	
9. Dementia/Alzheimer's Disease	
10. Delirium	
11. CVA/Post CCVA	
12. Other	
H. Genitourinary	
1. Urinary tract infection	
2. Pyelonephritis	
3. Abnormal pap	
4. Contraception	
5. Vaginitis	
a. yeast	
b. bacterial vaginosis	
c. nonspecific vaginitis	
d. atrophic vaginitis	
6. Sexually transmitted disease	
a. trichomonas	
b. genital warts/HPV	
c. chlamydia	
d. herpes	
e. gonorrhea	

Continued

	✓
f. HIV/AIDS	
g. syphillis	
h. nonspecific urethritis	
7. Breast	
a. masses	
b. tenderness	
c. discharge	
d. breast exam/SBE	
8. BPH	
9. Prostatitis	
10. Epididymitis	
11. Sexual dysfunction	
12. Gyn abd pain/R/O ectopic referral/follow up	
13. Bleeding/DUB	
14. Dysmenorrhea	
15. Amenorrhea	
16. Premenstrual syndrome	
I. Hematologic	
1. Iron deficiency	
2. Other/anemia	
3. B12 deficiency	
4. Hemochromatosis	
5. Abnormal WBC	
6. Other	
J. Diabetes & Diabetes Education	
1. Type 1	
2. Type 2	
K. Chronic pain	
L. Pediatrics/Prenatal	
1. Peds immunizations	
2. Well-child checkup/G&D	
3. Anticipatory guidance	
4. Initial prenatal checkup	
5. Drugs during pregnancy and breast-feeding	
6. Follow-up prenatal checkups	

	✓
7. Prenatal education	
8. Postpartum exam	
9. Other	
M. Psych mental health	
1. Anxiety	
2. Depression	
3. Substance abuse/referral	
4. Schizophrenia	
5. Other	
N. Health promotion	
1. Exercise	
2. Stress management	
3. Sleep	
4. Adult immunizations	
5. Prenatal referral	
6. Nutrition	
a. basic pyramid	
b. heart disease prevention/lipids	
c. anemia	
d. overweight	
e. diabetes	
f. hypertension	
g. gout	
h. osteoporosis prevention	
O. NAC Care (Natural/Alternative/Complementary Care)	
P. Procedures/Education	
1. Smoking cessation	
2. Infections in patient with other chronic illness (e.g., diabetes)	
3. Unna boot	
4. I&D of routine abscess/lesions	
5. Suturing	
6. Biopsy/Excision lesion	
Q. Lab/diagnostic ordering	

Continued

APPENDIX 1-1

	✓
1. Basic chest X-ray	
2. Mammogram	
3. R/O fracture X-ray	
4. Hematology	
5. Chemistry	
6. Urinalysis	
7. Basic bacteriology and virology	
8. UTS	
9. CT	
10. MRI	
11. EKG	
12. Specialty tests (list)	
IV. Forms, policies, and procedures to be familiar with by the end of the clinical experience:	
A. Mental Health Referral	
B. Outside referral to support groups—OA, AA, etc.	
C. Physical therapy referral	·
D. Referral to dietician and health educator	
E. Work excuse form	
F. Physician referral	
1. Within department—urgent and routine	
2. Subspecialty—urgent and routine	
G. Phone message slips	
1. Documentation of patient contact	
2. Call back	
H. Prescriptions	
1. Written	
2. Phone	
3. Protocols	
I. Cosign procedure for charts, lab, X-ray reports	
J. Appointment scheduling/changes	
K. Chart requests/chart transfer	
L. Release of medical information	
M. Knowledge of protocols for nursing staff	

	✓
N. Location of lab, X-ray, pharmacy, referral center, special care center	
O. Staffing pattern for department and role of registered nurse, nursing assistant, LPN, receptionist/appointment clerk	
P. Insurance forms, including Medicare/Medicaid	
Q. Workmen's compensation form	
V. Interpersonal skills	
A. Ethical dilemma handled well	
B. Multicultural encounters	
C. Competence verified	
D. Caring exhibited	
Reprinted with permission from the University of Wisconsin, Oshkosh College of Nursing	

Please use hash marks to indicate numbers

	ENT/ Sinus	Resp	Arth/ MS	Cardio Vasc	GI Abd	Integ	Endo, DM, Thy- roid	Eye	Periph Vasc	Neuro/ Fati- gue/ HA/ Dizzi- ness	Gyn/ GU	PN	Hem	Ment Hlth/ Psych/ Sub Abuse	HIV/ STD/ Infect Dis- ease	Hlth Promo	Well PE
Infant																	
Preschool																	
School age																	
Adolescent																	
Young adult																	
Middle adult																	
Older adult																	
Frail elderly																	

FAMILY TALLY SHEET

Please use a hash mark (✓) for each patient for each age seen

		Nursing 726	Nursing 727	Nursing 728
Newborn	0-1 mo			
Infant	1 mo- 1 yr			
Toddler	>1-2 yr			
Preschool	>2-4 yr			
School age	5-12			
Adolescent				
Young	13-15			
Old	15-18			
Young adult	>18-30			
Middle age	31-45			
Older middle age	45-64			
Gerontologic				
Young elderly	65-75			
Mid-elderly	76-85			
Frail elderly	86-95			
Frail elderly	96 & over			
Reprinted with permission from the University of Wisconsin, Oshkosh College of Nursing.				

State Board of Nursing Contact Information

Alabama
Alabama Board of Nursing
RSA plaza, Suite 250
770 Washington Avenue
Montgomery, AL 36104
Phone: (334)242-4060
Fax: (334)242-4360
Website: **www.abn.state.al.us**

Alaska
Alaska Board of Nursing
Department of Commerce and
Economic Development
Division of Occupational Licensing
550 West 7th Avenue, Suite 1500
Anchorage, AK 99501
Phone: (907)269-8161
Fax: (907)269-8196
Website: **www.dced.state.ak.us/ occ/pnur.htm**

American Samoa
Regulatory Board
LBJ Tropical Medical Center
Pago, Pago, AS 96799
Phone: (684)633-1222
Fax: (684)633-1869

Arizona
Arizona State Board of Nursing
1651 E. Morten Avenue, Suite 210
Phoenix, AZ 85020
Phone: (602)331-8111
Fax: (602)906-9365
Website: **www.azbn.org**

Arkansas
Arkansas State Board of Nursing
University Tower Building
1123 South University, Suite 800
Little Rock, AR 72204-1619
Phone: (501)686-2700
Fax: (501)686-2714
Website: **www.arsbn.org**

California
California Board of Registered Nursing
400 R. Street, Suite 4030
Sacramento, CA 94244-2100
Phone: (916)322-3350
Fax: (916)327-4402
Website: **www.rn.ca.gov**

Colorado
Colorado Board of Nursing
1560 Broadway, Suite 880
Denver, CO 80202
Phone: (303)894-2430
Fax: (303)894-2821
Website: **www.dora.state.co.us/ nursing**

Connecticut
Connecticut Board of Examiners
  for Nursing
Department of Public Health
410 Capitol Avenue, MS#13PH0
P.O. Box 340308
Hartford, CT 06134-0328
Phone: (860)509-7624
Fax: (860)509-7553
Website: **www.dph.state.ct.us/**

Delaware
Delaware Board of Nursing
861 Silver Lake Blvd.
Cannon Building, Suite 203
Dover, DE 19904
Phone: (302)739-4522
Fax: (302)739-2711
Website :
www.professionallicensing.
state.de.us/boards/nursing/
index.shtml

District of Columbia
District of Columbia Board of Nursing
Department of Health
825 N. Capitol Street, N.E.,
2nd Floor, Room 2224
Washington D.C. 20002
Phone: (202)442-4778
Fax: (202)442-9431
Website: **www.dcheath.dc.gov/**

Florida
Florida Board of Nursing
Mailing Address:
4052 Bald Cypress Way, BINC02
Tallahassee, FL 32399-3252
Phone: (850)245-4125
Fax: (850)245-4172
Physical Address
4042 Bald Cypress Way, Room 120
Tallahassee, FL 32399
Website: **www.doh.state.fl.us/ mqa/**

Georgia
Georgia Board of Nursing
237 Coliseum Drive
Macon, GA 31217-3858
Phone: (478)207-1640
Fax: (478)207-1660
Website: **www.sos.state.ga.us/**
plb/rn

Guam
Guam Board of Nurse Examiners
Regular Mailing Address
P.O. Box 2816
Agana, Guam 96932
Phone: (671)735-7411
Fax: (671)477-4733
Street address (for FedEx and UPS)
651 Legacy Square Commercial Complex
South Route 10
Mangilao, Guam 96913

Hawaii
Hawaii Board of Nursing
Professional & Vocational Licensing
Division
P.O. Box 3469
Honolulu, HI 96801
Phone: (808)586-3000
Fax: (808)586-2689
Website: **www.state.hi.us/dcca/**
pvl.areas_nurse.html

Idaho
Idaho Board of Nursing
280 N. 8th Street, Suite 210
P.O. Box 83720
Boise, ID 83720
Phone: (208)334-3110
Fax: (208)334-3262
Website: **www.state.id.us/ibn/**
ibnhome/htm

Illinois
Illinois Department of Professional
  Regulation
James R. Thompson Center
100 West Randolph, Suite 9-300
Chicago, IL 60601
Phone: (312)814-2715
Fax: (312)814-3145
Website: **www.dpr.state.il.us**

Indiana
Indiana State Board of Nursing
Health Professions Bureau
402 W. Washington Street, Room W066
Indianapolis, IN 46204
Phone: (317)234-2043
Fax: (317)233-4236
Website: **www.in.gov/hpb/boards/
isbn/appinst.html**

Iowa
Iowa Board of Nursing
River Point Business Park
400 S.W. 8th Street, Suite B
Des Moines, IA 50309-4685
Phone: (515)281-3255
Fax: (515)281-4825
Website: **www.state.ia.us/
government/nursing**

Kansas
Kansas State Board of Nursing
Landon State Office Building
900 S.W. Jackson, Suite 1051
Topeka, KS 6612
Phone: (785)296-4929
Fax: (785)296-3929
Website: **www.ksbn.org**

Kentucky
Kentucky Board of Nursing
312 Whittington Parkway, Suite 300
Louisville, KY 40222
Phone: (502)329-7000
Fax: (502)329-7011
Website: **www.kbn.ky.gov**

Louisiana
Louisiana State Board of Nursing
3510 N. Causeway Boulevard,
Suite 501
Metairie, LA 70002
Phone: (504)838-5332
Fax: (504)838-5349
Website: **www.lsbn.state.la.us/**

Maine
Maine State Board of Nursing
158 State House Station
Augusta, ME 04333
Phone: (207)287-1133
Fax: (207)287-1149
Website: **www.maine.gov/
boardofnursing/**

Maryland
Maryland Board of Nursing
4140 Patterson Avenue
Baltimore, MD 21215
Phone: (410)585-1900
Fax: (410)358-3530
Website: **www.mbon.org/
main.php**

Massachusetts
Massachusetts Board of
    Registration in Nursing
Commonwealth of
    Massachusetts
239 Causeway Street
Boston, MA 02114
Phone: (617)727-9961
Fax: (617)727-1630
Website: **www.mass.gov/
dpl/boards/rn/index.htm**

Michigan
Michigan CIS Bureau
Ottawa Towers North
611 W. Ottawa 1st Floor
Lansing, MI 48933
Phone: (517)335-0918
Fax: (517)373-2179
Website: **www.michigan.gov/
healthlicense**

Minnesota
Minnesota Board of Nursing
2829 University Avenue, S.E.,
Suite 500
Minneapolis, MN 55414
Phone: (612)617-2270
Fax: (612)617-2190
Website: **www.nursingboard.state.
mn.us/**

Mississippi
Mississippi Board of Nursing
1935 Lakeland Drive, Suite B
Jackson, MS 39216-5014
Phone: (601)987-4188
Fax: (601)364-2352
Website: **www.msbn.state.ms.us/**

Missouri
Missouri State Board
of Nursing
3605 Missouri Boulevard
P.O. Box 656
Jefferson City, MO 65102-0656
Phone: (573)751-0681
Fax: (573)751-0075
Website: **www.pr.mo.gov/
nursing.asp**

Montana
Montana State Board of Nursing
301 South Park
P.O. Box 200513
Helena, MT 59620-0513
Phone: (406)841-2340
Fax: (406)841-2343
Website: **www.discovering
montana.com/dli/bsd/license/
bsd_boards/nur_board/
board_page.asp**

Nebraska
Nebraska Health and Human Services
System
Dept. of Regulation and Licensure,
Nursing Section
301 Centennial Mall South,
P.O. Box 94986
Lincoln, N.E. 68509-4986
Phone: (402)471-4376
Fax: (402)471-1066
Website: **www.hhs.state.ne.us/crl/
nursing/nursingindex.htm**

Nevada
Nevada State Board of Nursing
Administration, Discipline &
Investigations
5011 Meadowood Mall #201
Reno, NV 89502-6547
Phone: (775)688-2620
Fax: (775)688-2628
Website: **www.nursingboard.
state. nv.us**
Nevada State Board of Nursing
License Certification and Education
4330 S. Valley View Blvd., Suite 106
Las Vegas, NV 89103
Phone: (702)486-5800
Fax: (702)486-5803

New Hampshire
New Hampshire Board of Nursing
P.O. Box 3898
78 Regional Drive, Bldg. B
Concord, NH 03302
Phone: (603)271-2323
Fax: (603)271-6605
Website: **www.state.nh.us.nursing/**

New Jersey
New Jersey Board of Nursing
P.O. Box 45010
Newark, NJ 07101
Phone: (973)504-6586
Fax: (973)648-3481
Website: **www.state.nj.us/lps/ca/
medical.htm**

New Mexico
New Mexico Board of Nursing
4206 Louisiana Boulevard, NE,
Suite A
Albuquerque, NM 87109
Phone: (505)841-8340
Fax: (505)841-8347
Website: **www.state.nm.us/
clients/nursing**

New York
New York State Board of Nursing
Education Building
89 Washington Ave.
2nd Floor West Wing
Albany, NY 12234
Phone: (518)474-3817 Ext. 120
Fax: (518)474-3706
Website: **www.nysed.gov/prof/
nurse.htm**

North Carolina
North Carolina Board of Nursing
3724 National Drive, Suite 201
Raleigh, NC 27612
Phone: (919)782-3211
Fax: (919)781-9461
Website: **www.ncbon.com/**

North Dakota
North Dakota Board of Nursing
919 South 7th Street, Suite 504
Bismark, ND 58504
Phone: (701)328-9777
Fax: (701)328-9785
Website: **www.ndbon.org/**

Northern Mariana Islands
Commonwealth Board of Nurse
    Examiners
P.O. Box 501458
Saipan, MP 96950
Phone: (670)664-4812
Fax: (670)664-4813

Ohio
Ohio Board of Nursing
17 South High Street, Suite 400
Columbus, OH 43215-3413
Phone: (614)466-3947
Fax: (614)466-0388
Website: **www.nursing.ohio.gov**

Oklahoma
Oklahoma Board of Nursing
2915 N. Classen Boulevard, Suite 524
Oklahoma City, OK 73106
Phone: (405)962-1800
Fax: (405)962-1821
Website: **www.youroklahoma.com/
nursing**

Oregon
Oregon State Board of Nursing
800 NE Oregon Street, Box 25
Suite 465
Portland, OR 97232
Phone: (503)731-4745
Fax: (503)731-4755
Website: **www.osbn.state.or.us/**

Pennsylvania
Pennsylvania State Board of Nursing
P.O. 2649
2601 N. 3rd St.
Harrisburg, PA 17101
Phone: (717)783-7142
Fax: (717)783-0822
Website: **www.dos.state.pa.us/
bpoa/cwp/**

Puerto Rico
Commonwealth of Puerto Rico
Board of Nurse Examiners
800 Roberto H. Todd Avenue
Room 202, Stop 18
Santurce, PR 00908
Phone: (787)725-7506
Fax: (787)725-7903

Rhode Island
Rhode Island Board
  of Nursing
Registration and Nursing
  Education
105 Cannon Building
Three Capitol Hill
Providence, RI 02908
Phone: (401)222-5700
Fax: (401)222-3352
Website: **www.health.ri.gov/hsr/**
professions/nurses.php

South Carolina
South Carolina State Board of Nursing
110 Centerview Drive, Suite 202
Columbia, SC 29210
Phone: (803)896-4550
Fax: (803)896-4525
Website: **www.llr.state.sc.us/POL/**
Nursing/

South Dakota
South Dakota Board of Nursing
4305 South Louise Ave., Suite 201
Sioux Falls, SD 57106-3115
Phone: (605)362-2760
Fax: (605)362-2768
Website: **www.state.sd.us/dcr/**
nursing/

Tennessee
Tennessee State Board of Nursing
425 Fifth Avenue North
1st Floor—Cordell Hull Building
Nashville, TN 37247
Phone: (615)532-5166
Fax: (615)741-7899
Website: **www.tennessee.gov/**
health

Texas
Texas Board of Nurse
  Examiners
333 Guadalupe, Suite 3-460
Austin, TX 78701
Phone: (512)305-7400
Fax: (512)305-7401
Website: **www.bne.state.tx.us/**

Utah
Utah State Board of Nursing
Heber M. Wells Bldg., 4th Floor
160 East 300 South
Salt Lake City, UT 84111
Phone: (801)530-6628
Fax: (801)530-6511
Website: **www.commercse.**
state.ut/us/

Vermont
Vermont State Board of Nursing
109 State Street
Montpelier, VT 05609-1106
Phone: (802)828-2396
Fax: (802)828-2484
Website: **www.vtprofessionals.org/**
opr1/nurses/

Virgin Islands
Virginia Islands Board of Nurse
  Licensure
Veterans Drive Station
St. Thomas, VI 00803
Phone: (340)776-7397
Fax: (340)777-4003

Virginia
Virginia Board of Nursing
6603 West Broad Street
5th Floor
Richmond, VA 23230-1712
Phone: (804)662-9909
Fax: (804)662-9512
Website: **www.dhp.state.va.us/**

Washington
Washington State Nursing Care Quality
  Assurance Commission
Department of Health
HPQA #6
310 Israel Rd SE
Tumwater, WA 98501-7864
Phone: (360)236-4700
Fax: (360)236-4738
Website: **www.fortress.wa.gov/
doh/hpqa2/hps6/nursing/
default.htm**

West Virginia
West Virginia State Board of Examiners
  for Registered Professional Nurses
101 Dee Drive
Charleston, WV 25311
Phone: (304)558-3596
Fax: (304)558-3666
Website: **www.wvrnboard.com**

Wisconsin
Wisconsin Department of Regulation
  and Licensing
1400 E. Washington Avenue
P.O. Box 8935
Madison, WI 53708
Phone: (608)266-0145
Fax: (608)261-7083
Website: **http://drl.wi.gov/
index.htm**

Wyoming
Wyoming State Board of Nursing
2020 Carey Avenue, Suite 110
Cheyenne, WY 82002
Phone: (307)777-7601
Fax: (307)777-3519
Website: **http://nursing.
state.wy.us/**

1-4

Family Nurse Practitioner Job Description

General Description

A family nurse practitioner (FNP) is a registered nurse who provides primary care. The FNP provides care to patients who have common acute illnesses and stable, chronic problems. The FNP will collaborate and consult with physicians and make referrals as needed.

Education

Graduate of an accredited school of nursing, current licensure as a registered nurse, and completed a preceptorship. Certification as a nurse practitioner in the state of Michigan is required.

Work Experience

1 year of experience as a family nurse practitioner

Responsibilities

Assesses the health status of the individual using a holistic framework.

- Conducts a complete history and physical examination.
- Assesses physical and psychosocial parameters.

Identifies patient problems.

- Clearly identifies problems.
- Recognizes emergent and urgent situations and acts accordingly.
- Includes patient and family/significant other in needs identification and problem resolution.

Plans care and intervenes as appropriate.

- Collaborates with appropriate health care professionals.
- Includes patient, family/significant other in plan.
- Addresses physical/psychological and social factors.
- Orders appropriate laboratory and diagnostic tests with attention to cost effectiveness.

- Facilitates continuing care through appropriate agency referrals.
- Sets patient educational goals and demonstrates achievement.

Evaluates and documents plan of care at each visit.

- Tracks diagnoses and referrals.
- Collaborates and consults with health care providers.
- Involves patients and families in modifying plans of care.
- Documents clearly and completely.

Documents clearly and consistently.

- Charts in a timely manner.
- Documents patient progress.
- Documents nursing interventions and patient outcomes.

Demonstrates leadership.

- Serves as a role model for professional conduct and practice.
- Serves as a preceptor for students.
- Assists in presenting inservices.
- Designs quality improvement programs and follows through.
- Maintains open communication.
- Participates in peer review.
- Participates in schedules screening clinics.

Acts as a professional.

- Maintains current practice.
- Remains accountable for time, materials, and human resources.
- Acts as a patient advocate.
- Develops policies and procedures.
- Acts as a member of the team.
- Is a positive force in the office.
- Is active in professional organizations.

Accidents of Health Hazards

Requires exposure to communicable disease and/or body fluids, toxic substances, medicinal preparations, and other conditions common to a clinic environment.

Essential Functions

1. Ability to hear conversational voice and read, write, and interpret English.
2. Ability to communicate effectively.
3. Ability to see clearly in an environment that is equipped with "normal" lighting.
4. Ability to perform manual tasks that require the use of the fine muscle motor skills.

5. Ability to walk up to 5 miles per day.
6. Ability to lift up to 75 pounds as needed each work day and to bend and stretch freely.
7. Ability to work in a latex rich environment, practice universal precautions as needed, and tolerate frequent hand washing as needed.
8. Ability to move from one office location to another via mobile transport.

Self-Assessment Scale

Self-Assessment Scale

Rate your level of confidence with regard to your ability to perform the skill listed in each statement by circling one appropriate number below each statement. 1 indicates the least amount of confidence; 6 indicates the most amount of confidence.

	Least				Most	
1. Know the difference between subjective and objective data.	1	2	3	4	5	6
2. Know the component parts of a health history.	1	2	3	4	5	6
3. Obtain a complete health history.	1	2	3	4	5	6
4. Know age-appropriate modifications for the health history.	1	2	3	4	5	6
5. Evaluate history for completeness, organization, and clarity	1	2	3	4	5	6
6. Use communication skills appropriate to age of client.	1	2	3	4	5	6
7. Use communication skills appropriate to type of data collection.	1	2	3	4	5	6
8. Recognize and respond to verbal cues presented by the client.	1	2	3	4	5	6
9. Recognize and respond to nonverbal cues presented by the client.	1	2	3	4	5	6
10. Differentiate between normal and abnormal heart sounds.	1	2	3	4	5	6
11. Perform a respiratory system examination.	1	2	3	4	5	6
12. Perform an abdominal examination.	1	2	3	4	5	6
13. Perform a musculoskeletal examination.	1	2	3	4	5	6
14. Perform a neurological examination.	1	2	3	4	5	6
15. Perform a pelvic examination.	1	2	3	4	5	6
16. Perform an examination of the head and neck.	1	2	3	4	5	6
17. Perform an examination of the skin.	1	2	3	4	5	6
18. Perform a breast examination.	1	2	3	4	5	6
19. Perform a lymphatic system examination.	1	2	3	4	5	6
20. Perform a complete physical examination.	1	2	3	4	5	6
21. Know the observation component of the physical examination.	1	2	3	4	5	6
22. Know the palpation component of the physical examination.	1	2	3	4	5	6
23. Know the percussion component of the physical examination.	1	2	3	4	5	6
24. Know the auscultation component of the physical examination.	1	2	3	4	5	6
25. Present physical findings in descriptive terms using the POMR (problem-oriented medical record) format.	1	2	3	4	5	6
26. Relate knowledge of anatomy and physiology to the physical examination.	1	2	3	4	5	6

27. Describe the role and functions of a nurse practitioner.	1	2	3	4	5	6
28. Perform a DDST (Denver Developmental Screening Test).	1	2	3	4	5	6
29. Develop a definition of health congruent with a conceptual model of nursing practice.	1	2	3	4	5	6
30. Analyze nursing and medical models in the delivery of primary care.	1	2	3	4	5	6
31. Assume leadership responsibility in collaboration with other providers to establish standards for health care management.	1	2	3	4	5	6
32. Apply knowledge of change theory in acting as a client advocate.	1	2	3	4	5	6
33. Apply knowledge of life-span physical and psychosocial factors to the delivery of primary care.	1	2	3	4	5	6
34. Develop protocols for nursing management for selected risk factors.	1	2	3	4	5	6
35. Evaluate protocols for selected risk factors.	1	2	3	4	5	6
36. Plan nursing management strategies for selected risk factors across the age span.	1	2	3	4	5	6
37. Apply a conceptual nursing model to nursing management of risk factors.	1	2	3	4	5	6
38. Evaluate lay literature on health care.	1	2	3	4	5	6
39. Analyze use of over-the-counter medications as part of nursing management.	1	2	3	4	5	6
40. Utilize a comprehensive database in the delivery of primary care.	1	2	3	4	5	6
41. Initiate or perform laboratory examinations.	1	2	3	4	5	6
42. Apply knowledge of therapeutic nutrition across the age span in nursing management of clients.	1	2	3	4	5	6
43. Incorporate knowledge of pharmacological agents in nursing management of clients.	1	2	3	4	5	6
44. Ability to clearly state my philosophy of nursing.	1	2	3	4	5	6
45. Ability to clearly state my philosophy of primary care.	1	2	3	4	5	6
46. Ability to prepare my resumé.	1	2	3	4	5	6
47. Negotiate for position and salary.	1	2	3	4	5	6
48. Analyze current licensure and credentialing laws.	1	2	3	4	5	6
49. Know nurse practice act in state where I practice.	1	2	3	4	5	6
50. Describe various means of reimbursement for nurse practitioner services.	1	2	3	4	5	6
51. Utilize several methodologies in implementing change.	1	2	3	4	5	6
52. Utilize concepts of power and authority.	1	2	3	4	5	6
53. Educate clients and other providers as to the role of the nurse practitioner.	1	2	3	4	5	6
54. Analyze supports and obstacles to the role of the nurse practitioner.	1	2	3	4	5	6
55. Plan strategies to change or diminish obstacles to role implementation.	1	2	3	4	5	6
56. Plan research as part of role implementation.	1	2	3	4	5	6
57. Plan a demonstration project for health care delivery to a selected group of clients.	1	2	3	4	5	6
58. Evaluate total role of nurse practitioner.	1	2	3	4	5	6

59. Describe methods of audit and quality assurance.	1	2	3	4	5	6
60. Incorporate communication theory and group process into role.	1	2	3	4	5	6
61. Describe assertiveness techniques and evaluate use for nurse practitioner role.	1	2	3	4	5	6
62. Utilize nursing model in role implementation.	1	2	3	4	5	6
63. Analyze financial aspects of the role of nurse practitioner as employee and/or independent practitioner.	1	2	3	4	5	6
64. Apply teaching-learning theory to a variety of teaching situations.	1	2	3	4	5	6
65. Evaluate the effectiveness of my teaching.	1	2	3	4	5	6

SUMMARY

This self-assessment assists in identifying your strengths and areas for growth. Those items that you rated as a 6 are areas you are comfortable with. The items you rated as a 1, 2, or 3 are growth opportunities.

Developed by Janice A. Thibodeau, RN, C, EdD, FAAN, Professor Emerita, University of Connecticut School of Nursing, and Joellen W. Hawkins, RNC, PhD, FAAN, Professor, Boston College, William F. Connell School of Nursing.

Attitudes and Values Scale

Attitudes and Values Scale

Read each statement carefully. Indicate your agreement with each statement by circling the appropriate number. 1 indicates the least agreement with the statement. 6 indicates the most agreement with the statement. NP=Nurse practitioner

	Least				Most	
1. The physical examination is the most important part of the database.	1	2	3	4	5	6
2. NPs are physician extenders.	1	2	3	4	5	6
3. A psychosocial history is the most important part of the database.	1	2	3	4	5	6
4. Health is harmony of the mind, body, and spirit.	1	2	3	4	5	6
5. NPs should receive third party payments as independent practitioners.	1	2	3	4	5	6
6. The client should be expected to comply with a plan of care prescribed by the NP.	1	2	3	4	5	6
7. The NP role is best enhanced by collaborative practice with other NPs.	1	2	3	4	5	6
8. The goal of health care is to cure illness.	1	2	3	4	5	6
9. Care of physical problems should receive priority over psychosocial problems.	1	2	3	4	5	6
10. NPs should base their practice on a conceptual model of nursing practice.	1	2	3	4	5	6
11. The NP can practice independently within the scope of nurse practice acts.	1	2	3	4	5	6
12. Physical examination skills are more important than interviewing skills.	1	2	3	4	5	6
13. NPs should know how to perform laboratory procedures such as lumbar punctures and jugular punctures.	1	2	3	4	5	6
14. All education for NPs should take place within schools of nursing.	1	2	3	4	5	6
15. Health is the absence of abnormalities of structure and function.	1	2	3	4	5	6
16. NPs should know how to read and interpret x-rays.	1	2	3	4	5	6
17. NPs learn the role best from nurse preceptors.	1	2	3	4	5	6
18. NPs should know how to suture and perform other minor surgical procedures.	1	2	3	4	5	6
19. Nursing management strategies should flow from one's model of nursing practice.	1	2	3	4	5	6
20. For NPs to be effective, they must include medical management in their practices.	1	2	3	4	5	6

21. A nursing model directs the NP as to what data to collect.	1	2	3	4	5	6
22. NPs should not practice without medical back-up.	1	2	3	4	5	6
23. Physicians should participate in the education of NPs.	1	2	3	4	5	6
24. A medical model is most congruent with the NP role.	1	2	3	4	5	6
25. NPs need to develop their own protocols for practice.	1	2	3	4	5	6
26. It is essential that all NPs function as client advocates.	1	2	3	4	5	6
27. Health maintenance is the prime component of the NP role.	1	2	3	4	5	6
28. The NP must be skilled in differential diagnosis of all common illnesses.	1	2	3	4	5	6
29. Health teaching is the primary component of the NP role.	1	2	3	4	5	6
30. Protocols should be developed for NPs by their physician preceptors.	1	2	3	4	5	6
31. NPs in practice with physicians have more status.	1	2	3	4	5	6
32. The NP must utilize knowledge of nursing research in the delivery of care.	1	2	3	4	5	6
33. The physician should be the team leader with the NP designated certain clients to manage.	1	2	3	4	5	6
34. Leadership within the nursing profession is central to the role of the NP.	1	2	3	4	5	6
35. Physicians should participate in the evaluation of NPs.	1	2	3	4	5	6
36. NPs are responsible for contributing to nursing knowledge through research.	1	2	3	4	5	6
37. NPs are responsible for quality assurance and evaluation of their practice.	1	2	3	4	5	6

This scale may assist you in identifying and assessing your attitudes and values about professional nursing practice.

———

Developed by Janice A. Thibodeau, RN, C, EdD, FAAN, Professor Emerita, University of Connecticut School of Nursing, and Joellen W. Hawkins, RNC, PhD, FAAN, Professor, Boston College, William F. Connell School of Nursing.

Five Categories of Controlled Substances and Sample DEA Application for Registration

Controlled substances are placed into one of five categories based on the drug's usefulness, potential for harm, and the potential for abuse or addiction. Schedule I consists of the most dangerous drug considered to have no medicinal indications (peyote, PCP, etc.). Schedule II drugs have a high risk of dependence, and include oxycodone and cocaine. Schedule III drugs include pentobarbital and ketamine, whereas Schedule IV drugs include diazepam, lorazepam, and chloral hydrate. Schedule V drugs are drugs that are considered the least likely to cause harm or addiction (cough syrup with codeine and the like).

Listed below are examples of the schedules with assigned drug code numbers. If you are in need of additional information, see 21 cfr 1308 or contact the DEA Office serving your area.

SCHEDULE I

NARCOTIC & NON NARCOTIC BASIC CLASSES

	CODE
Acetorphine	
Acetylmethadol	
Allyprodine	
Alphacetylmethadol (except LAAM)	
Bufotenine	
Dextromoramide	
Diethyltryptamine (DET)	
2,5-Dimethoxyamphetamine (DMA)	
Dimethyltryptamine (DMT)	
Etorphine (except HCL)	
Heroin	
Ibogaine	
Ketobemidone	
Lysergic acid diethylamide (LSD)	
Marihuana	
Mescaline	
Methaqualone	
3,4-Methylenedioxyamphetamine (MDA)	
3,4-Methylenedioxymethamphetamine (MDMA)	
N-Ethyl-1-Phenylcyclohexylamine (PCE)	
Peyote	
1-(1-Phenylcyclohexyl)pyrrolidine (PCPy)	
Psilocybin	
Psilocyn	
Tetrahydrocannabinols (THC)	
1-[-1-(2-Thienyl)-cyclohexyl]-piperidine (TCP)	

SCHEDULE II

NARCOTIC BASIC CLASSES

	CODE
Alphaprodine	9010
Anileridine	9020
Cocaine	9041
Codeine	9050
Dextropropoxyphene (bulk)	9273
Diphenoxylate	9170
Diprenorphine (M50-50)	9058
Ethylmorphine	9190
Etorphine Hydrochloride (M-99)	9059
Glutethimide	2550
Hydrocodone	9193
Hydromorphone	9150
Levo-alphacetylmethadol (LAAM)	9648
Levorphanol	9220
Meperidine	9230
Methadone	9250
Morphine	9300
Opium, powdered	9639
Opium, raw	9600
Oxycodone	9143
Oxymorphone	9652
Poppy Straw	9671
Poppy Straw Concentrate	9670
Thebaine	9333

NON NARCOTIC BASIC CLASSES

	CODE
Amobarbital	2125
Amphetamine	1100
Methamphetamine	1105
Methylphenidate	1724
Pentobarbital	2270
Phencyclidine (PCP)	7471
Phenmetrazine	1631
Phenyacetone	8501
Secobarbital	2315

SCHEDULE III

NARCOTIC BASIC CLASSES

	CODE
Codeine up to 90mg/du + other ingred.	9804
Dihydrocodeine up to 90mg/du + other	9807
Ethlmorphine up to 15mg/du + other	9808
Hydrocodone up to 15mg/du + other	9806
Morphine up to 50mg/100ml or gm + other	9810
Opium up to 500mg/100ml + other active ingred.	9809

NON NARCOTIC BASIC CLASSES

	CODE
Anabolic Steroids	4000
Benzphetamine	1228
Butalbital	2100
Dronabinol Pharmaceutical Product	7369
Ketamine	7285
Methyprylon	2575
Pentobarbital + noncontrolled active ingred.	2271
Pentobarbital suppository	1615
Phendimetrazine	2316
Secobarbital + noncontrolled active ingred.	2316
Secobarbital suppository	2329
Thiopental	2335
Vinbarbital	

SCHEDULE IV

NARCOTIC BASIC CLASSES

	CODE
Dextropropoxyphene du	9278
Difenoxin 1mg/25ug atropine SO4/du	9167

NON NARCOTIC BASIC CLASSES

	CODE
Alprazolam	2882
Barbital	2145
Chloral Hydrate	2465
Chlordiazepoxide	2744
Clorazepate	2768
Diazepam	2765
Diethylpropion	1610
Fenfluramine	1670
Flurazepam	2767
Halazepam	2762
Lorazepam	2885
Mazindol	1605
Mebutamate	2800

SCHEDULE IV (cont'd)

	CODE
Mephobarbital	2250
Meprobamate	2820
Methohexital	2264
Midazolam	2884
Oxazepam	2835
Paraldehyde	2585
Pemoline	1530
Pentazocine	9709
Phenobarbital	2285
Phentermine	1640
Prazepam	2764
Quazepam	2881
Temazepam	2925
Triazolam	2887
Zolpidem	2783

SCHEDULE V

	CODE
Buprenorphine	9064
Codeine Cough Preparation	9100

Sample DEA Application Instructions

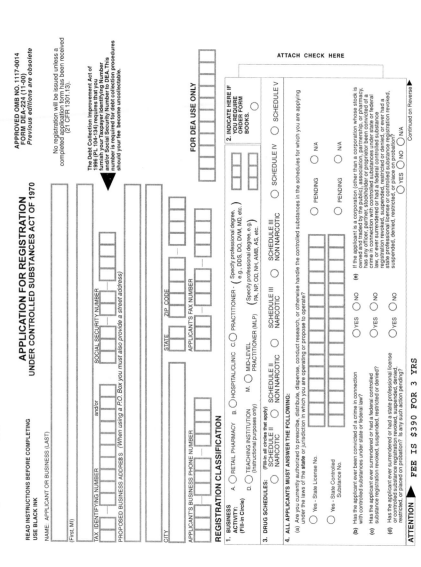

READ INSTRUCTIONS BEFORE COMPLETING
USE BLACK INK

APPROVED OMB NO. 1117-0014
FORM DEA-224 (11-00)
Previous editions are obsolete

APPLICATION FOR REGISTRATION
UNDER CONTROLLED SUBSTANCES ACT OF 1970

No registration will be issued unless a
completed application form has been received
(21 CFR 1301.13).

The Debt Collection Improvement Act of
1996 (PL 104-134) requires that you
furnish your Taxpayer Identifying Number
and/or Social Security Number to DEA. This
number is required for debt collection procedures
should your fee become uncollectable.

NAME: APPLICANT OR BUSINESS (LAST)

(First, MI)

TAX IDENTIFYING NUMBER   and/or   SOCIAL SECURITY NUMBER

PROPOSED BUSINESS ADDRESS *(When using a P.O. Box you must also provide a street address)*

CITY   STATE   ZIP CODE

APPLICANT'S BUSINESS PHONE NUMBER   APPLICANT'S FAX NUMBER

FOR DEA USE ONLY

**2. INDICATE HERE IF
YOU REQUIRE
ORDER FORM
BOOKS.** ◯

REGISTRATION CLASSIFICATION

**1. BUSINESS
ACTIVITY:**
(Fill-in Circle)

A. ◯ RETAIL PHARMACY   B. ◯ HOSPITAL/CLINIC   C. ◯ PRACTITIONER - Specify professional degree, e.g., DDS, DO, DVM, MD, etc.

D. ◯ TEACHING INSTITUTION
(Instructional purposes only)

M. ◯ MID-LEVEL
PRACTITIONER (MLP)   (Specify professional degree, e.g.,
PA, NP, OD, NH, AMB, AS, etc.

3. DRUG SCHEDULES: (Fill-in all circles that apply)

◯ SCHEDULE II
NARCOTIC   ◯ SCHEDULE II
NON NARCOTIC   ◯ SCHEDULE III
NARCOTIC   ◯ SCHEDULE III
NON NARCOTIC   ◯ SCHEDULE IV   ◯ SCHEDULE V

4. ALL APPLICANTS MUST ANSWER THE FOLLOWING:

(a) Are you currently authorized to prescribe, distribute, dispense, conduct research, or otherwise handle the controlled substances in the schedules for which you are applying
under the laws of the **state** or jurisdiction in which you are operating or propose to operate?   ◯ YES ◯ NO

◯ Yes - State License No.

◯ Yes - State Controlled
Substance No.

(b) Has the applicant ever been convicted of a crime in connection
with controlled substances under state or federal law?   ◯ YES ◯ NO

(c) Has the applicant ever surrendered or had a federal controlled
substance registration revoked, suspended, restricted or denied?   ◯ YES ◯ NO

(d) Has the applicant ever surrendered or had a state professional license
or controlled substance registration revoked, suspended, denied,
restricted, or placed on probation? Is any such action pending?   ◯ YES ◯ NO

(e) If the applicant is a corporation (other than a corporation whose stock is
owned and traded by the public), association, partnership, or pharmacy,
has any officer, partner, stockholder or proprietor been convicted of a
crime in connection with controlled substances under state or federal
law, or ever surrendered or had a federal controlled substance
registration revoked, suspended, restricted or denied, or ever had a
state professional license or controlled substance registration revoked,
suspended, denied, restricted, or place on probation?
◯ PENDING ◯ N/A
◯ PENDING ◯ N/A
◯ YES ◯ NO ◯ N/A

ATTENTION ▶ **FEE IS $390 FOR 3 YRS**

Continued on Reverse ▶

ATTACH CHECK HERE

4. CONTINUED

(f) MLP only: Applicant is authorized to engage in the following controlled substance activities by the **state** in which applicant practices. (Fill-in all circles that apply.)

	Prescribe	Administer	Dispense	Procure*
SCHEDULE II NARCOTIC	○	○	○	○
SCHEDULE II NON NARCOTIC	○	○	○	○
SCHEDULE III NARCOTIC	○	○	○	○
SCHEDULE III NON NARCOTIC	○	○	○	○
SCHEDULE IV	○	○	○	○
SCHEDULE V	○	○	○	○

*Procure means to individually obtain controlled substances by purchase or receipt of samples from a manufacturer or distributor. It does not include receipt of controlled substances from, or pursuant to an order from a collaborating or supervising physician.

5. EXPLANATION FOR ANSWERING "YES" TO ITEM(S) 4(b), (c), (d), OR (e). Applicants who have answered "YES" to item(s) 4(b), (c), (d), or (e) are required to submit a statement explaining such response(s). The space provided below should be used for this purpose. If additional space is needed, use a separate sheet and return with application.

6. PAYMENT METHOD (Fill-in only one circle)

○ VISA   ○ MASTER CARD   ○ CHECK

FEES ARE NOT REFUNDABLE

CREDIT CARD NUMBER

EXPIRATION DATE

SIGNATURE OF CARD HOLDER

7. CERTIFICATION FOR FEE EXEMPTION (Fill-in Circle)

○ FILL-IN CIRCLE IF APPLICANT NAMED HEREON IS A FEDERAL, STATE, OR LOCAL GOVERNMENT OPERATED HOSPITAL, INSTITUTION, OR OFFICIAL. The undersigned hereby certifies that the applicant named hereon is a federal, state or local government operated hospital, institution, or official, and is exempt from payment of the application fee.

SIGNATURE OF CERTIFYING OFFICIAL (Other than applicant)   DATE

PRINT OR TYPE NAME OF CERTIFYING OFFICIAL   PRINT OR TYPE TITLE OF CERTIFYING OFFICIAL

8. APPLICANT SIGNATURE (must be an original signature in ink) ► Remove form from package before signing

SIGNATURE   DATE

I hereby certify that the foregoing information furnished on this application is true and correct.

Print or Type Name

Print or Type Title (e.g., President, Dean, Procurement Officer, etc...)

RETURN COMPLETED APPLICATION WITH FEE IN ATTACHED ENVELOPE

MAKE CHECK OR MONEY ORDER PAYABLE TO

DRUG ENFORCEMENT ADMINISTRATION

UNITED STATES DEPARTMENT OF JUSTICE
DRUG ENFORCEMENT ADMINISTRATION
P. O. BOX 530295
ATLANTA, GA 30348-0295

For information, call 1 (800) 882-9539
See "Privacy Act" Information on last page of application.

MAKE A COPY FOR YOUR RECORDS.

DEA OFFICES (800, 877 and 888 are toll free numbers)

ATLANTA DIVISION OFFICE
Attn: Registration
75 Spring Street, SW, Room 740
Atlanta, GA 30303

Georgia	(888) 219-7898
North Carolina	(888) 219-8689
South Carolina	(888) 219-8689
Tennessee	(888) 219-7898

BOSTON DIVISION OFFICE
JFK Federal Bldg., Room E-400
15 New Sudbury Street
Boston, MA 02203-0131

Connecticut	(617) 557-2200
Maine	(617) 557-2200
Massachusetts	(617) 557-2200
New Hampshire	(617) 557-2200
Rhode Island	(617) 557-2200
Vermont	(617) 557-2200

CARIBBEAN DIVISION OFFICE
P.O. Box 2167
San Juan, PR, 00922-2167

Puerto Rico	(787) 775-1766
U.S. Virgin Islands	(787) 775-1766

CHICAGO DIVISION OFFICE
230 S. Dearborn Street, Suite 1200
Chicago, IL 60604

Illinois	(312) 353-1234
Indiana	(312) 353-1236
Minnesota	(312) 353-9166
North Dakota	(312) 353-9166
Wisconsin	(312) 353-1236

DALLAS DIVISION OFFICE
10160 Technology Blvd, East
Dallas, TX 75220

Oklahoma	(888) 336-4704
Texas (Northern)	(888) 336-4704

DENVER DIVISION OFFICE
115 Inverness Drive East
Englewood, CO 80112

Colorado	(800) 326-6900
Montana	(800) 326-6900
Utah	(800) 326-6900
Wyoming	(800) 326-6900

DETROIT DIVISION OFFICE
431 Howard Street
Detroit, MI 48226

Kentucky	(800) 230-6844
Michigan	(800) 230-6844
Ohio	(800) 230-6844

HOUSTON DIVISION OFFICE
1433 West Loop South, Suite 600
Houston, TX 77027

New Mexico	(800) 743-0595
Texas (South + Central)	(800) 743-0595

LOS ANGELES DIVISION OFFICE
255 East Temple Street, 20th Floor
Los Angeles, CA 90012

California (So. Central)	(888) 415-9822
Hawaii	(888) 415-9822
Nevada	(888) 415-9822
Trust Territory	(213) 621-8960

MIAMI DIVISION OFFICE
8400 N.W. 53rd Street
Miami, FL 33166

Florida	(800) 667-9752

NEWARK DIVISION OFFICE
80 Mulberry Street
Newark, NJ 07102

New Jersey	(888) 356-1071

NEW ORLEANS DIVISION OFFICE
Three Lake Way
3838 N. Causeway Boulevard, Suite 1800
Metairie, LA 70002

Alabama	(888) 514-7302 or 8051
Arkansas	(888) 514-7302 or 8051
Louisiana	(888) 514-7302 or 8051
Mississippi	(888) 514-7302 or 8051

NEW YORK DIVISION OFFICE
99 Tenth Avenue
New York, NY 10011

New York	(877) 883-5789

PHILADELPHIA DIVISION OFFICE
William J Green Federal Building
600 Arch Street, Room 10224
Philadelphia, Pa 19106

Delaware	(888) 393-8231
Pennsylvania	(888) 393-8231

PHOENIX DIVISION OFFICE
3010 N. 2nd Street, Suite 301
Phoenix, AZ 85012

Arizona	(800) 741-0902

SAN DIEGO DIVISION OFFICE
4560 Viewridge Avenue
San Diego, CA 92123-1672

California (Southern)	(800) 264-1152

SAN FRANCISCO DIVISION OFFICE
450 Golden Gate Avenue
P.O. Box 36035
San Francisco, CA 94102

California (Northern)	(888) 304-3251

SEATTLE DIVISION OFFICE
400 Second Avenue West
Seattle, WA 98119

Alaska	(888) 219-4261
Idaho	(888) 219-4261
Oregon	(888) 219-4261
Washington	(888) 219-1418

ST LOUIS DIVISION OFFICE
United Missouri Bank Building
7911 Forsyth Boulevard, Suite 500
St. Louis, MO 63105

Iowa	(888) 803-1179
Kansas	(888) 803-1179
Missouri	(888) 803-1179
Nebraska	(888) 803-1179
South Dakota	(888) 803-1179

WASHINGTON, D.C. DIVISION OFFICE
Techworld Plaza
800 K Street, N.W., Suite 500
Washington, D.C. 20001

District of Columbia	(877) 801-7974
Maryland	(410) 962-7580
Virginia	(877) 801-7974
West Virginia	(410) 962-7580

HEADQUARTERS
United States Department of Justice
Drug Enforcement Administration
Central Station
P.O. Box 28083
Washington, D.C. 20038-8083

(800) 882-9539

NOTE: Additional information can be found on the Internet, www.deadiversion.usdoj.gov

Title 21, United States Code, Section 827(g) requires all registrants to report any changes of professional or business address to the DEA. Notification of address changes must be made in writing to the DEA office which has jurisdiction for your registered location. Direct requests for the following actions to the address listed for your state. 1. Request a modification to your DEA Registration (address change), 2. Request order form books, 3. Status of pending application.

PRIVACY ACT INFORMATION

AUTHORITY: Section 302 and 303 of the Controlled Substances Act of 1970 (PL 91-513) and Debt Collection Improvement Act of 1996 (PL 104-134.) (for federal taxpayer identifying number and/or social security number).

PURPOSE: To obtain information required to register applicants pursuant to the Controlled Substances Act of 1970.

ROUTINE USES: The Controlled Substances Act Registration Records produces special reports as required for statistical analytical purposes. Disclosures of information from this system are made to the following categories of users for the purposes stated:
A.   Other federal law enforcement and regulatory agencies for law enforcement and regulatory purposes.
B.   State and local law enforcement and regulatory agencies for law enforcement and regulatory purposes.
C.   Persons registered under the Controlled Substances Act (PL 91-513) for the purpose of verifying the registration of customers and practitioners.

EFFECT: Failure to complete form will preclude processing of the application

Item 1 Business Activity (choose "midlevel practitioner" and furnish the professional degree in the space provided).

Item 2 Order Form Books (indicate only if you intend to purchase or transfer Schedule II substances).

Item 3 Drug Schedules (indicate schedule[s] of controlled substance[s] pertaining to your business activity and those you intend to handle).

Item 4 State Licensure. Federal registration is based on the applicant being in compliance with applicable state and local laws. If your state requires a separate controlled substance license, this number must be provided. If state-licensing authority is not required, indicate N/A. All applicants must answer items 4 (c), (d), (e), and (f), if you answer YES to any of these, you must give a detailed answer to these in item 5. Item 5 requires no explanation for answering YES to Item(s) 4 (c), (d), (e), or (f).

Item 6 Method of Payment. The federal government accepts checks, credit card (VISA or MasterCard) (include signature and expiration dates), but does not accept checks drawn on foreign banks. Application fees are not refundable

Item 7 Fee Exemption. Limited to federal, state, or local government operated hospitals, clinics, institutions, or officials. Supervisor's title, signature and address of the affiliated government entity must be included on the application.

Item 8 Application Signature. Must be original and in ink.

Collaborative Agreement

(If you are required to write a collaborative agreement, some of the information presented may be useful in satisfying this requirement.)

It is the intent of this document to set forth the collaborative practice agreement between Mary Smith, RN, MSN, FNP, and Jane Doe, MD, to provide direct primary care of families and family members throughout the life span. This is done in accordance to state law and covers the overlapping scope of practice between advanced nursing practice and medical functions where such services shall be performed in collaboration with a physician.

FOCUS OF CARE

Services to be provided: primary care of families and family members that includes identification and management and/or referral of health conditions to include health promotion, disease prevention, health maintenance, and disease management, including acute and stable chronic problems. Care will be provided at "Health Sources" located at 100 Main Street, Anywhere, USA, as well as in the patients' homes. Focus of care will include coordination of care, comprehensive assessment, and advocacy for the patient and family. Care will be delivered within an interdisciplinary model, utilizing the expertise of pharmacists, physical therapists, physicians, and other medical specialties.

ELEMENTS OF CARE

- Assessing families and family members for health status and illness conditions, responses to treatment, and identification of health behaviors through ongoing history, physical, and laboratory assessment.
- Diagnosing actual and potential health problems.
- Intervening to assist the patient and families to achieve the highest level of wellness, and to cope with altered health patterns. Interventions may include direct care, ordering of medications and treatments, consultation with Jane Doe, MD, or consultation or referral to other health care providers.
- Evaluation of the effectiveness of care individually, as well as through institutional quality assurance activities.

CONSULTATION

Consultation will occur as needed in the form of direct on-site discussion, via telephone, fax transmission, or otherwise by written document. All consultations and collaborations will be documented in the health care record. Clinicians will be expected to seek consultation or collaboration when a condition occurs outside their prior education or scope of practice. A random monthly chart review of 10 charts will be conducted and discussed each month.

COLLABORATION FOR PRESCRIPTIVE PRACTICE

Nurse practitioners through this agreement will be authorized to prescribe medications that are congruent with existing state law. Authority will be delegated by Jane Doe, MD, to Mary Smith, RN, MSN, and FNP to include controlled substances, Schedules II-V. References for prescriptions will be the current *Physicians' Desk Reference* and/or the monthly *Nurse Practitioner/ Physician Monthly* or *Quarterly Prescribing Guide.*

Collaborating Parties Signatures:

_____ Jane Doe, MD

_____ Mary Smith, RN, MSN, FNP

Approval Date _____

Renewal Date _____

Sample Protocol

Nurse practitioners working for Primetime Care shall practice in accordance with protocols developed in collaboration with and signed by a licensed physician. Each protocol will address established protocols for the management of common presenting problems in this medical practice, and will designate the degree of collaboration, independent action, and supervision needed in the assessment, diagnosis, treatment, and evaluation of clients with commonly presenting medical problems.

Diagnosis and Management of Acute Pharyngitis

This guideline applies to patients 3 years of age or older who present to the clinic with complaints of a sore throat. The purpose of the protocol is to provide care that will achieve the following patient outcomes:

- Prevention of complications
- Prevention of rheumatic fever
- Prevention of the spread of group A beta-hemolytic streptococcal infection
- Relief of clinical signs and symptoms
- Decreased use of inappropriate antibiotic.

Clinicians should be aware that 10% to 20% of patients presenting with sore throat will have group A beta-hemolytic streptococcal infection. Although some may have sore throats caused by other bacteria (group C strep, *Chlamydia*) or disease processes, the majority will have a sore throat secondary to a viral etiology, and will benefit from treatment of symptoms alone.

Symptoms/Signs that Increase the Suspicion of Strep

Age 3-14

- Recent fever >38°C
- Absence of a cough
- Exudate on tonsils
- Anterior cervical adenitis
- Current strep in the community
- Recent exposure to strep.

Symptoms/Signs that Decrease the Suspicion of Strep

- Age 45 or older
- No fever
- Cough or hoarseness
- Conjunctivitis
- Oral lesions
- Diarrhea.

RECOMMENDATION 1: Throat Swab

A throat swab should be taken when a diagnosis of strep throat is suspected from the clinical signs and symptoms. If the rapid strep test is positive, antibiotics should be prescribed. All negative rapid strep tests will be cultured. After 24 hours, if the culture is positive, patients will then be placed on antibiotics. All other patients will be treated with symptomatic treatment alone.

RECOMMENDATION 2: Antibiotics

First line: Penicillin V (250 mg PO tid/qid for 10 days).
Recommended alternative for penicillin-allergic patients: Erythromycin (30-40 mg/kg/day divided bid/tid for 10 days).

RECOMMENDATION 3: Symptomatic Treatment

Includes gargling with saltwater, use of lozenges, use of antipyretics such as Tylenol, drinking plenty of fluids, and rest.

RECOMMENDATION 4

For patients presenting with a sore throat and hepatosplenomegaly, a monospot test should be performed. Consultation with a physician should be made for all positive Monospot tests.

RECOMMENDATION 5

Patients presenting with simple pharyngitis or strep pharyngitis may be treated independently. Nurse practitioners should seek a consult for any patient presenting with signs of airway compromise or inability to swallow secretions.

Example of Cost Considerations for a Capitation Model

In a capitated model of reimbursement, it is imperative that you recognize the actual costs and resources needed to provide the service. To set up the model, you need to know the number of covered lives you will be responsible for, the disease or wellness makeup of this group of lives, and the projected number of visits per client per year. In the following example, 1000 lives will be covered with a projected number of three visits per year.

Next, you need to consider the expense of providing the service intended to this group of clients. The largest single expense will be for the staff's salary and fringe benefits. The model of care provided will give clues about the types and number of staff required. For example, nurse-managed centers often hire nurse practitioner providers in lieu of physician providers to direct patient care. This expense may be less than that for physician counterparts. Nurse-managed centers value the role of the nurse and often hire RNs as ancillary staff instead of medical assistants with less knowledge and experience.

Other expenses include office lease expense, office supplies and services, clinical supplies and services, malpractice insurance costs, collaborating physician expense, and laboratory and radiology services expenses. Many other expenses may be included in the model depending on the individual circumstance you are considering. It is important to poll a number of individuals close to the operation so that all expected and/or projected expenses are captured. When negotiating capitation payment, you need to ensure that the expenses inherent to provide services within the model of care are compensated. It may be helpful to seek assistance from an individual with a strong financial background to determine that revenue will indeed cover expenses.

Expenses projected for the annual period are then totaled. The number of member months are divided into the total expense to arrive at the per-member per-month expense. Then the amount of revenue per month to cover expenses is calculated. This amount gives a basis for contract negotiation considering the desired margin of profit or the "break-even" status desired.

In the example, the total expense of caring for 1000 members in a primary care model for 12 months equals $360,000. The per-member per-month (PMPM) amount of $30 is arrived at by dividing the total expense by the total member months. It is calculated that $30,000 revenue per month will be required to cover the cost of the services provided.

Capitation Model for Primary Care Services

Assumptions: 1000   Members
              12,000   Member months (members × 12)
              3,000   Visits per year (3 visits/yr avg)
                        12-Month proposal

Staffing:	FTE	Salary/FTE	Total (12 months)

Salary:

Nurse practitioner(s)
Office manager
RN staff
Clinical assistant(s)
Clerical assistant(s)
Billing staff
Others?

Fringe Benefits:

According to staff allocated above

Total Salary and Fringe Benefit Expense _____

(Salaries will vary according to the employee category and geographic variation. You may contact a local NP chapter or gather local market rates for NP salaries and contact local health care agencies for salary rates for ancillary staff.)

Office Lease

Per square foot (sf) charge × number of sf × 12 months

Supplies & Services; General Expense

Office equipment: computers, printers, fax, copier, telephones, pagers, etc.
Office supplies: medical record folders and dividers, paper, miscellaneous office supplies
Office services: computer support, equipment maintenance contracts, answering service, telephone charges.

Clinical Expenses

Medications including immunizations
Supplies for direct patient care
Equipment for direct patient care
Malpractice insurance: Liability coverage for all providers annually
Physician collaboration expense: Hours per week × salary/fringe benefits annualized

APPENDIX 6-1

Radiology services: estimated number of procedures × average expense per procedure annualized

Laboratory services: estimated number of procedures × average expense per procedure annualized

CALCULATING YOUR MONTHLY REVENUE

Add up your total expenses (in our example, $360,000) and divide that number by your total member months (12 × total members [1000] = 12,000) to calculate the total PMPM amount ($30). Multiply the PMPM amount by the number of members to calculate a monthly revenue of $30,000.

Total Annual Expenses	$360,000
Total Member Months	12,000
Total PMPM:	$30
MONTHLY REVENUE:	$30,000

Information Necessary to Start the Nurse Practitioner Credentialing Process

Legal Name: _____

Home Address: _____

Home Phone: _____

Daytime Phone/Pager #: _____

Fax Number: _____

Date of Birth: _____

Place of Birth: _____

Country of Birth Place (if applicable): _____

Social Security Number: _____

Any Foreign Languages Spoken (list): _____

State License Number: _____Expiration Date: _____

Federal DEA #: _____Expiration Date: _____

Medicare Provider ID Number: _____Medicare UPIN #: _____

Current Medicare Carrier (name of the carrier): _____

State Medicaid Provider ID Number: _____

Specialty: _____Subspecialty: _____

Board Certified: Yes_____No_____

Specialty you are certified in: _____

Certification Number: _____Exp. Date: _____

Date Issued: _____Recertification Date: _____

Name of Issuing Board: _____

Undergraduate Education

College/University: _____Degree: _____

Address: _____

Dates Attended: From: _____ To: _____Date of Degree: _____

Graduate/Professional Education

College/University: _____Degree: _____
Specific Program: _____
Address: _____
Dates Attended: From: _____ To: _____Date of Degree: _____

Additional Training

Location: _____
Address: _____
Specific Program: _____
Dates Attended: From_____ To: _____

Teaching Appointments

Institution: _____
Address: _____
Specific Program: _____
Dates Attended: From_____ To: _____

Hospital/Facility Affiliations

Name: _____
Address: _____
Staff Category: _____Chairperson: _____
Department/Specialty: _____
Dates: From_____To_____

Name: _____
Address: _____
Staff Category: _____Chairperson: _____
Department/Specialty: _____
Dates: From_____To_____

Name: _____
Address: _____
Staff Category: _____Chairperson: _____
Department/Specialty: _____
Dates: From_____To_____

Work History (List Most Current First)

Practice Name: _____
Address: _____

Phone Number: _____ Fax Number: _____
Contact Person: _____
Dates: From_____ To_____

Practice Name: _____
Address: _____
Phone Number: _____ Fax Number: _____
Contact Person: _____
Dates: From_____ To_____

Practice Name: _____
Address: _____
Phone Number: _____ Fax Number: _____
Contact Person: _____
Dates: From_____ To_____

Malpractice Data (For the Past 10 Years)

Liability Carrier_____ Telephone Number_____
Address_____
Amount of Coverage $_____ Policy Number_____
Effective Dates: From _____ To_____
Specialty Coverage_____

Liability Carrier_____ Telephone Number_____
Address_____
Amount of Coverage $_____ Policy Number_____
Effective Dates: From _____ To_____
Specialty Coverage_____

Documentation Needed

State License
Federal DEA Controlled Substance Registration Certificate
Controlled Substance License
Copies of all malpractice insurance face sheets
Wall copies of **all** diplomas
Board certification diplomas OR letters of eligibility
CV (complete and up to date)
Complete details of any malpractice cases (include case numbers, settlement
   information, insurance carriers involved, etc.)

————

Used with permission from Audrey Westdorp, Partner, Certified Healthcare Business Consultant, Enrolled Agent, Grand Management Group, 96 Monroe Centre NW, Suite 300, Grand Rapids, MI 49503

Sample Business Plan

Title Page

Community-Based Family Health Center
4759 East Elmwood Street
Baldwin, Michigan 47984
Phone: (616)555-9726
Fax: (616)555-1092

Mary Smith, RN, FNP

Table of Contents

Executive Summary

The proposed Community-Based Family Health Center will be a primary care office that specializes in the care of individuals, groups, and families in the Baldwin Community. The purpose of the community-based family health center is to provide a holistic model of nursing care to the community. The objectives of the health center are to increase access of health care to the Baldwin community and to offer convenient, community-based health care services. It is located in a rural community at 4759 East Elmwood Street in Baldwin, Michigan. The primary care center (building) is owned and will be operated by Mary Smith, who is an experienced nationally certified family nurse practitioner and nurse manager of ambulatory services. A collaborative agreement has been signed with Jack Markitz, M.D. Susan Fisher, a nationally certified FNP, is excited to work in the clinic. The Baldwin area was chosen for the community-based family center because of the lack of primary care clinics and services offered in a 75-mile area radius.

The scheduled opening date for this primary care center is August 1, 2006. A mailed survey has been conducted and town meetings have been held, both of which demonstrate a need for a primary care center in this rural location. Individuals, families, business owners, and church leaders have provided letters of support for the initiation of the center and volunteer assistance for renovations. There is strong support for the Community-Based Family Health Center being located in Baldwin to increase access within a reasonable distance from individual residences for primary health care services. Marketing efforts will focus on maintaining and strengthening the connections with community agencies, schools, and churches. Quarterly free health and wellness seminars will be held.

The demand for health care services is great in the Baldwin area. It is anticipated that the Community-Based Family Health Center will have many patients transferring care to the new center due to close access and availability of appointments. Revenue projections for Year 1 are strong and show a profit of $64,292. The Community-Based Family Health Center operation will need $200,000 for start-up costs.

Vision, Mission, and Value Statements

Vision

To provide affordable, accessible, quality community-based primary care.

Mission

The Community-Based Family Health Center's mission is to provide community-based, holistic, comprehensive quality primary care to individuals, groups, and families.

Value Statements

- Each individual has the right to primary care services, regardless of the ability to pay.
- Each patient will receive high-quality, cost-effective primary health care.

Market Analysis

A simple market survey was conducted by mailing post cards to Baldwin residents to determine the name of their health care provider, type of health insurance coverage, the distance traveled for a clinic visit, and the desirability of changing to a health care provider in town. Of the 250 individuals sampled (80% response rate), 85% indicated that they traveled more than 70 miles to their health care provider and that they would switch providers if there was a health care center in town. According to national statistics, an individual will make 2.1 visits per year to his or her primary care provider. The geographical area from which we will draw clients is a radius around Baldwin of approximately 40 miles. The population in this area is 15,000. There are no other health care providers for a 75-mile radius, so the competition is limited. Health insurance providers in this area include Medicare, Medicaid, Blue Cross & Blue Shield, PPOM, MESA, and Aetna.

The strengths of this proposal are that there are no health care providers in the local geographical area and there is a strong desire by residents of the town to initiate a local clinic. The two FNPs are respected and trusted in the local community. The weaknesses of the proposed venture are the amount of capital required to start the health center and the lack of existing patients to ensure a continuous revenue stream. The opportunities include establishing a comprehensive community-based primary care center in Baldwin to provide access and convenient, comprehensive, holistic, quality care to residents. The threats include the possibility of a low patient volume when the center initially opens and the possibility that another health care provider would start a health care clinic in Baldwin diluting the patient base between two clinics. These threats are important, but with 15,000 residents in the immediate service area and a survey that indicates 85% may be willing to transfer to a local health care center, the number of patients may exceed capacity with two providers and an additional FNP may need to be added to the practice. Once the health center is established, it will have the competitive advantage over a new clinic because patients will be established and quality care will be ensured through peer review and patient satisfaction questionnaires routinely collected and improvements made based on data collected.

Product Design

The services that will be provided in the Community-Based Family Health Center include health promotion, risk reduction, disease prevention, and the diagnosis and treatment of common acute problems and chronic stable conditions. A holistic approach to the provision of patient care will be used and a functional assessment format will be the foundation of the database for each patient. The office will open on August 1, 2004, for primary care services. The hours for operation of the center will be 40 hours per week. The hours will be 9:00 a.m. to 5:00 p.m. on Monday, Wednesday, and Friday and 10:00 a.m. to 7:00 p.m. on Tuesday and Thursdays. The center will be closed on major holidays.

Simple procedures will be performed at the health center. Examples of procedures include, but are not limited to, nebulizer treatments, blood glucose monitoring, hemoglobin assessment, simple laceration repairs, uncomplicated mole removals, medication injections (allergy shots, Rocephin injections), pulse oximetry, spirometry, cerumen irrigation, anoscopy, Pap smear collection, and collection of specimens (hemoccult analysis, simple urine dip, strep screening).

A quality improvement plan has been discussed and is in place for implementation. This plan includes the distribution of a patient satisfaction survey on the first day of each month. Results will be tabulated and presented at the monthly staff meeting to discuss systems improvements. Other clinical quality indicators will include monitoring immunization status, cervical screening, mammograms, and digital rectal examinations on males older than age 40. Chart audits will be done quarterly on 20 random charts per provider. These results will be shared at the provider meeting.

A collaborative physician agreement has been negotiated and signed with Jack Markitz, M.D., for the Community-Based Family Health Center. This agreement was developed for the purpose of establishing a prescriptive authority agreement, developing a referral system, designing a consultation system, and establishing an on-call plan. Letters of agreement are being sent to physician groups for the purpose of hospital admissions for needed services. The goal is to have pediatric and adult hospital admissions available with physician groups for the nearest hospital 75 miles south of Baldwin in Satchataw. On-call services will be provided when the clinics are closed so as to triage individuals in need of emergent care. A 7-day-a-week, 24-hour-per-day on-call plan will be in effect for individuals needing this service.

Operational Development

Mary Smith will be a full time FNP and work 32 hours of direct patient care and 8 hours of administration. Susan Fisher, FNP, will also work full time 40 hours per week in direct patient care. A full-time receptionist, two full-time medical assistants, and a 20-hour-per-week coder and biller will be hired. Dr. Markitz has signed a collaborative agreement with Smith and Fisher. A cleaning agency will be contracted with for housekeeping services. Accounting services (bookkeeping and auditing services) have been arranged through a local CPA (Brian Sandar) and a lawyer (Jeff Small) has agreed to handle clinic legal issues for reviewing contracts. Marketing activities will be conducted by clinic personnel.

Initial equipment expenditures will include the following items:

Computer (2)	$5,470
Microscope	$1,450
Anoscope	$50
Nebulizer	$110
EKG machine	$6,900
Suturing sets	$100
Pelvic light source	$150
Speculums	$50
Thermometer	$325
Cryofreeze equipment	$325
Tympanogram	$2,180
Hemoque	$125
Glucometer	$120
Adult scale	$350
Baby scale	$350
Oto/ophthalmoscopes (3)	$400
Peak flow meter	$100
BP cuff (A/P/L)	$300
Refrigerator/freezer	$700
TOTAL INITIAL EQUIPMENT COST	$19,555

Marketing Plan

Based on the mission of the Community-Based Family Health Center, marketing efforts will focus on alerting individuals, groups, and families to the community-based, holistic, comprehensive, quality primary care services that are offered. The goal of the marketing campaign is to get the message that the Community-Based Family Health Center is available to all age groups and provides comprehensive services. Specific objectives of the marketing plan are to (1) inform businesses, schools, and community agencies of the opening and services provided at the Community-Based Family Health Center; (2) provide free community-based health promotion seminars to the public; (3) provide basic health and wellness services to the community such as flu immunization clinics and school-based sports physicals; and (4) collaborate with existing community programs to promote the health and welfare of citizens in Baldwin.

To accomplish the objectives, the following marketing activities will be planned, implemented, and evaluated by clinic staff. An open house will be hosted the weekend prior to the opening of the health center. Balloons, coffee, and popcorn will be available at the open house for the health center. All staff members will be available to tour guests and the FNPs will be holding free health seminars throughout the day in the conference room. Local merchants have offered to put brochures about the Community-Based Family Health Center on their bulletin boards. The Baldwin Public School will send brochures home with each child and the local church groups will post brochures on the bulletin board and make announcements at social functions. Mary Smith, FNP, has contacted the local chamber of commerce, church groups, and local health department and has offered to host free educational sessions. The Community-Based Family Health Center will also conduct sports physicals for $23.00 per child at the public school and provide each participant with a brochure. A flu vaccination clinic will be held in October at the health center with a fee of $15.00 per flu vaccination. This flu clinic may be the first contact a patient has with the health center. Tours of the facility will be provided on request. The Chamber of Commerce welcome center has agreed to place a brochure about the health center in their welcome packet to visitors and new residents.

Maintaining community ties and relationships will be very important. Attendance at Chamber of Commerce meetings and communication with the public school and church groups will be ongoing. Free health care seminars will be offered quarterly in the community.

Organizational Plan

The administrator and owner of the clinic is Mary Smith. Mary will handle the managerial aspects of the business and spend part of her time in direct patient care. Susan will work full time as a FNP providing direct patient care. Susan will manage day-to-day operations when Mary is on vacation or out of the office for conferences or illness. Dr. Jack Markitz will be the collaborating

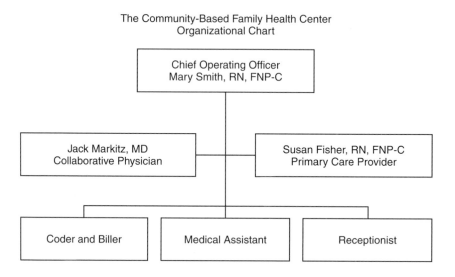

The Community-Based Family Health Center
Organizational Chart

physician and will schedule a monthly meeting to review charts and consult on select cases. The coder and biller, receptionist, and medical assistants will report to Mary, but will also be responsible to Susan for day-to day operational issues. Mary and Susan will hold an hour-long weekly team meeting to review personnel, staffing, patient issues, administrative initiatives, and quality assurance activities. The figure on the previous page illustrates the organizational chart for the Community-Based Family Health Center.

Development Schedule

The table on the following page provides a visual representation of a year of planning, implementation, and evaluation activities.

Community-Based Family Health Center Project Activities

ACTIVITY	May-05	Jun-05	Jul-05	Aug-05	Sep-05	Oct-05	Nov-05	Dec-05	Jan-06	Feb-06	Mar-06	Apr-06
Sign collaborative agreement	X											
Sign accountant agreement	X											
Lawyer reviews contracts	X											
Obtain Medicare numbers	X											
Obtain Medicaid numbers	X											
Obtain other insurance provider numbers												
• Blue Cross & Blue Shield	X											
• MESA	X											
• PPOM	X											
• Aetna	X											
Obtain CLIA laboratory waiver	X											
Obtain hazardous license permit		X	X									
Purchase equipment		X										
Hire staff												
• Receptionist		X										
• Two medical assistants		X										
• Coder/biller		X										

Activity												
Orient staff		X	X									
Marketing activities	X	X	X		X	X	X	X	X	X	X	X
Quality improvement activities												
• Patient satisfaction questionnaire distribution				X	X	X	X	X	X	X	X	X
• Immunization reviews						X		X	X		X	X
• Pap & pelvic reviews						X		X	X		X	X
• Digital rectal exam reviews						X		X	X		X	X
• Mammography reviews						X		X	X		X	X
Health & wellness community programs	X			X		X		X	X			
Develop policies & procedures												
• OSHA		X										
• Clinical		X										
• Personnel		X										
Begin investigating electronic medical record cost and implementation		X	X	X	X	X						

Financial Plan

Anticipated Costs

Personnel:	2.0 FTE FNP	$140,000
	2.0 FTE MA	$44,000
	1.0 FTE Receptionist	$20,000
	0.5 FTE Biller	$14,000
Contracts and Expenses:	Physician:	$20,000
	CLIA	$200
	Biohazard	$75
	Malpractice Insurance	$3,500
	Accountant Fee	$3,500
	Attorney Fee	$1,500
	Housekeeping Fee	$1,500
	Marketing Costs	$3,000
Annual Patient Care Supplies:		$1,800
Annual Office Supplies		$3,000
Other Expenses: Phone Toll		$1,000
	Data Lines	$840
Office Management Systems		$5,000
Computer Support		$1,500
	FAX Costs	$250
	Copying	$1,000
	Postage	$500
Total Start-Up Equipment Costs:		$19,555
First-Year Mortgage Expense:		$17,000
Annual Maintenance (Equipment Purchases, Building Repair, Equipment Repair)		$12,000
TOTAL FIRST-YEAR OPERATIONAL COSTS:		$314,720
	(fringe benefits)	+ $71,940
		$386,660

Revenue Projections

Visit Types: All visits may be either with an existing or new patient. Reimbursement rates are higher for new patients due to the documentation requirements, intensity, and data collection required at each level.

Projected service numbers are based on a projection of one-half typical provider volume per FNP. Susan has 5 days per week at 20 open visits per day and Sharon has 4 days per week at 20 open visits per day. Based on a 46-week work year (6 weeks vacation/personnel days), the total possible number of patient visit slots ($\frac{1}{2}$ load) is 90 patient visits per week × 46 weeks = 4140 visits.

In Year 2, when the clinic has been operational for 1 year, we anticipate a full patient visit slot per day. The mix of new patients will still be approximately the same as Year 1 because new patients will be transferring to the Community-Based Family Health Center. In this scenario it is anticipated that Susan would work 5 days per week with 20 open visit slots per day, and Sharon would have 4 days per week at 20 open visit slots per day. Based on the 46-week work year with 180 patient visits per week = 8,280 visits.

In Year 3, we anticipate a full schedule based on community demand with 8,280 visits. The difference here will be that the number of existing patients will be greater than that of new patients. Based on our initial survey data for demand, we may consider adding a third provider to handle new patients. This decision will be made during Year 2.

- Level 1 visit – basic visit, simple service provision, health teaching may be presented at this visit. Often coded for nurse visits such as simple BP check or a visit for a urinary tract infection
- Level 2 – minor, uncomplicated visit and service provision
- Level 3 – moderately complex visit and service provision
- Level 4 – complex visit and service provision
- Level 5 – intensive, comprehensive service provision.

Visit Type	Expected Volume/ Year 1	Average/ Charge/ Service	Total
99211/Existing Patient Level 1 Visit	120	$26	$3,120
99212/Existing Patient Level 2 Visit	550	$36	$19,800
99213/Existing Patient Level 3 Visit	700	$65	$45,500
99214/Exisitng Patient Level 4 Visit	200	$96	$19,200
99201/New Patient Level 1 Visit	125	$36	$4,500
99202/New Patient Level 2 Visit	550	$48	$26,400
99203/New Patient Level 3 Visit	700	$97	$67,900
99204/New Patient Level 4 Visit	200	$129	$25,800
99381/Preventive visit, new infant	10	$107	$1,070
99382/Preventive visit, new, age 1-4	57	$117	$6,669
99383/Preventive visit, new ages 5-11	57	$117	$6,669
99384/Preventive visit, new, 12-17	67	$127	$8,509
99385/Preventive visit, new, 18-39	100	$146	$146,000
99386/Preventive visit, new, 40-64	101	$176	$17,776
99387/Preventive visit, new 65 & older	135	$186	$25,110

Continued

Visit Type	Expected Volume/ Year 1	Average/ Charge/ Service	Total
99391/Preventive visit, established infant	10	$96	$960
99392/Preventive visit, established, age 1-4	57	$107	$6,099
99393/Preventive visit, established, age 5-11	57	$107	$6,099
99394/Preventive visit, established, age 12-17	67	$117	$7,839
99395/Preventive visit, established, age 18-39	100	$127	$12,700
99396/Preventive visit, established, age 40-64	101	$136	$13,736
99397/Preventive visit, established, age 65 & older	76	$146	$11,096
Total Services	**4,140**		**$506,252**

Common Procedures	Number of Procedures	Revenue Projection
Strep screen ($20)	250	$5,000
Urinalysis ($16)	250	$4,000
Nebulizer treatment ($37)	75	$2,775
Spirometry ($49)	35	$1,715
Pulse oximetry ($16)	65	$1,040
Flu vaccine ($15)	650	$9,750
Total Services	**1,325**	**$24,280**

Total Revenues	$530,532
15% Industry Write-Off for Uninsured	$79,580
Total Collectable Revenues	$450,952
Total First-Year Expenses	$386,660
Total Projected Profit* Year 1	$ 64,292
Goal for Rainy Day Fund for Unexpected Expenditures	$100,000

SUMMARY

In summary, I feel that the Community-Based Family Health Center is a viable, critical primary care service offered to the Baldwin community. Residents of Baldwin will have improved access, 24-hour-per-day, 7-day-a-week access via clinic or triage service. The projected revenue and expenditures illustrate that a profit can be made in the first year based on market projections and will continue for each subsequent year in operation.

――――

*Profits will be paid to staff when Rainy Day Fund, mortgage and future expenditures are funded. Staff will receive a $1,000 bonus and Susan will receive a bonus of $1,500 or 15% of revenues she generates, whichever is greater.

Sample Basic Grant Application with Introductory Cover Letter

Date

Michigan Campus Compact
31 Kellogg Center
East Lansing, MI 48824-1022

Dear Michigan Campus Compact Personnel:

I have enclosed a copy of a grant proposal for a project entitled "Health and Fitness K-12." This proposal provides an opportunity for Community Health Nursing Students to provide needed community services to school-age children. This program is intended to increase students' awareness of the need to volunteer and provide essential services to the community. It will also develop a partnership between State County Health Department, Anytown Public Schools, and the School of Nursing.

Proposal originator's name:
Mary Smith, R.N., Ph.D., FNP-C
Professor of Nursing
College of Nursing
State University
Anytown, MI 49401
(616)555-3558

Person who will advise the project and budget:
Susan Carey, Director of Student Life
Student Life Office, School of Nursing
State University
Anytown, MI 49401
(616)555-2345

Thank you for your consideration of this proposal.

Sincerely,

Mary Smith, RN, PhD
Professor of Nursing

Title Page
Health and Fitness K-12
Mary Smith, RN, PhD, FNP-C
Professor of Nursing
College of Nursing
State University

Abstract

Health and Fitness for K-12

The Health and Fitness for K-12 grant is an initiative by the College of Nursing to facilitate student involvement in community projects as part of their community health clinical rotation. The grant will assist students in selecting teaching projects focusing on health and fitness for students in grades K-12 and strengthen working relationships with the State County Health Department. The Health Department personnel will identify those schools in the Grand Rapids area that are in need of teaching interventions for health and fitness activities. The faculty in the Community Health Nursing Clinical Rotations will meet, coordinate, integrate, and evaluate this project. The addition of a community school teaching project for health and fitness for K-12 students will be a valuable component and learning activity in the undergraduate student nursing program.

Table of Contents

Introduction

Health and Fitness for K-12 is an initiative by the College of Nursing at State University to facilitate student involvement in community projects as part of their community health clinical nursing rotation. The proposed project activities are (1) to assist students to select teaching projects focusing on health and fitness for students in grades K-12; and (2) to work with the County Health Department to identify schools in the Grand Rapids area that need teaching interventions from nursing students for health and fitness activities.

The intended outcome of the proposed project is to increase students' awareness of the need to volunteer and provide services to the community. A second outcome is to provide needed services to the Grand Rapids community. While most of the Grand Raids public schools employ a nurse to cover basic health problems, one nurse may cover up to seven schools, making it nearly impossible to provide first aid, coordinate health activities, and implement routine health teaching. In addition, most private and parochial schools in this area do not employ a nurse and rely on the County Health Department for consultation. Because of the nurses' assignments at the County Health Department, they may not be able to provide routine teaching on health and fitness to all of the students in the private and parochial schools. Therefore, in the K-12 grades in the Grand Rapids area there is a need for school-age children to receive teaching on health and fitness.

Background

The U.S. Public Health Service has published the *Healthy People 2010* document (U.S. Department of Health and Human Services, 2000) and established national health goals. The purpose of establishing nationwide goals is to provide support for improving the health of children and adults in America. Specifically, the goal for children is to optimize health through education and health care. Families are often the primary providers of care and developing healthy habits, but communities have responsibilities to promote health and fitness. The development of community-based programs is essential to meet the goals of the U.S. Public Health Service. Examples of community-based programs to improve health and fitness include health fairs, bicycle safety helmet campaigns, and programs on healthy lifestyles. An important role of the community health nurse is to link needed services with the school system to improve the health of school-age children. The goal of our proposed program is to provide health and fitness education to children in K-12 to help fill a need in our community.

A problem in providing needed community services is the lack of coordination of programs. We intend to work closely with the County Health Department to identify those schools and grade levels that are in desperate need of health and fitness education. In this way the Community Health Nursing Faculty in the College of Nursing will build a link with schools and the County Health Department in providing services to those who need them.

In the United States health problems have resulted from limited exercise, increased amounts of junk food consumption, and excessive television viewing. Michigan is listed among the top 10 states whose citizens have limited exercise patterns and have a disproportionate number of obese children and adults. Research shows that prevention of health problems and improving healthy lifestyles for children and adults result in significant cost savings. Therefore, money spent on health and fitness for children is a sound investment.

Proposal Description

The project is intended to increase student nurses' awareness of volunteerism, to design, implement, and evaluate a teaching program, and to facilitate student participation in a community teaching activity. Health and Fitness for K-12 is vital to the child establishing a healthy life pattern. As part of the students' community health clinical rotation, a teaching project targeting grades K-12 will be required. The clinical experience will be community based and facilitate the students' involvement in community work.

There are three community health clinical rotations in the fall semester lasting 7 weeks for a total of 45 students. The community health team has agreed to implement a teaching project focusing on three to four grades per each of the three clinical rotation sites. Therefore, the three community health nursing faculty at three different community health nursing sites will require their students to complete a teaching project. The students will be able to select the grade and health topic of their choice using a developmentally appropriate topic for the specific age and target population in conjunction with the Health Department and college personnel. A list of schools will be prepared by the community health faculty in collaboration with the Health Department to be distributed to the students to select a school and grade that needs health and fitness teaching.

Project Timeline

The health teaching aids will be purchased during the summer so that materials for teaching grades K-12 will be readily available to students in the Learning Resource Laboratory at the College of Nursing on a sign-out basis. During the summer months, community health nursing faculty will work with the County Health Department Educational Coordinator to establish a list of schools and grade levels that are in need of health educational programs.

At the end of the summer semester we will call a team meeting for community health nursing clinicals, review the school list, and discuss our school targets (so that we don't choose the same schools for health teaching). In fall and winter terms we will schedule a health education program for three different schools involving nine grades.

Probable Effects of this Project on the Identified Problem

1. Community and student awareness of the importance of health and fitness education in K-12
2. Student interaction with community, faculty, teachers, students, and principles about health education
3. Student awareness and commitment to the importance of volunteerism in the community
4. Improved health promotion in select K-12 grades
5. Experience in designing, implementing, and evaluating a teaching program.

Anticipated Impact of this Project

1. The students involved in the project:
   a. Increased knowledge of the development levels of students at different grade levels
   b. Interaction of students with school personnel to organize and coordinate a successful health education program
   c. Development of presentation and speaking skills
   d. An awareness of the health teaching needs of students in the County and the role they can play in meeting these needs
   e. An opportunity for personal growth in planning, conducting, and meeting a need in the community
   f. Increased skill in designing, implementing and evaluating a teaching program.
2. The campus:
   a. The program will build links between schools, the County Health Department, and the College of Nursing.
   b. The program will provide positive interactions and university recognition for providing essential services to the community.
   c. This program may serve as a model for other disciplines to include community projects in their academic programs.
3. The community:
   a. The program will build positive working relationships between schools, the County Health Department, and the College of Nursing.
   b. Students who reside in this community will experience community service and may continue their efforts in volunteerism in the future.

Project Evaluation

Based on the developmental level of the students we present health and fitness education to, we will either verbally for elementary grades or written for secondary grades elicit their understanding of the material. We will send home with the students a letter explaining what we have taught to their son or daughter and written materials on each topic encouraging their parents or caregivers to reinforce this material. We will speak with the teachers and have them evaluate the programs and offer suggestions for improvement.

Supporting Letter

Date

Michigan Campus Compact
31 Kellogg Center
East Lansing, MI 48824-1022

Dear Grant Committee Members:

I am in full support of the "Health and Fitness K-12" proposal currently before your committee. This community-based project will provide students in their Community Health Nursing Clinical rotation with the opportunity to provide needed community service to school-age children. It will strengthen links between the County Health Department, Grand Rapids schools, students, and faculty of the College of Nursing.

I appreciate your consideration of the "Health and Fitness K-12" proposal.

Sincerely,

Jane Fryer
Dean, College of Nursing

Susan Baker
Coordinator, County Health Department

References

U.S. Department of Health and Human Services. (2000). *Healthy people 2010: National health promotion and disease prevention objective* (Conference edition in two volumes). Washington, DC: U.S. Government Printing Office.

Description of Project Personnel

Principal Investigator: Mary Smith, RN, PhD, FNP-C, Professor of Nursing at the College of Nursing

Community Health Nursing Faculty: June Freer, RN, MSN, and Deb Angle, RN., MSN

Dr. Mary Smith will be responsible for coordinating and holding team meetings with the Community Health Nursing Faculty.

Dr. Mary Smith, Professor Freer, and Professor Angle will work together to plan, coordinate, implement, and evaluate this project. The team will meet with the County Health Department coordinator to develop a list of schools in need of health teaching. Each faculty member will make the appropriate contacts with the area schools and work with the nursing students to design, implement, and evaluate the teaching projects.

Budget for Health and Fitness K-12

Material Resources

1. Health Edco Company
   a. Mr. Clean Mouth Teaches Oral Hygiene
      i. D079148 Mr. Clean Mouth — $84.95
      ii. D054034 Giant Toothbrush — $14.95
      iii. D079161 Carrying Case — $27.95
   b. D079647 Consequences of AIDS — $295.00
   c. D050525 Brush, Comb, Scrub — $3.95
   d. Staying Clean & Healthy: Creative Activities for Teaching Basic Personal Hygiene Habits
      i. D079242 Staying Clean & Healthy Set — $19.95
      ii. D041166 Staying Clean & Healthy Workbook — $9.95
      iii. D089389 Set of 4 Posters — $15.95
      iv. D090389 Set of 4 Posters — $23.95
      v. D090387 Don't Bring Germs to Dinner — $6.95
      vi. D090386 Did You Wash Your Hands? — $6.25
      vii. It's No Secret .. Bath — $6.25
      viii. D090388 This Prince.. Teeth — $6.25
   e. D041144 Self-Esteem — $100.00
   f. D041342 Nutrition — $100.00
   g. D085300 Healthy Sticker Messages — $100.00
   h. D085501 Pyramid Game and Nutrition Flash Cards — $89.95
   i. D054250 The Heart of America — $297.00
   j. D054457 Lung Model — $207.00
   k. D054604 Mini Skeleton with Skull — $215.00
2. ABCO – Medical Products Catalog
   a. Dopler Abco Pocket DOP II 080500 Unit w/5 MHz Vascular Probe — $635.00
3. 9810PL Classification and Appearance of Burns — $21.95
4. 9820PL First Aid for Burns — $21.95
5. 9830PL Smoke Inhalation and Inhalation Injuries — $21.95
6. ZAD-2F Zaadi Dolls to Teach Children About Their Bodies — $249.95
7. The Fat Case TFC 2 — $89.95
8. Dental Hygiene Kit — $295.00
9. First Aid Kit — $275.00
10. D079116 Crash Kramer Seat Belt Demonstration & Replacement (D079119) — $135.00 / $14.95
11. D085002 Our Teeth: A multilayered puzzle — $21.95
12. Microscope — $175.00
13. TOTAL EXPENSES: — $3,622.05

Common Terms and Definitions Used in the Coding and Billing Process

Term	Definition
International Classification of Diseases, 9th edition	A system designed to standardize health care diagnoses for reimbursement purposes
Fee for service	Health care providers charge patients separately for each service
Capitation	Prepayment for services on a per-member per-month basis.
Copayment	Portion of claim or expense that the member must pay out of own pocket
Coinsurance	A provision in insurance that limits amount of coverage to a certain percentage (80%)
Deductible	Amount the member must pay before any insurance coverage applies
Adverse selection	Situation where the insurance carrier has a disproportionate enrollment risk
Community rating	Setting premiums based on an average cost for a service in a given area
Experience rating	Rate setting based on average cost of service by various group characteristics
Global budgeting	Overall budget limit on health care services, regardless of where funds originate
Current Procedural Terminology Code	A system designed by the American Medical Association to reimburse specific units of health care services
Omnibus Budget Reconciliation Act	Congressional acts that frequently have legislation related to health care
Resource-based relative value scale	Complex federal regulations that rate health care activities for Medicare Part B reimbursement

Health Care Financing Agency (HCFA)	Federal agency that determines rules and regulations for health care reimbursement policy
Relative value unit	A unit of health care that is specifically reimbursed according to rates set by HCFA; varies according to level of care and geographical area
Skilled nursing facility	A facility such as a nursing home; nursing reimbursement is permitted under specific regulations
Diagnostic-related groupings	A predetermined payment to a hospital based on the patient diagnosis
Tax Equity and Fiscal Responsibility Act	Federal regulation that allows states to reimburse health care for special populations according to their needs through a system of waivers
Physician Payment Review Commission	Agency that determines Medicare reimbursement rates and regulations
Primary care providers	Health care professionals who are in ongoing relationships with the patients
Prospective payment system	A capitated reimbursement plan that provides payment based on designated amount per enrollee per year
Civilian Health and Medical Program of the United States	Plan that provides health care to military personnel and their families and reimburses NPs
Federal Employee Health Benefit Plan	Group insurance plan of federal employees and their dependents that recognizes APNs as providers
Prepaid Medical Assistance Program	Managed care system for Medicare populations that includes all services such as prevention, care, transportation, and interpreter services
Federally designated clinics or federally qualified health clinics	Clinics located in urban or rural underserved areas to improve access to care for specific populations

Source: From APN Reimbursement Module, University of Minnesota, School of Nursing. Available at *www.nursing.umn.edu/professional/reimbursement/index2.html*; Bodenheimer, T.S., & Grumbach, K. (2002). *Understanding health policy: A clinical approach* (3rd ed.). New York: Lange.; Sheehy, C.M., & McCarthy, M.C., (1998). *Advanced practice nursing: Emphasizing common roles.* Philadelphia: F.A. Davis.

Coding Case Study

T.C., a 50-year-old African-American female (new office visit) presents with BP elevation in the Occupational Health Services after complaining of a headache while at work.

Subjective

CC: C/O HTN, no care for the past 10 years, no primary care provider
HPI: Diagnosed in 1991 with HTN, without medicine past 10 years because she did not feel she needed them. She stated "I felt fine until the last couple of months." No prescriptive or OTC medications, denies use of any herbal products. She has had dizziness and headache intermittently for the past 2 months. Denies CP, SOB, palpitations, blurred vision, edema. Episodes of syncope once a week for 3 weeks; no LOC. States she feels "dizzy when going from sitting to standing position." Denies blackouts, bowel or bladder incontinence.

ALLERGIES: None known
PMH: Asthma as adolescent, no current meds
PAST SURGICAL HISTORY: Denies any surgery
FAMILY HISTORY: Father 77, alive, HTN, MI 1993 at age of 70
                       Mother 75, alive, HTN, Alzheimer's
                       Grandparents: Unknown
                       Siblings, all healthy, 2 sisters, ages 52 , 54; no known medical problems

SOCIAL HISTORY: Tobacco: 30 packs per year; no desire to quit, no previous attempts to quit. ETOH: 2 drinks per week
Denies any use of marijuana or other street drugs.
Exercise: Walks approx. about one mile/day at work. No exercise outside work.
Nutrition: 2 meals/day, breakfast and dinner. One fried meal per day. Caffeine, one cup per day

PSYCHOLOGICAL: Single, never married, lives alone, owns home. No current stressors. No abuse history. Works full time in Medical Records at Hometown Hospital.

ROS: Neuro: 3-4 HA/week × two months. Denies visual changes
CV and RESP: Denies SOB, palpitations, pedal edema, or chest discomfort

RENAL: Denies dysuria, hematuria, CVA tenderness, or nocturia
Denies personal or family history of disease. Reports no polyuria, polydipsia, or polyphagia.

Objective

Well appearing, overweight AA female NAD
Ht: 5 feet; Wt: 164; BMI: 32.1; right arm sitting 194/120, HRR 98
Repeat BP: R sitting 178/115, supine 194/122; Left standing 191/110
Eyes: PERRLA, EOMI, no AV nicking, hemorrhaging, exudates
Neck: Lt JVD, 1-2 cm, no bruits, no thyromegaly, no lymphadenopathy
Chest: Inspiratory wheezing, bilateral anterior upper airways, posterior clear
Heart: S1S2, Grade II/VI systolic murmur at LSB nonradiating, RRR at 78
Abdomen: Soft. Nontender, nondistended, BS×4 no femoral bruits, no hepato-splenomegaly
Extremities: Warm, 2+ pulses radial, DP, PT no edema or varicosities
EKG: Done in office diagnosed the left ventricular hypertrophy (LVH)

Assessment

Uncontrolled HTN, Stage III with LVH (ICD–9: 401.9 and 401.10, 402.90 for LVH)
Knowledge Deficit CV disease process and HTN (NANDA-I: 00126)
Nicotine dependence: Precontemplation Stage (No ICD-9 or NANDA-I code exists)
Imbalanced nutrition (NANDA-I: 00001)

Plan

Labs: Lytes, BUN, creatinine, TSH, CBC, Multistick U/A (81000) Urine creatinine, protein, microalbumin, coronary risk profile, lipid profile (venipuncture in office: 36415)
Meds: Clonidine 0.1 mg by mouth once a day.
       HCTZ 25 mg once daily
Tests: 12-Lead EKG (CPT 93005)
Health education (NIC: 5510): Side effects and precautions re: medication.
Teaching, prescribed diet, disease information (NIC: 5614) 2 gram sodium diet, use salt substitute examples provided. Informed about HTN as "Silent Killer"; brochure given.
Anticipatory guidance (NIC: 5210) re: risk associated with smoking and CV disease.
Behavior modification (NIC: 4360) encouraged to consider quitting and setting quit date, brochures provided.
Patient agrees to read and consider the plan.

Other: Off work 3 days, pending improved blood pressure
Follow Up: RTO 3-5 days for complete PE—patient agrees

Summary of coding processes:
E&M Code: 99203, detailed history, detailed exam, and low complexity decision making

ICD–9, Diagnosis Code(s):
401.9 Uncontrolled Hypertension
401.10402.90 Left Ventricular Hypertrophy
305.1 Nicotine Dependence

NANDA-I Code(s)
Deficient Knowledge r/t CV disease process and HTN (NANDA-I 00126)
Nicotine Dependence: Precontemplation Stage (No code)
Imbalanced nutrition (NANDA-I 00001)

CPT Code(s)
EKG: 93005
Multistick UA: 81000
Venipuncture in office: 36415

NIC Codes:
Anticipatory guidance (5210)
Behavior modification (4360)
Health Education (5510)
Teaching, Prescribed Diet (5614)

Payers and Basic Rules and Regulations for APN Billing

Payer/Billing Mechanism	Rules and Regulations for APN Billing
Medicaid recognition by statute	Type of APN recognized in statute varies by state (e.g., for Michigan it includes CNMs, FNP, PNP, ANP).
Medicaid recognition through regulations	Recognition approved in all states; amount reimbursed varies by state and type of APN (e.g., for Michigan regulations exist for 100% for NPs, 65% for CNMs).
Private reimbursement laws	Some states have written regulations mandating private insurers to directly reimburse APNs.
Medicare reimbursement allowed with state practice act that allows for collaboration	Direct Medicare reimbursement is allowed for APN services if it is allowed by state statute and it varies by type of APN who can be reimbursed. The rate is set at 85% per the federal government (e.g., in Michigan, direct reimbursement is allowed at 85% for NPs only).
Medicare "Incident to" reimbursement allowed	"Incident to" Medicare reimbursement is allowed for APN services if it is allowed by state statute. The rate is set at 100% per the federal government, but specific rules and regulations surround the billing of APN services on an "Incident to" basis (e.g., in Michigan, direct reimbursement is allowed at 100% for APNs given the rules are applied).
Direct managed care organization reimbursement	Few MCOs have allowed for direct reimbursement to APNs due to restrictions placed on policies for the empanelling of providers. (e.g., in Michigan only three organizations have developed policies for APNs and only three NP groups have been reimbursed).

CHAMPUS	All APNs can be directly reimbursed for their services. The percentage of reimbursement varies by type of APN and the service delivered (e.g., in Michigan, NPs can be reimbursed at 100%).
FQHC, RHC reimbursement	All APNs can be directly reimbursed for their services. The percentage of reimbursement varies by type of APN and the service delivered (e.g., in Michigan, NPs can be reimbursed at 100%). Rates are set by the federal government and vary by designation (i.e., FQHC versus RHC).
Indemnity insurance companies	Although few currently exist, some companies will directly reimburse for services (e.g., in Michigan Blue Cross and Blue Shield will directly reimburse NPs at 85% and CNMs at 65%). Separate union-negotiated contracts may exclude these reimbursement policies for APNs.

Examples of Superbills

Example 1: Family Practice Superbill

Any Family Practice
1111 Central Avenue • Metropolis, MI 49008 • (616) 789-9876

Code	$	Description	Code	$	Description	Code	$	Description
		Office Tests			**Injections**			**X-Rays**
82075		Alcohol - Breath	90782		Admin.			
82055		Alcohol - Urine	20610 & J7320		Synvisk Inj. (includes aspiration)			
92551		Audio Test	J1020		Depomedral 20 Mg			
93000		EKG	J1030		Depomedral 40 Mg			
93230		Holter	J1040		Depomedral 80 Mg			
94010		PFT	95115		Allergy			
92567		Tympanogram	J3301		Aristocort ___ MG			
92081		Vision	J0702		Celestone ___ CC			
			J05		CR Bicillin ___ Units			
		Fractures	J1000		Estrogen			
27808		Ankle Bimallerlar	J1760		Iron-Infed			
25622		Carpal	J0696		Rocephin ___			
23500		Clavical	X9253		Stadol			
27230		Femur	J1080		Testosterone			
27780		Fibula	J1885		Toradol ___ MG			
24500		Humeral Shaft	J3410		Vistaril ___ MG			**P.M. Exam**
26600		Metacarpal	J3420		Vitamin B-12	OB		OB visit No Charge
28470		Metatarsal R & L				NC		No Charge Follow Up
28400		os Calais (Heel)			**Procedures**	99211		Suture Removal
26720		Phalanges	57454		Colposcopy	99381		New Phys Exam Infant under Age 1
25600		Radial Distal	57511		Cyro Cervix	99382		New Phys Exam Age 1-4
25500		Radial Shaft	58100		Endometrial Biopsy	99383		New Phys Exam Age 5-11
25560		Radial Ulnar	59426		New OB	99384		New Phys Exam Age 12-17
21800		Rib FX	94760		Pulse Ox- Simple	99385		New Phys Exam Age 18-39
27750		Tibia	20550		Trigger Point Inj.	99386		New Phys Exam Age 40-64
27800		Tibia & Fibula				99387		New Phys Exam Age 65+
24670		Ulna-Proximal			**Immunizations**	99391		Est. Phys Exam Infant under Age 1
25530		Ulna-Shaft	90659		Flu HD	99392		Est. Phys Exam Age 1-4
			90700		DPT/ DTAP HD	99393		Est. Phys Exam 5-11
		Labs	90744		Hepatitis B 0 to 17 HD	99394		Est. Phys Exam 12-17
85024		CBC	90746		Hepatitis B 18 & Older HD	99395		Est. Phys Exam 18-39
DS		Drug Screen	90645		HIB HD	99396		Est. Phys Exam 40-64
DSC		Drug Screen Collection	90713		IPV HD	99397		Est. Phys Exam Age 65+
82962		Glucose -fingerstick	90707		MMR HD			
82950		Glucose Tolerance 1 hr.	90712		OPV HD			
86308		Mono Spot	90669		Prevnar HD			
82270		Occult Blood	86580		TB HD			
81025		Pregnancy	90716		Varicella HD			
87880		Strep Screen	95115		Immun Admin, single inj HD			
81001		Urinalysis W/ Micro	95117		Immun Admin, 2 oz + inj HD			
81003		Urinalysis W/O Micro						
36415		Venipuncture Fee			**Ultrasounds/**			
G0001		Venipuncture MCR			**Bone Density**			
85610		Protine	76075		Bone Density			
			76700		ABD			
		EM Codes	93925		Arterial Duplex			
99211		EST PT/ Supervisio n/ Minimal	76645		Breast			
99212		EST PT/ Prob focus/ Limited	93880		Carotid Dup Limited			
99213		EST PT/ Exp Focus/ Low to Mod.	93882		Carotid Dup Unlimited			
99214		EST PT/ Detailed/ Mod. To High	76775		Gallbladder			
99215		EST PT/ Comp/ High Complexity	76805		OB Complete			
99201		New PT/ Prob Focus/ Limited	76815		OB Limited			
99202		New PT/ Exp Focus/ Low to Mod.	76856		Pelvic			
99203		New PT/ Detailed/ Mod. To Sever.	93970		Verous Dup, Bilateral			
99204		New PT/ Comp/ Mod. To High Sev.	93971		Verous Dup Uni or Limited			
99205		New PT/ Comp/ High Complexity						

Previous Balance: ___

Today's Charges: ___

Paid on Account: ___

Method of Payment: Cash Check CC

TOTAL

DUE ___

NEXT APPOINTMENT:

Days ___ Weeks ___ Months ___

PROCEDURE: ___

TESTS/PROCEDURES TO BE SCHEDULED: ___

Example 2: Speciality Superbill

Any Gynecology Practice
1111 Midwest Lane
Rural, Michigan 49000

CODE	$	DESCRIPTION – OFFICE	CODE	$	DESCRIPTION – SURGICAL	CODE	$	DESCRIPTION – PATH & LAB
			11400		Exc B lesion trunk,arm,leg 0.5 or			
		Office Visits						*Pathology & Laboratory*
99201		NP, Foc Prob, Strt	11401		0.6 cm – 1.0 cm	81002		Urinalysis
99202		NP, Exp Prob, Strt	11402		1.1 cm – 2.0 cm	82270		Guaiac Stool Test
99203		NP, Det H&P, Low Comp	11420		Exc B lesion genit, scalp etc 0.5	84703		Pregnancy Test
99204		NP, Det H&P, Mod Comp	11421		0.6 cm – 1.0 cm	85018		Hemoglobin
99205		NP, Det H&P, High Comp	11422		1.1 cm – 2.0 cm	86585		TB Test
99211		Est. PT, Minimal Service	11975		Norplant Insertion	86588		Streptococcus, screen, direct
99212		Est PT, Prob Foc, H&P Strt	11976		Norplant Removal	57210		Wet Mount
99213		Est. PT, Exp H&P, Low Comp	19000		Breast Cyst, Aspiration			
99214		Est. PT, Det H&P, Mod Comp	56420		I & D Bartholin Abscess			
								Radiology
99215		Est. PT, Comp H&P, High Com	56501		Condylomata Mult Chem	76075		Bone Density Scan, axial Skeleton
			56600		Cervical Polyp Removal	76076		Bone Density Scan, append Skel.
		Preventive Medicine						
99384		New Patient, Age 12-17	56605		Vulva Biopsy, first lesion	76805		Echography, OB, complete
99385		New Patient, Age 18 – 39	56606		Each additional lesion	76810		Echography, OB, comp, mult gest.
99386		New Patient, Age 40 – 64	57061		Destruction Vaginal Lesion	76815		Echography, OB, limited
99387		New Patient, Age 65 & Over	57170		Diaphragm Fitting	76816		Echography, OB, repeat/ follow-up
99394		Est. Patient, Age 12 – 17	57452		Colposcopy			
99395		Est. Patient, Age 18 – 39	57454		Colposcopy with Biopsy			
								Obstetrics
99396		Est. Patient, Age 40 – 64	57520		Cervical Biopsy, single/multiple	X4850		VBAC
99397		Est. Patient, Age 65 & Over	57505		Endocervical Curettage	X4853		PN per Visit
G0101		Pap, Pelvic, Breast Exam	57510		Cervical Cauterization	X4854		High Risk Prenatal
			57511		Cryosurgery-Cervix	X4855		High Risk PN, Per Visit
		Office/Out Patient Consults						
99241		Prob Foc H&P, Strt	57520		Conization of Cervix (LEEP)			
99242		Exp Prob Foc H&P, Strt	58120		D & C			
99243			58100		Endometrial Biopsy			*Hospital*
		Det H&P, Low Comp						
99244		Comp H&P, Mod Comp	58300		IUD Insertion	54160		Circumcision
99245		Comp H&P, High Comp	58301		IUD Follow-up/Removal	57700		Colpotomy; w/Exploration
			58340		Hysterosalpingogram	58605		PP Sterilization, OB
		Surgical Procedures						
10060		I & D Boil, Skin, Abscess				59000		Amniocentesis
11100		Skin Biopsy, first lesion	99070		Supplies * Specify	59160		D & C After Delivery
11101		Each additional lesion				59400		Routine OB Care, Package - Vaginal
11200		Removal Skin Tags 1 - 15				59410		Vaginal Delivery & PP care
					Injections			
11201		Each additional 10 lesions	90718		Tetanus & Diphtheria, Adult	59412		External Ceplialic Version
11300		Shaving lesion trunk,arm,leg 0.5	90782		Administration Fee, Injection	59420		Antepartum Care Only
11301		0.6cm – 1.0 cm	J0970		Delestrogen	59430		Postpartum Care Only
11305		Shaving lesion genit, scalp etc 0.5	J1050		Depo Provera	59510		Routine OB Care, Package – C-Section
11306		0.6 cm – 1.0 cm	J1739		Hydroxprogester 500 MG	59515		Cesarean Section & PP Care
11310		Shaving lesion face, ears etc 0.5	J1741		Hydroxprogester 250 MG			
11311		0.6 cm – 1.0 cm						

DIAGNOSIS:

Primary Insurance:	Policy #:	**Total This Visit: $**
Secondary Insurance:	Policy #:	**Amount Paid: $**
		Balance Due: $
NEXT APPOINTMENT:	1 2 3 4 5 6 Days Weeks Mths Year	**Method of PMT:** ___ Case___ Check__ Cr. Card
	(Circle One) (Circle One)	
SPECIAL INSTRUCTIONS/ORDERS:		

Sample Appeal Letter

Date

[Name], APRN, BC
Address

RE: Refusal to authorize/make for [name of therapy] for [xyz] malignancy
Patient: [patient name]
Date(s) of Service: [date]
Date of Denial: [date]
Services Denied: [services]
HIC #: [number]

Dear Dr. [Medical Director's Name],

On behalf of the above beneficiary, I have received your letter dated [date of letter] denying payment for [name of drug] for the treatment of [diagnosis] for [patient name]. I would like to appeal that decision. I believe that the treatment should be approved because the use of [name of drug] for [diagnosis] is supported by [USP DI or AHFS]. The basis for coverage of any service or supply is the medical necessity of that service or supply. I believe that in [patient name]'s case, the medical necessity and the efficacy of the [name of drug] therapy is borne out by the reference in the [USP DI or AHFS].

The Medicare Carriers Manual requires coverage for uses of FDA-approved drugs used in anti-cancer chemotherapeutic regimens supported by one or more citations in at least one of the drug compendia.

[Provider should cite specific examples from the patient's medical record here that attests to the benefit that this particular patient can/will receive from this particular treatment.]

In light of these facts, I would like you to reconsider your decision to deny the use of [name of drug] therapy for Mr./Mrs. [patient name].

Thank You

Sincerely,

[APRN name]

[Attach copy of AHFS or USP DI monograph]

Commonly Used Medical Abbreviations

AA	Alcoholics Anonymous; African American
AAA	abdominal aortic aneurysm
AB	antibody; abortion
ABD	abdomen
ABG	arterial blood gas
ABI	ankle brachial index
ABX	antibiotics
AC	anterior chamber; acromioclavicular; before meals
ACE-I	angiotensin-converting enzyme inhibitor
ACL	anterior cruciate ligament
ACLS	advanced cardiac life support
ACS	acute coronary syndrome
ADA	American Diabetes Association
ADL	activities of daily living
ADR	adverse drug reaction
AF	atrial fibrillation; afebrile
AFB	acid-fast bacterium
AI	aortic insufficiency
AIDS	acquired immunodeficiency syndrome
AKA	above-knee amputation; also known as
ALL	acute lymphocytic leukemia
ALS	amyotrophic lateral sclerosis; advanced life support
AMA	against medical advice
AMI	acute myocardial infarction; anterior myocardial infarction
AMS	altered mental status
ANGIO	angiography
A&O	alert and oriented
AP	anterior-posterior
A/P	assessment and plan
APC	atrial premature contraction
APPY	appendectomy
APS	adult protective services
ARB	angiotensin receptor blocker
ARDS	acute respiratory distress syndrome
ARF	acute renal failure

AS	aortic stenosis; also ankylosing spondylitis
ASA	aspirin
ASD	atrial septal defect
A/V Nicking	arteriolar/venous nicking
AVSS	afebrile, vital signs stable
B	bilateral
BBB	bundle branch block
BCC	basal cell carcinoma
BCG	bacille Calmette-Guérin
BE	bacterial endocarditis; barium enema
BET	benign essential tremor
BIB	brought in by
bid	twice a day
BKA	below-knee amputation
BL CX	blood culture
BM	bone marrow; bowel movement
BMI	body mass index
BP	blood pressure
BPV	benign positional vertigo
BR	bed rest
BRB	bright red blood
BRBPR	bright red blood per rectum
BRP	bathroom privileges
BS	bowel sounds; breath sounds and blood sugar
BUN	blood urea nitrogen
BX	biopsy
C	with
C DIF	*Clostridium difficile*
CABG	coronary artery bypass graft
CAD	coronary artery disease
CATH	catheterization
CB	cerebellar
C/B	complicated by
CBC	complete blood count
CBD	common bile duct; closed bag drainage
CBI	continuous bladder irrigation
CC	chief complaint
CCB	calcium channel blocker
CCE	clubbing, cyanosis, edema
CCK	cholecystectomy
C/D	cup-to-disk ratio
CDI	clean dry intact
CEA	carcinoembryonic antigen
chemo	chemotherapy

CHF	congestive heart failure
CHI	closed head injury
chole	cholecystectomy
CIC	clean intermittent catheterization
CK	creatine kinase
Cl	chloride
CM	cardiomegaly
CMP	cardiomyopathy
CMT	cervical motion tenderness
CMV	cytomegalovirus
CN	cranial nerves
CNS	central nervous system
CO	cardiac output
C/O	complains of
COPD	chronic obstructive pulmonary disease
CPAP	continuous positive airway pressure
CPR	cardiopulmonary resuscitation
CPS	child protective services
CRFs	cardiac risk factors
CRI	chronic renal insufficiency
CRP	C-reactive protein
CSF	cerebral spinal fluid
CT	cat scan; chest tube; cardiothoracic
CTA	clear to auscultation
CVA	cerebral vascular accident
CVL	central venous line
CVP	central venous pressure
C/W	consistent with; compared with
CX	culture
CXR	chest X-ray
D	diarrhea; disk
DBP	diastolic blood pressure
DC	discharge; discontinue; doctor of chiropractics
D&C	dilatation and curettage
DD	differential diagnosis
DF	dorsiflexion
DFE	dilated fundus examination
DIC	disseminated intravascular coagulopathy
DIF	differential
DIP	distal interphalangeal
DJD	degenerative joint disease
DKA	diabetic ketoacidosis
DM	diabetes mellitus
DNR	do not resuscitate

D/O	disorder
DP	dorsalis pedis
DPL	diagnostic peritoneal lavage
DPOA	durable power of attorney
DR	diabetic retinopathy
DRE	digital rectal exam
D/T	due to
DTR	deep tendon reflex
DTs	delirium tremens
DU	duodenal ulcer
DVT	deep venous thrombosis
DX	diagnosis
EBL	estimated blood loss
EBM	evidence-based medicine
EBV	Epstein-Barr virus
ECG	electrocardiogram (also known as EKG)
ECHO	echocardiography
ED	erectile dysfunction
EEG	electroencephalogram
EF	ejection fraction (in reference to ventricular function)
EGD	esophagogastroduodenoscopy
EJ	external jugular
EKG	electrocardiogram (also known as ECG)
EMG	electromyelogram
EMS	emergency medical system
EMT	emergency medical technician
E/O	evidence of
EOMI	extraocular muscles intact
eos	eosinophils
EPO	erythropoietin
ER	external rotation; emergency room
ERCP	endoscopic retrograde cholangiopancreatography
ES	epidural steroids
ESI	epidural steroid injection
ESLD	end-stage liver disease
ESR	erythrocyte sedimentation rate
ESRD	end-stage renal disease
ESWL	extracorporeal shock-wave lithotripsy
ETOH	alcohol
ETT	exercise tolerance test; endotracheal tube
EWCL	extended-wear contact lens
EX FIX	external fixation
EX LAP	exploratory laparotomy
EXT	extremities

FB	foreign body
F/B	followed by
FBS	fasting blood sugar
Fe	iron
FEM	femoral
FEV1	forced expiratory volume 1 second
FFP	fresh frozen plasma
flex sig	flexible sigmoidoscopy
flu	influenza
FNA	fine-needle aspiration
FOOSH	fall on outstretched hand
FOS	full of stool; force of stream
FP	family practitioner
FRC	functional residual capacity
FSG	finger-stick glucose
FSH	follicle-stimulating hormone
FTT	failure to thrive
F/U	follow-up
FUO	fever of unknown origin
FX	fracture
G	guaiac (followed by + or −)
GA	general anesthesia
GAD	generalized anxiety disorder
GAS	Group A strep; guaiac all stools
GB	gall bladder; Guillain-Barré
GBS	Group B strep
GC	gonorrhea
GCS	Glasgow Coma Scale
GERD	gastroesophageal reflux disease
GERI	geriatrics
GET	general endotracheal
GI	gastrointestinal
GIB	gastrointestinal bleeding
GLC	glaucoma
GMR	gallops, murmurs, rubs
GN	glomerulonephritis
GNR	gram-negative rod
GOO	gastric outlet obstruction
GP	general practitioner
G#P#	gravida # para #
GS	Gram stain
GSW	gunshot wound
GTT	glucose tolerance test
G-tube	gastric feeding tube

GU	genitourinary; gastric ulcer
H FLU	*Haemophilus influenzae*
H2	histamine 2
HA	headache
HAART	highly active antiretroviral therapy
HACE	high-altitude cerebral edema
HAPE	high-altitude pulmonary edema
HCC	hepatocellular carcinoma
HCG	human chorionic gonadotropin
HCL	hard contact lens
HCM	health care maintenance
HCT	hematocrit
HCV	hepatitis C virus
HD	hemodialysis
HDL	high-density lipoprotein
HEENT	head, ears, eyes, nose, throat
HEME/ONC	hematology/oncology
HGB	hemoglobin
HH	hiatal hernia
H&H	hemoglobin and hematocrit
HI	homicidal ideation
HIB	*Haemophilus influenzae* B vaccine
HIV	human immunodeficiency virus
HL	heparin lock
HOB	head of bed
HOH	hard of hearing
HPI	history of present illness
HPV	human papilloma virus
HR	heart rate
HRT	hormone replacement therapy
HSM	holosystolic murmur; hepatosplenomegaly
HSV	herpes simplex virus
HTN	hypertension
HX	history
I–	without ionic contrast (in reference to a cat scan)
I+	with ionic contrast (in reference to a cat scan)
IA	intraarticular
IABP	intraaortic balloon pump
IBD	inflammatory bowel disease
IBS	irritable bowel syndrome
IBW	ideal body weight
ICD	implantable cardiac defibrillator
ICH	intracranial hemorrhage
ICP	intracranial pressure

ID	infectious diseases
I&D	incision and drainage
IDDM	insulin-dependent diabetes mellitus
IFN	interferon
IH	inguinal hernia (usually preceded by *l* or *r*)
IJ	internal jugular
IL	interleukin; indirect laryngoscopy
IM	intramuscular; intramedullary
IMI	inferior myocardial infarction
IMP	impression
INR	international normalized ratio
I&O	intake and output
IOL	intraocular lens
IOP	intraocular pressure
IP	interphalangeal
IR	interventional radiology; internal rotation
IRB	indications risks benefits; institutional review board
ITP	idiopathic thrombocytopenia
IUD	intrauterine device
IUP	intrauterine pregnancy
IV	intravenous
IVC	inferior vena cava
IVDU	intravenous drug use
IVF	intravenous fluids; in vitro fertilization
IVP	intravenous pyelogram
JP	Jackson Pratt
J-tube	jejunal feeding tube
JVD	jugular venous distention
JVP	jugular venous pressure
K	potassium
KCAL	kilocalories
KUB	kidneys, ureters, and bladder
KVO	keep vein open
L	left
LA	left atrium
LAC	laceration
LAD	left anterior descending; left axis deviation
LAP	laparoscopic; laparotomy
LBBB	left bundle branch block
LBO	large bowel obstruction
LBP	low back pain
LCL	lateral collateral ligament
LCX	left circumflex
L&D	labor and delivery

LDH	lactate dehydrogenase
LDL	low-density lipoprotein
LE	lower extremity; leukocyte esterase
LFT	liver function test
LH	leuteinizing hormone; left-handed; light-headed
LHC	left heart cath
LHRH	leuteinizing hormone releasing hormone
LLE	left lower extremity
LLL	left lower lobe; left lower lid
LLQ	left lower quadrant
LM	left main coronary artery
LMN	lower motor neuron
LMP	last menstrual period
LMWH	low-molecular-weight heparin
LN	lymph node; liquid nitrogen
LND	lymph node dissection
LOA	lysis of adhesions
LOC	loss of consciousness
LP	lumbar puncture
LPN	licensed practical nurse
LS	lumbosacral
LT	light touch
LUE	left upper extremity
LUL	left upper lobe; also left upper lid
LUQ	left upper quadrant
LVEDP	left ventricular end diastolic pressure
LVF	left ventricular function
LVH	left ventricular hypertrophy
lytes	electrolytes
MAC	monitored anesthesia care
MCL	medial collateral ligament
MCP	metacarpal-phalangeal
MCV	mean corpuscular volume
MDRTB	multi-drug-resistant tuberculosis
meds	medicines
MFM	maternal-fetal medicine
MI	myocardial infarction
MICU	medical intensive care unit
M&M	morbidity and mortality
MMP	multiple medical problems
MMR	measles, mumps, and rubella vaccine
MOM	milk of magnesia
MR	mitral regurgitation
MRCP	magnetic resonance cholangiopancreatography

MRI	magnetic resonance imaging
MRSA	methicillin-resistant *Staphylococcus aureus*
MS	mental status; mitral stenosis; multiple sclerosis; morphine sulfate
MSSA	methicillin-sensitive *Staphylococcus aureus*
MTP	metatarsal-phalangeal
MVP	mitral valve prolapse
MVR	mitral valve replacement
N	nausea
NA	not available
NABS	normal active bowel sounds
NAD	no apparent distress; no acute distress; no acute disease
NC/AT	normocephalic atraumatic
NCS	nerve conduction study
NEB	nebulizer
NGT	nasogastric tube
NGU	nongonococcal urethritis
NH	nursing home
NICU	neonatal intensive care unit
NIDDM	non–insulin-dependent diabetes mellitus
NKDA	no known drug allergies
NOS	not otherwise specified
NP	nurse practitioner
NPO	nothing by mouth
NS	normal saline
NSBGP	nonspecific bowel gas pattern
NSR	normal sinus rhythm
NT	nontender
NTD	nothing to do
NUCS	nuclear medicine
NYHA	New York Heart Association
OA	osteoarthritis
OB	occult blood (followed by + or –)
OCD	obsessive compulsive disorder
OCP	oral contraceptive pill
OD	right eye
OE	otitis externa
OM	otitis media
ON	optic nerve; overnight
OOB	out of bed
O&P	ovum and parasites
O/P	oropharynx
ORIF	open reduction with internal fixation
OS	left eye

OSA	obstructive sleep apnea
OT	occupational therapy
OTC	over the counter
OTD	out the door
OU	both eyes
O/W	otherwise
P	pulse; pending; after
P VAX	pneumococcal vaccination
PA	posterior-anterior; physician's assistant
PACU	postanesthesia care unit
PAD	peripheral arterial disease
PALS	pediatric advanced life support
PC	after meals
PCA	patient-controlled analgesia
PCI	percutaneous coronary intervention
PCL	posterior cruciate ligament
PCM	pacemaker
PCOD	polycystic ovarian disease
PCP	primary care physician; pneumocystic pneumonia
PCWP	pulmonary capillary wedge pressure
PD	Parkinson's disease; personality disorder; peritoneal dialysis
PDA	patent ductus arteriosus
PE	physical exam; pulmonary embolism
PERRLA	pupils equal, round, reactive to light
PET	positron emission tomography
PF	peak flow; plantar flexion
PFO	patent foramen ovale
PFTs	pulmonary function tests
PICC	peripherally inserted central catheter
PICU	pediatric intensive care unit
PID	pelvic inflammatory disease
PIH	pregnancy-induced hypertension
PIP	proximal interphalangeal
PLT	platelets
PMD	primary medical doctor
PMH	past medical history
PMI	point of maximum impulse
PMN	polymorphonuclear leukocytes
PMRS	physical medicine and rehabilitation service
PN	progress note
PNA	pneumonia
PNBX	prostate needle biopsy
PND	paroxysmal nocturnal dyspnea; postnasal drip
PNS	peripheral nervous system

PO	by mouth
POP	popliteal
PP	pin prick
PPD	purified protein derivative
PPH	primary pulmonary hypertension
PPI	proton pump inhibitor
PPN	peripheral parenteral nutrition
PPTL	postpartum tubal ligation
PR	per rectum
PRBCs	packed red blood cells
prn	refers to treatments or medications patient can receive on an "as needed" basis
PSA	prostate specific antigen
PSH	past surgical history
PT	physical therapy; posterior tibial; prothrombin time; patient
PTA	prior to admission; peritonsillar abscess
PTCA	percutaneous transluminal coronary angioplasty
P-thal	Persantine thallium
PTSD	post-traumatic stress disorder
PTT	partial thromboplastin time
PTX	pneumothorax
PUD	peptic ulcer disease
PV	polycythemia vera; portal vein
PVC	premature ventricular contraction
PVD	peripheral vascular disease; posterior vitreous detachment
PVR	post void residual
q	every
qhs	every night
qid	four times per day
QNS	quantity not sufficient
R	right
RA	right atrium
RAD	right axis deviation; reactive airways disease
R/B	referred by; relieved by
RBBB	right bundle branch block
RBC	red blood cell
RCA	right coronary artery
RCT	randomized controlled trial; rotator cuff tear
RD	retinal detachment; registered dietician
RF	rheumatoid factor; risk factor
RFA	radio-frequency ablation; right femoral artery
RHC	right heart cath
RHD	rheumatic heart disease
rheum	rheumatology

R/I	rule in
RIG	rabies immunoglobulin
RLE	right lower extremity
RLL	right lower lobe; right lower lid
RLQ	right lower quadrant
RML	right middle lobe
R/O	rule out
ROM	range of motion
ROMI	rule out myocardial infarction
ROS	review of systems
RPR	rapid plasma reagin
RR	respiratory rate
RRR	regular rate and rhythm
RSD	reflex sympathetic dystrophy
RSV	respiratory syncytial virus
RT	respiratory therapy
RTC	return to clinic
RUE	right upper extremity
RUG	retrograde urethrogram
RUL	right upper lobe; right upper lid
RUQ	right upper quadrant
RV	right ventricle; residual volume
RVAD	right ventricular assist device
RVG	right ventriculogram
RVR	rapid ventricular response
RX	treatment
S	without
SA	sinoatrial; *Staphylococcus aureus*
SAB	spontaneous abortion
SAH	subarachnoid hemorrhage
SBE	subacute bacterial endocarditis
SBO	small bowel obstruction
SBP	spontaneous bacterial peritonitis; systolic blood pressure
SC	subcutaneous
SCCA	squamous cell cancer
SCL	soft contact lens
SEM	systolic ejection murmur
SFA	superficial femoral artery
SFV	superficial femoral vein
SI	suicidal ideation
SIADH	syndrome of inappropriate antidiuretic hormone secretion
SICU	surgical intensive care unit
SIDS	sudden infant death syndrome
SK	seborrheic keratosis; streptokinase

SL	sublingual
SLE	systemic lupus erythematosus; slit-lamp exam
SLR	straight leg raise
SNF	skilled nursing facility
S/P	status post; suprapubic
SPF	sun protection formula
SQ	subcutaneous
SSI	sliding scale insulin
SSRI	selective serotonin reuptake inhibitor
STAT	immediately
STI	sexually transmitted infection
STS	soft-tissue swelling
STX	stricture
SVC	superior vena cava
SVG	saphenous vein graft
SW	social work; stab wound
SX	symptoms
SZ	seizure
T	temperature
T&A	tonsillectomy and adenoidectomy
TAA	thoracic aortic aneurysm
TAB	threatened abortion; therapeutic abortion
TAH	total abdominal hysterectomy
TB	tuberculosis; total bilirubin
TC	current temperature
T&C	type and cross
TCA	tricyclic antidepressant
TD	tetanus and diphtheria vaccination; tardive dyskinesia
TDWBAT	touch down weight bearing as tolerated
TEE	Trans-Esophageal Echocardiogram
TFs	tube feeds
TG	triglycerides
THA	total hip arthroplasty
THR	total hip replacement
TIA	transient ischemic attack
TIBC	total iron binding capacity
tid	three times per day
TIPS	transvenous intrahepatic porto-systemic shunt
TKA	total knee arthroplasty
TKR	total knee replacement
TLC	triple lumen catheter; total lung capacity
TM	tympanic membrane; maximum temperature
TMJ	temporomandibular joint
TMN	tumor metastases nodes

TNF	tumor necrosis factor
TOA	tubo-ovarian abscess
TOX	toxicology
TOXO	toxoplasmosis
TP	total protein
TPA	tissue plasminogen activator
TPN	total parenteral nutrition
TR	tricuspid regurgitation
TRUS	transrectal ultrasound
T&S	type and screen
TSH	thyroid-stimulating hormone
TTE	trans-thoracic echocardiogram
TTP	tender to palpation
TURBT	transurethral resection bladder tumor
TURP	transurethral prostatectomy
TV	tidal volume
TVC	true vocal cord
TX	transfusion; treatment
UA	urinalysis; uric acid
UC	ulcerative colitis
UCC	urgent care center
UCX	urine culture
UE	upper extremity
UFH	unfractionated heparin
UMBO	umbilical
UMN	upper motor neuron
UNSA	unstable angina
UO	urine output
URI	upper respiratory tract infection
US	ultrasound
UTD	up to date
UTI	urinary tract infection
UV	ultraviolet
V	vomiting
VA	visual acuity
VAX	vaccine
VBAC	vaginal birth after cesarean section
VBG	venous blood gas
VC	vital capacity; vocal cord
VCUG	voiding cystourethrogram
VF	ventricular fibrillation
VP	ventriculoperitoneal
V&P	vagotomy and pyloroplasty
VS	vital signs

VSD	ventricular septal defect
VSS	vital signs stable
VT	ventricular tachycardia
VWF	von Willebrand factor
WBAT	weight bearing as tolerated
WBC	white blood cells
WDWN	well developed, well nourished
WNL	within normal limits
W/O	without
W/U	workup
X	except
XLR	crossed leg raise
XRT	radiation therapy
ZE	Zollinger Ellison

Source: University of California at San Diego website. (2004). *A practical guide to clinical medicine.* Available at *http://medicine.ucsd.edu/clinicalmed/abbreviation.htm* (accessed January 25, 2004).

Examples of Preprinted Progress Notes

ACUTE ILLNESS

Name: _____ Date: _____

Subjective: Wt: T: BP: P: R:

Onset/duration:	Allergies:
Symptoms:	Medications:
☐ Fever/chills:	
☐ Headache:	
☐ Sinus pain:	
☐ Facial/tooth pain:	Self-care:
☐ Sore throat:	
☐ Difficulty swallowing:	Chronic diseases:
☐ Nasal congestion/rhinnitis:	
☐ Ear pain/congestion:	
☐ Myalgias:	Tobacco:
☐ Fatigue/malaise:	
☐ Nausea/vomiting:	Occup. exposure:
☐ Abdominal pain:	
☐ Diarrhea:	
☐ Cough:	Other:
☐ SOB/dyspnea:	
☐ Other:	
☐ Exposure to illness:	

OBJECTIVE:	WNL	See note	Comments
General:			
Eyes:			
Ears:			
Nose:			
Sinuses:			
Mouth/pharynx:			
Lymph nodes:			
Lungs:			
Heart:			
Abdomen:			

Assessment:

Plan:

☐ Shared findings/mgmt options   **Medications:**   **Education:**
☐ Mgmt of symptoms/illness

☐ Increase fluids

☐ Action/SE of meds

☐ Increase humidity

☐ Other:

☐ Rest

☐ Return to work/school: Follow-up:

☐ Prevention of spread

Referral:

☐ Other:

Provider: _____

APPENDIX 9-2

History and Physical Form

Name: _____ Date: _____

Ht: Wt: B/P:	Allergies:
BS:	
Urine: pH: pro: ket: gluc:	Medications:
leuk est: nitrite: blood:	

Habits

Tob: Exercise:
ETOH:
Drugs: Nutrition:
Safety: Calcium
  Seatbelts   Caffeine
  Smoke detector
  Falls risk

CC/HPI

PMH

FMH

Social history

Review of systems

	WNL	Notes
Gen		
Eyes		
Ears		
Nose		
Mouth		
Teeth		
Throat		
Skin		
Endo		
Resp		
Cardiac		
GI		
GU		
Gyn		

MS		
Neuro		
Mental		
Sleep		
Stress		
Heme/Lym		
Allergy		

Physical exam

	WNL	See note	Findings
Gen			
Head			
Eyes			
ENT/Mouth			
Neck			
Lymph			
Chest			
Breast			
Heart			
Abdo			
Pelvic			
Genital			
Rectal			
Extrem			
Spine			
Neuro			
Skin			
Mental			
MMSR	–/30		

Assessment:

1. Health maintenance/screening (age, gender, ethnicity)

2. Health risks: (family history, lifestyle, inadequate screening)

Plan:

Diagnostics:
- [ ] CBC
- [ ] LIPIDS
- [ ] LFTs
- [ ] ProT
- [ ] Chem 18
- [ ] HgA1C
- [ ] FBS
- [ ] UA
- [ ] Urine C&S
- [ ] PSA
- [ ] Pap
- [ ] Mammo
- [ ] BMD
- [ ] CXR
- [ ] EKG
- [ ] Echo
- [ ] TM
- [ ] Doppler
- [ ] U/S
- [ ] Colonoscopy
- [ ] Hemocult X 3
- [ ] Other:

Immunizations:
- [ ] Tetanus
- [ ] Influenza
- [ ] Pneumovax
- [ ] TB test

Other:

Medications:

Education:

Exercise

Nutrition:
- [ ] Cholesterol
- [ ] Weight loss
- [ ] Diabetic

Smoking cessation:

Medication(s) use/side effects

Stress/coping counseling:

Other:

RTC:

Provider _____

Hypertension
Progress Note

Name: _____ Date: _____

Subjective: Wt: 　　T: 　　BP: 　(sitting) 　(standing) 　(supine) 　P: 　R:

Symptoms:	Allergies:
☐ Chest pain:	Medications/compliance:
☐ Headache:	
☐ TIA:	
☐ Paresthesia:	
☐ DOE:	Diet:
☐ Fatigue/malaise:	Other chronic diseases:
☐ Nausea/vomiting:	Habits:
☐ Abdominal pain:	☐ Tobacco:
☐ PND/cough:	☐ ETOH:
	☐ Exercise:
☐ SOB:	
☐ Other:	

Objective:	WNL	See note	Comments
General:			
Neck/carotids:			
Lungs:			
Heart:			
Abdomen/bruits			

Assessment:

1. Hypertension (normal, uncontrolled stage 1, stage 2)

2. Compliance with treatment regimen: (low, moderate, high)

3. End organ consequences (cardiac, renal, vascular)

4. Other:

Plan:

☐ Shared findings/mgmt options   Medications: Education:

☐ Lifestyle modification   ☐ Mgmt of Symptoms/illness

☐ Increase exercise   ☐ Action/SE of meds

☐ Low salt and fat diet   ☐ Other:

☐ Decrease ETOH: Follow-up:

☐ Smoking cessation advice   Referral:

☐ Other:

Provider: _____

9-4

Evaluation and Management Documentation Guide

HISTORY	Chief C/O	HPI	ROS	PSFH
Problem focused	Establish	Brief (1-3 components)	NA	NA
Expanded Problem focused	Establish	Brief (1-3 components)	Problem Pertinent (1 system)	NA
Detailed	Establish	Extended (4 components)	Extended (2-9 systems)	Pertinent (1 element)
Comprehensive	Establish	Extended (4 components)	Complete (≥10 systems)	Complete (2-3 elements)

Components	Systems	Past History	Family History	Social History
Location	Constitutional	Prior major illnesses/injuries	Health status/cause of death of parents, siblings, children	Marital status/living arrangements
Severity	Eyes	Prior surgeries	Specific diseases in family that relate to patient's current problem	Current employment
Duration	Ears, nose, mouth, throat	Prior hospitalizations	Hereditary diseases	Occupational history
Timing	Cardiovascular	Current medications		Use of drugs, alcohol, tobacco
Precipitating factors (context)	Respiratory	Allergies (food and drugs)		Sexual history
Modifying factors	Gastrointestinal	Chemical dependency		Other relevant social factors
Associated signs	Genitourinary	Behavioral/functional history		
	Musculoskeletal	Age-correct immunization status		
	Integumentary (skin/breast)	Age-correct feeding and dietary status		
	Neurologic	Any other relevant past history		
	Psychiatric			
	Endocrine			
	Hematologic/lymphatic			
	Allergic/immunology			

EXAMINATION	System	Other symptomatic or related organ systems	# Elements included
Problem focused	Limited to affected organ/system	NA	1-5
Expanded PF	Affected organ/system	Include	At least 6 in 1 or more system
Detailed	Extended exam of organ/system	Include (at least 6)	2 Elements from 6 systems OR 12 elements in 2 or more systems
Comprehensive	Complete single system exam OR complete multi-system exam		At least 2 bullets in at least 9 systems

MEDICAL DECISION MAKING

Diagnoses/ management options	Number X	Pts =	Type of Data	Pts =	Medical decision (complexity)	# Diagnoses/ management options	Data to be reviewed	Risk of complications, morbidity/ mortality (table of risk on back)
Self-limited, minor	(Max = 2)	1	Review and/or order clinical lab tests	1	Straightforward	Minimal (1)	Minimal (1)	Minimal (1)

			Low	Limited (2)	Limited (2)	Low (2)
Est. prob; stable, improved	1	1				
Est. prob; worsening	2	1				
New prob; no add'l workup (Max = 1)	3	1	Moderate	Multiple (3)	Moderate (3)	Moderate (3)
New prob; add'l workup planned	4	2				
TOTAL		1	High	Extensive (4+)	Extensive (4+)	High (4)
		2				

Data reviewed	Points
Review and/or order tests in 7xxxx per CPT coding manual	1
Review and/or order tests in 9xxxx per CPT coding manual	1
Discuss test results with performing MD	1
Independent review of image, tracing, or specimen	2
Decision to obtain old records and/or obtain history from others	1
Review and summarize old records and/or obtain records	2

Examination Requirements for E&M Documentation

	Multisystem	Eyes	ENT	CV	Resp	GU(Male)	GU (Female)	MS	Neuro	Skin	Psych	H/A/I
CONSTITUTIONAL		N/A										
Measurement 3 out of 7 VS: (1) sitting/standing BP; (2) supine BP; (3) pulse rate and regularity; (4) respiration; (5) temperature; (6) height; (7) weight	x		x	x	x	x	x	x	x	x	x	x
General appearance of patient (development, nutrition, habitus, deformities, grooming)	x		x	x	x	x	x	x	x	x	x	x
Assessment of ability to communicate (e.g., use of sign language or other communication aids) and quality of voice			x									
EYES					N/A	N/A	N/A	N/A			N/A	
Visual acuity		x										
Visual fields by confrontation		x										
Ocular motility including primary gaze alignment		x	x									
Inspection of bulbar and palpebral conjunctivae		x										
Inspection of conjunctivae and lids	x			x						x		x

Continued

	Multisystem	Eyes	ENT	CV	Resp	GU(Male)	GU (Female)	MS	Neuro	Skin	Psych	H/A/I
Exam of ocular adnexae including lids, lacrimal glands, lacrimal drainage, orbits, and preauricular lymph nodes		x										
Exam of pupils and irises including shape, direct/consensual reaction, size, morphology	x	x										
Slit-lamp exam of corneas including epithelium, stroma, endothelium, and tear film		x										
Slit-lamp exam of anterior chambers including depth, cells, and flare		x										
Slit-lamp exam of lenses including clarity, anterior and posterior capsule, cortex, nucleus		x										
Measurement of intraocular pressures		x										
Ophthalmoscopic exam through dilated pupils of optic discs including size, C/D ratio, appearance, nerve fiber layer	x	x							x			
Posterior segments including retina and vessels (exudates, hemorrhages)	x	x							x			

HEAD AND FACE	N/A										
Inspection of head and face (overall appearance, scars, lesions, masses)	x										x
Palpation/percussion of face (sinus tenderness)	x										x
Exam of salivary glands	x										
Assess facial strength	x	N/A				N/A	N/A	N/A	N/A	N/A	
EARS, NOSE, MOUTH, AND THROAT	N/A					N/A	N/A	N/A	N/A	N/A	
Otoscopic exam of external auditory canals and tympanic membranes	x										x
Otoscopic exam of external auditory canals and TMs including pneumo-otoscopy with notation of mobility of membranes	x										
Assessment of hearing with tuning forks and clinical speech reception thresholds (e.g., whispered voice, finger rub)	x										
External inspection of ears and nose (e.g., overall appearance, scars, lesions, masses)	x				x						
Inspection of nasal mucosa, septum, turbinates	x				x						x
Inspection of lips, teeth, gums	x				x				x	x	x
Exam of oropharynx: oral mucosa, salivary glands, hard/soft palates, tongue, tonsils, posterior pharynx (e.g., asymmetry, lesions, hydration of mucosal surfaces)	x				x				x	x	x

Continued

	Multisystem	Eyes	ENT	CV	Resp	GU(Male)	GU (Female)	MS	Neuro	Skin	Psych	I/V/H
Inspection of pharyngeal walls and pyriform sinuses (e.g., pooling of saliva, asymmetry, lesions)			x									
Inspection of oral mucosa with notation of presence of pallor or cyanosis			x	x								
Exam by mirror of larynx including condition of epiglotis, false vocal cords, true vocal cords, mobility of larynx			x									
Exam by mirror of nasopharynx including appearance of mucosa, adenoids, posterior choanae, and Eustachian tubes			x									
NECK		N/A						N/A	N/A		N/A	
Exam of neck (masses, overall appearance, symmetry, tracheal position, crepitus)	x		x		x	x	x					
Exam of thyroid (enlargement, tenderness, mass)	x		x	x	x	x	x			x		x
Exam of jugular veins (e.g., distention; a, v, or cannon a waves)				x	x							x

							N/A	N/A	N/A	N/A
RESPIRATORY	N/A									
Inspection of chest with notation of symmetry and expansion		x	x							x
Assessment of respiratory effort (e.g., intercostals retractions, accessory muscle use, diaphragmatic movement)	x	x	x	x	x					
Percussion of chest (e.g., dullness, flatness, hyperresonance)	x		x							
Palpation of chest (e.g., tactile fremitus)	x		x							
Auscultation of lungs (e.g., breath sounds, adventitious sounds, rubs)	x	x	x	x	x					x
CARDIOVASCULAR	N/A									
Palpation of heart (e.g., location, size, and forcefulness of PMI, thrills, lifts, palpable S3 or S4)	x	x	x							
Auscultation of heart including sounds, abnormal sounds, and murmurs	x	x	x	x	x			x		x
Measurement of blood pressure in two or more extremities (aortic dissection, coarctation)		x	x							
Exam of carotid arteries (waveform, pulse amplitude, bruits, apical-carotid delay)	x		x					x		

Continued

	Multisystem	Eyes	ENT	CV	Resp	GU(Male)	GU (Female)	MS	Neuro	Skin	Psych	H/A/I
Abdominal aorta (size, bruits)	x			x								
Femoral arteries (pulse amplitude, bruits)	x			x								
Pedal pulses (pulse amplitude)	x			x								
Exam of extremities for peripheral edema and/or varicosities	x			x								
Peripheral vascular system by observation (e.g., swelling, varicosities) and palpation (e.g., pulses, temperature, edema, tenderness)			x		x	x	x	x	x	x		x
CHEST		N/A	N/A	N/A	N/A				N/A	N/A	N/A	N/A
Inspection of breasts (symmetry, nipple discharge)	x											
Palpation of breasts and axillae (masses or lumps, tenderness)	x											
ABDOMEN		N/A	N/A					N/A	N/A		N/A	
Exam of abdomen with notation of presence of masses or tenderness	x				x	x	x					x
Exam of liver and spleen	x			x		x	x			x		x
Exam for presence/absence of hernia	x					x	x					

Examination Element										
Exam of anus, perineum, rectum, including sphincter tone, presence of hemorrhoids, rectal masses	x									
Exam of anus for condyloma and other lesions								x		
Obtain stool sample for occult blood test when indicated	x		N/A	N/A	x	x				
GENITOURINARY (MALE)	N/A		N/A	N/A			N/A	N/A	N/A	N/A
Inspection of anus and perineum					x					
Exam (with/without specimen collection of smears and cultures): Scrotum (e.g., lesions, cysts, rashes)	x				x					
Epididymides (e.g., size, symmetry, masses)					x					
Testes (e.g., size, symmetry, masses)					x					
Urethral meatus (e.g., size, location, lesions, discharge)					x					
Penis (e.g., lesions, presence/absence of foreskin, foreskin retractability, plaque, masses, scarring, deformities)	x				x					
Digital rectal exam including prostate gland (e.g., size symmetry, nodularity, tenderness)	x				x					
Seminal vesicles (e.g., symmetry, tenderness, masses, enlargement)					x					
Sphincter tone, presence of hemorrhoids, rectal masses					x					

Continued

	Multisystem	Eyes	ENT	CV	Resp	GU(Male)	GU (Female)	MS	Neuro	Skin	Psych	H/A/I
GENITOURINARY (FEMALE)		N/A	N/A	N/A	N/A			N/A	N/A	N/A	N/A	N/A
Includes at least 7 of the following 11 elements: inspection and palpation of breasts (e.g., masses/lumps, tenderness, symmetry, nipple discharge)	x						x					
DRE including sphincter tone, presence of hemorrhoids, rectal masses							x					
Pelvic exam (with or without specimen collection for smears/cultures):							x					
External genitalia (e.g., general appearance, hair distribution, lesions)												
Urethral meatus (e.g., size, location, lesions, prolapse)							x					
Urethra (e.g., masses, tenderness, scarring)	x						x					
Bladder (e.g., fullness, masses, tenderness)	x						x					
Vagina (e.g., general appearance, estrogen effect, discharge, lesions, pelvic support, cystocele, rectocele)							x					

Cervix (e.g., general appearance, lesions, discharge)	x							x	
Uterus (e.g., size contour position, mobility, tenderness, consistency, descent or support)	x							x	
Adnexa/parametria (e.g., masses, tenderness, organomegaly, nodularity)	x							x	
Anus and perineum								x	
LYMPHATIC	N/A	N/A							
Palpation of lymph nodes in neck, axillae, groin, or other location	2 + areas		N/A	x	x	x	N/A	x	x
MUSCULOSKELETAL	N/A	N/A		N/A	N/A				
Exam of gait and station	x		x	x		x	x	x	
Inspection and/or palpation of digits and nails (e.g., clubbing, cyanosis, inflammatory conditions, petechiae, ischemia, infections, nodes)	x		x	x		x	x	x	x
Exam of back with notation of kyphosis or scoliosis			x						
Exam of joint(s), bone(s) and muscle(s)/tendon(s) of 4 of following 6 areas: (1) head and neck; (2) spine, ribs, pelvis; (3) right upper extremity; (4) left upper extremity; (5) right lower extremity; (6) left lower extremity	x					x			

Continued

	Multisystem	Eyes	ENT	CV	Resp	GU(Male)	GU (Female)	MS	Neuro	Skin	Psych	H/A/I
The exam of a given area includes: Inspection, percussion and/or palpation with notation of misalignment, asymmetry, crepitation, defects, tenderness, masses or effusions	x							x				
Assessment of ROM with notation of any pain, crepitation, contracture	x							x				
Assessment of stability with notation of any dislocation, subluxation, laxity	x							x				
Assessment of muscle strength in upper and lower extremities	x			x	x			x	x		x	
Assessment of muscle tone (e.g., flaccid, cog wheel, spastic, atrophy, abnormal movements)	x			x	x			x	x		x	
NOTE: For the comprehensive level of exam, all four of the elements identified by a bullet must be performed and documented for each of four anatomic areas. For the three lower levels of exam, each element is counted separately for each body area (e.g., assessing ROM in 2 extremities = 2 elements)												

SKIN					N/A		N/A	N/A	
Palpation of scalp and inspection of hair of scalp, eyebrows, face, chest, pubic area (when indicated), and extremities								x	
Inspection of skin and subcutaneous tissue (e.g., rashes, lesions, ulcers) in 8 of following 10 areas: (1) head including face; (2) neck; (3) chest, including breasts and axillae; (4) abdomen; (5) genitalia, groin, buttocks; (6) back; (7) right upper extremity; (8) left upper extremity; (9) right lower extremity; (10) left lower extremity	x	x	x	x		x		x	x
Palpation of skin and subcutaneous tissue (rashes, lesions, ulcers, susceptibility to and presence of photo damage) in 8 of following 10 areas: (1) head including face; (2) neck; (3) chest, including breasts and axillae; (4) abdomen; (5) genitalia, groin, buttocks; (6) back; (7) right upper extremity; (8) left upper extremity; (9) right lower extremity; (10) left lower extremity	x	x	x	x		x		x	x
NOTE: For comprehensive level, exam must include at least eight anatomic areas; for the three lower levels of exam, each body area is counted separately.									

Continued

	Multisystem	Eyes	ENT	CV	Resp	GU(Male)	GU (Female)	MS	Neuro	Skin	Psych	H/A/I
Inspection of eccrine and apocrine glands of skin and subcutaneous tissue with identification and location of any hyperhidrosis, chromhidrosis, or bromhidrosis.										x		
NEUROLOGICAL		N/A									N/A	
Evaluation of higher integrative functions including: Orientation to time, place, person									x			
Recent and remote memory									x			
Attention span and concentration									x			
Language (naming objects, repeating phrases, spontaneous speech)									x			
Fund of knowledge (awareness of current events, past history, vocabulary)									x			
Test the following cranial nerves (CNs): 2nd CN (visual acuity, visual fields, fundi)	x		x						x			
3rd, 4th, and 6th CNs (pupils, eye movements)	x		x						x			

Examination element			
5th CN (facial sensation, corneal reflexes)	x	x	
7th CN (facial symmetry, strength)	x	x	
8th CN (hearing with tuning fork, whispered voice, and/or finger rub)	x	x	
9th CN (spontaneous or reflex palate movement)	x	x	
11th CN (shoulder shrug strength)	x	x	
12th CN (tongue protrusion)	x	x	
Exam of sensation (touch, pin, vibration, proprioception)		x	
Exam of DTRs in upper and lower extremities with notation of pathological reflexes (Babinski)	x	x	
Test coordination (finger/nose, heel/knee/shin, rapid alternating movements in upper and lower extremities, evaluation of fine-motor coordination in young children)		x	
PSYCHIATRIC			
Description of speech, including rate, volume, articulation, coherence, and spontaneity with notation of abnormalities (perseveration, paucity of language)			x
Description of thought processes, including rate of thoughts, content of thoughts (logical vs. illogical, tangential), abstract reasoning and computation			x

Continued

	Multisystem	Eyes	ENT	CV	Resp	GU(Male)	GU (Female)	MS	Neuro	Skin	Psych	H/A/I
Description of associations (loose, tangential, circumstantial, intact)											x	
Description of abnormal or psychotic thoughts including hallucinations, delusions, preoccupation with violence, homicidal or suicidal ideation, obsessions		x									x	
Description of patient's judgment (concerning everyday activities and social situations) and insight (concerning psychiatric condition)											x	
Complete mental status examination including: Orientation to time, place, person	x	x	x	x	x	x	x	x		x		x
Recent and remote memory	x							x	x	x	x	
Attention span and concentration									x		x	
Language (naming objects, repeating phrases)									x		x	
Fund of knowledge (awareness of current events, past history, vocabulary)									x		x	
Mood and affect (depression, anxiety, agitation, hypomania, lability)	x	x	x	x	x	x	x	x	x	x	x	x

Sample Documentation of Patient Encounter

	E&M Coding Criteria
SUBJECTIVE John D., 45 yo, AAM **CC:** Weight loss and fatigue during past 30 days **HPI:** Noted onset weight loss and fatigue 1 month ago, muscles ache all over, doesn't feel rested on awakening in am. Sleeps 6-8 hours per night, interrupted 2-3 times by awakening to void. Able to resume sleep readily. Notes blurred vision especially on arising, slowly clears during day somewhat. Loss of 30# past month without change in activity or diet. Often forgets to take Metformin, fatigue is worse on those days. Notes increased hunger and thirst, and increased frequency of urination without dysuria or hematuria noted. Denies chest discomfort, shortness of breath. Denies fever or chills. **ROS:** *General:* See HPI: + wt loss, fatigue, weakness (-) fever *Eyes:* Wears corrective lenses, last eye exam 6 years ago *ENT:* Denies head congestion, PND, nasal discharge *Heart:* Denies CP, palpitations *Chest/Lung:* Denies SOB, wheezing, hemoptysis, cough *GI:* Denies blood in stools, no hx hemorrhoids, denies heartburn *GU:* Denies dysuria, hematuria, weakened stream (+) frequency *MS:* occ LBP after long work hours, no known injury, no hx fractures or other injuries; notes occ stiffness of L knee after prolonged sitting, relieves on own with slow ambulation *Skin:* Increased dryness during past 1-2 months, uses moisturizer daily *Neuro:* Notes slight tingling in toes both feet; notes generalized weakness, which is progressively worsening over past 2 weeks; denies dizziness *Psychiatric:* Denies s/s current depression	History: Comprehensive Chief C/O: present HPI: Extended (4+) ROS: Complete PSFH: Complete

	E&M Coding Criteria
Endocrine: (+) polyuria/polydipsia/polyphagia, (-) heat intolerance Hematologic/lymphatic: Denies hx anemia Allergic/immunology: Denies seasonal, environmental, drug allergies Medications: Lisinopril 10 mg daily Verapamil 120 mg daily Metformin 500 mg every evening MVI daily Allergies: PCN (rash) **Past Health History:** Appy age 10 Cholecystectomy age 39 HTN × 8 years DM × 6 months **Family Medical History:** Mother deceased @ 68: DM, HTN, CVA Father deceased @ 52: MVA, HTN Brother 42, HTN Sister 44, DM Son, 17, A+W **Social History:** Married × 25 years, lives in own home with wife and son, works as electrician in large paper mill × 20 years, denies excess stress in life Tob: 1 ppd × 30 years ETOH: 1 Pint scotch/week Drugs: Past use marijuana, none × 10 years	
OBJECTIVE *Gen*: 45 yo AAM, WD, NAD *Vital signs*: B/P: 135/78, P: 92, R: 20, T: 97.8, Ht: 5'9" Wt 225 # (last documented weight 3 months ago: 260#) Random blood sugar (finger stick): 305 mg/dL. *Eyes*: PERLA, fundi benign bilaterally. *ENT*: TMs clear bil, nasal mucosa pale, dry, buccal mucosa pale pink without lesion, posterior pharynx benign. *Neck*: Supple, trachea midline, thyroid nontender/not enlarged. *Chest/Lungs*: Unlabored respirations, resonant percussion throughout, breath sounds CTA throughout. *Heart*: Regular rhythm and rate, grade 2/6 early to midsystolic low-pitched murmur loudest @ 3ICS@LSB, radiates throughout precordium, carotid arteries without bruits bilaterally, 1+ pitting edema bil feet and ankles, extending to midcalf.	Examination: Comprehensive Contains 2 bulleted items from 10 systems

	E&M Coding Criteria
Abdomen: Obese, doughy, nontender, normoactive BS, no masses or organomegaly, percussion tympanic throughout, rectal exam with sl enlarged prostate, nontender, no nodules noted; hemoccult (-). *Musculoskeletal*: Joints of back, both upper extremities, both lower extremities without deformity, redness, warmth, or tenderness, FROM all joints, muscle tone 5/5 bilateral UEs and LEs. *Neuro*: CN II-XII grossly intact, DTR's 2+ bilaterally and symmetrical. *Mental*: Alert and oriented × 3, appropriate responses to questions, calm.	
Assessment: HTN, controlled DM, Type 2, uncontrolled Altered nutrition: more than body requirements RT excessive intake or insulin resistance due to Type 2 DM Tobacco Dependence: Precontemplation stage	
Plan: Dx: CBC, HgbA1c, Chemistry 18, PSA, lipid profile Therapeutic: Lisinopril to 10 mg daily #30, RF X 1 Verapamil 120 mg bedtime #30, RF X 1 Metformin 500 mg bid #60, RF X 1 Glucometer with test strips / lancets, test blood sugar BID Education: Discussed self-management of diabetes (diet, exercise, blood glucose testing), and pathophysiology of diabetes and complications. Diet: Discussed carbohydrate counting ADA 2400 calorie diet, handouts provided. Discussed importance of decreasing cigarette use and risks associated with DM. Exercise: Recommended starting walking program, handout given. Medications: Discussed importance of daily use, suggested strategies to decrease missing doses. Return visit: 1 Week to recheck status of blood sugar (bring record of home testing to visit for review).	Medical Decision Making: Moderate # dx / mgmt options: multiple est. problem stable = 1 est. problem, worsening =2 data to review: minimal risk: moderate # diagnoses: moderate procedures: minimal management: moderate

Table of Risk

Level of Risk	Presenting Problem(s)	Diagnostic Procedure(s) Ordered	Management Options Selected
Minimal	One self-limited or minor problem, e.g., cold, insect bite, tinea corporis	Laboratory tests requiring venipuncture Chest X-rays EKG/EEG UA US, echocardiography KOH prep	Rest Gargles Elastic bandages Superficial dressings
Low	Two or more self-limited or minor problems One stable chronic illness, well-controlled (HTN, Type 2 DM, BPH) Acute uncomplicated illness or injury (cystitis, allergic rhinitis, simple sprain)	Physiologic tests not under stress (PFTs) Noncardiovascular imaging studies w/contrast (barium enema) Superficial needle biopsies Clinical lab tests requiring arterial puncture Skin biopsies	OTC drugs Minor surgery PT OT IV fluids w/o additives
Moderate	One or more chronic illnesses with mild exacerbation, progression, or side effects of treatment Two or more stable chronic illnesses Undiagnosed new problem with uncertain prognosis (lump in breast) Acute illness with systemic symptoms (pyelonephritis, pneumonitis, colitis) Acute complicated injury (head injury with brief loss of consciousness)	Physiologic tests under stress (cardiac stress test, fetal contraction stress test) Diagnostic endoscopies with no identified risk factors Deep needle or incisional biopsy Cardiovascular imaging studies with contrast and no identified risk factors (arteriogram, cardiac cath) Obtain fluid from body cavity (lumbar puncture, thoracentesis, culdocentesis)	Minor surgery with identified risk factors Elective major surgery (open percutaneous or endoscopic) with no identified risk factors Prescription drug management Therapeutic nuclear medicine IV fluids with additives Closed treatment of fracture or dislocation without manipulation

Continued

Level of Risk	Presenting Problem(s)	Diagnostic Procedure(s) Ordered	Management Options Selected
High	One or more chronic illnesses with severe exacerbation, progression, or side effects of treatment Acute or chronic illnesses or injuries that pose a threat to life or bodily function (multiple trauma, acute MI, progressive severe rheumatoid arthritis, psychiatric illness with potential threat to self or others) An abrupt change in neurological status (seizure, TIA, sensory loss)	Cardiovascular imaging studies with contrast with identified risk factors Cardiac electrophysiological tests Diagnostic endoscopies with identified risk factors Discography	Elective major surgery (open, percutaneous or endoscopic) with identified risk factors Emergency major surgery (open, percutaneous, or endoscopic) Parenteral controlled substances Drug therapy requiring intensive monitoring for toxicity Decision not to resuscitate or to de-escalate care because of poor prognosis

Referral Letter

July 6, 2005

Dr. Harry Brown, MD
Endocrinology Associates, PC
3600 West Adams Avenue
NewCastle, MI 55055

Dear Dr. Brown:

I am referring my patient, Alice Arbor (DOB 5-9-65), to you for further evaluation and management of her hyperthyroidism. She was seen in my office on 6-30-06 for complaints of palpitations, tremors, amenorrhea, and fatigue during the previous month. Current medications are loratadine 10 mg daily and Ibuprofen 600 mg q8h prn menstrual cramps. She has no allergies. She has no previous history of thyroid disorder or other chronic disease.

Examination revealed an enlarged and mildly tender thyroid without discrete masses, sinus tachycardia, dry and warm skin, normal abdominal exam and pelvic exam. She has lost 12 pounds since her last visit 3 months ago. Thyroid function studies done 6-30-05 revealed TSH: 0.02, Total T4:18, T3: 245, T3U: 40%. Serum HCG was negative, CBC was within normal limits, renal and hepatic functions were normal as well.

She was started on Inderal 20 mg bid and instructed to continue with her routine medications and to keep her appointment with you, scheduled for July 10, 2005.

If you have further questions regarding this patient, please do not hesitate to contact me directly at 555-555-1000, extension 29. Thank you for your consideration in evaluating and managing Ms. Arbor's thyroid disorder.

Sincerely,

Mary P. White, ANP

Consultation Letter

July 6, 2005

Mary White, NP
Primary Care Associates
3400 West Adams Avenue
NewCastle, MI 55055

Dear Mary:

Thank you for your kind referral of Bridget Martin (DOB 3-9-75), for further evaluation of her abnormal Pap smear.

Her past medical history is significant for treatment of a CIN I via cervical conization in 1999. Her Pap smears since then have been within normal limits until the Pap test done in your office 6-12-05, which indicated LSIL. She denies any vaginal discharge, postcoital bleeding, dyspareunia, change in her normal menstrual pattern. She is sexually active with the same male partner for the past 4 years. She uses oral contraceptives for birth control, and her partner does not use condoms.

Colposcopy with biopsies on 6-22-05 revealed CIN I. A LEEP was performed on 6-30-05 without complications.

She will return for a repeat Pap smear in 3 months, and has been advised to have a Pap test every 3 months for the next year. Please contact me with any questions or concerns regarding the care of this patient. You can reach me directly at 555-555-1010.

Thank you again for your kind referral.

Sincerely,

Jane Smithe, CNM

Asthma Handout

Basic Asthma **Information**

Asthma Keys

- Develop an Asthma Action/Management Plan with your doctor. Go over it with your doctor or asthma specialist until you are comfortable with it. Update it often.
- Avoid your triggers.
- Know when and how to use your medications. Take them as directed.
- Check your peak flow daily, if your doctor tells you to.
- Have your quick relief medications handy at all times.
- Watch for early warning signs of an asthma attack.

What is Asthma?

Asthma is a lifelong, chronic breathing problem caused by swelling (inflammation) of the airways in the lungs. It cannot be cured, but it can be prevented and controlled. When you have asthma, your airways are super sensitive, or "twitchy." They may react to many things. These things are called triggers. People who have asthma may wheeze or complain of feeling "tight" in the chest. They may also cough a lot when their asthma is not under control.

Is Asthma a Serious Disease?

Asthma is a serious disease, and can kill if it is not treated the right way. When it is treated the right way, people with asthma can live normal, active lives.

What are the Symptoms of Asthma?

Not all people with asthma have the same symptoms, however, the most common symptoms are:

- Shortness of breath, chest "tightness"
- Wheezing

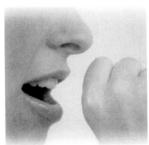

- Cough lasting more than a week, or that happens during the night or after exercise
- Chronic cough (sometimes coughing is the only symptom you will have)
- When you have a cold, it lasts for more than 10 days, and goes into your chest

Who Gets Asthma?

Anyone can get asthma, at any age. Sometimes it starts in infancy, other times it starts later in childhood. Although some children seem to "outgrow" asthma, the disease never really goes away; there is just a time when you are not having any breathing problems. Asthma can also start at any time during adulthood, including the senior years. Some people start having asthma symptoms after a bad cold or flu. Other people develop asthma after a work-related exposure. If you suspect that you have asthma, see your doctor or health care provider.

What is an Asthma Attack?

An asthma "attack" or episode is a time of increased asthma symptoms. The symptoms can be mild or severe. Anyone can have a severe attack, even a person with mild asthma. The attack can start suddenly or slowly. Sometimes a mild attack will seem to go away, but will come back a few hours later, and the second attack will be much worse than the first. Severe asthma symptoms need medical care right away.

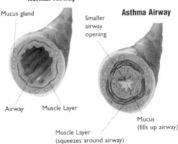

Normal Airway

Mucus gland

Smaller airway opening

Asthma Airway

Airway   Muscle Layer

Muscle Layer (squeezes around airway)

Mucus (fills up airway)

During an asthma attack, the lining of the airways in the lungs swells. The muscles around the airways tighten and make the airways narrower. All of these changes in the lungs block the flow of air, making it hard to breathe. Knowing what is happening in the lungs during an asthma attack will help you to know why it often takes more than one medicine to treat the disease.

Basic Asthma Information

What Can Be Done During an Asthma Attack?

The best time to plan for an asthma attack is long before one happens, at the doctor's office. There, the doctor, the person with asthma and their family can make an **Asthma Action Plan** that will tell them what to do if asthma symptoms start.

Along with following the Asthma Action Plan, here are some other helpful hints:

1. Stay calm, and try to relax. It isn't easy! But the more you panic, the worse your breathing will get.

2. Tell someone that you are having asthma symptoms. Get help if you need it.
Don't try to tough it out alone!

3. Take the quick-relief medication as your Asthma Action Plan tells you to. Not sure which medication is the quick-relief one? Ask your doctor, asthma counselor, or pharmacist about it before you need it in an emergency!

4. If the quick-relief medicine hasn't helped in 5-10 minutes, call the doctor or 911.

5. Keep taking the quick-relief medicine every 5-10 minutes until the ambulance arrives.

Never adjust your asthma medications or change how much you take unless your doctor has written it in your Asthma Action Plan or told you to do so over the phone.

What Can You Expect from Your Asthma Treatment?

With proper treatment for your asthma, you should be able to:

- Stay active and symptom free
  (this includes exercising and playing sports)

- Reduce or even prevent asthma symptoms

- Maintain normal functioning

  - No missed school or work because of asthma

  - No or minimal need for emergency department visits or hospitalizations

  - Sleep through the night without having asthma symptoms

- Have no or very few side effects from asthma medicines

- Have normal or near normal lung function

- Be satisfied with your asthma care

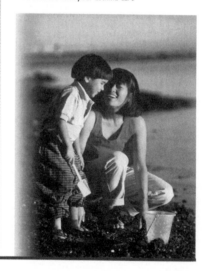

11-1

Electronic Health (Medical) Record Software Companies

The following is a list of Electronic Health (Medical) Record Software companies adapted from Bates, Ebell, Gotlieb, Zapp, and Mullins, "A proposal for electronic medical records in the U.S. primary care" (2003). The author does not endorse any one particular company.

List of Electronic Health (Medical) Record Software Companies	
Charting Plus	www.medinotes.com
ChartWare	www.chartware.com
ComChart	www.comchart.com
Dossier	www.ptf.com/dossier
Dr. Notes Program	www.drnotes.com/drnotes.htm
ENTITY	www.hcds.com/Products/ENTITY/medicalrecs.asp
EpicCare	www.epicsystems.com
Health Probe Patient Information Manager	www.healthprobe.com/
HealthMatics	www.a4healthsystems.com/electronic-medical-record/
Logician/Logician Internet	www.medicalogic.com/
MedicWare	www.medicware.com
NextGen	www.nextgen.com/?OVRAW=nextgen%20emr&OVKEY=emr&OVMTC=standard
Partner	www.pmsi.com/pr/patientrecords.htm?ovchn=OVR&ovcpn=overture&ovcrn=emr&ovac=PPC&OVRAW=partner%20emr&OVKEY=emr&OVMTC=standard
Patient Records QD Clinical	www.statsystems.com/
Physician Practice Solution	www.ergopartners.com/
PowerMed EMR	www.powermed.com/

Practice Partner	*www.pmsi.com/news/05192004.htm*
SoapWare	*www.docs.com/*
Versaform	*www.versaform.com/*
Welford Chart	*www.emirj.com/WelfordChartNotes.html*

Source: Data from Bates, D., Ebell, M., Gotlieb, E., Zapp, J., & Mullins, H. C. (2003). A proposal for electronic medical records in the U.S. primary care. *Journal of the American Medical Infomatrics Association* 10 (1), 1-10.

The following is a good site for all products.

- Society of Teachers in Family Medicine. Medical record software. Retrieved July 14, 2004, from *www.fammed.usouthal.edu/stfm/SWEMRFrame.htm*

The following is the Executive Learning, Inc., website, which provided the process improvement seminars.

- *www.elinc.com/*

The following article provides a comparison between different electronic medical record systems.

- Rehm, S., & Kraft, S. (2001). Electronic medical records: The FPM vendor survey. *Family Practice Management, 1,* 45-54.

13-1

Patient Internet Information Letter

Dear Patient,

I want to work with you to help you maintain the best of health. Many people these days are taking the initiative to learn more about responsible self-care for themselves and family members. If you're doing so, I commend you and offer this handout to support your efforts.

Some books, articles, and online information services are reliable, but many are not. You need to distinguish what is helpful from what is harmful. It's important to be aware that many of the online health services were created by companies whose main goal is to make money. Don't be duped by something that serves as an advertisement, even if it doesn't look like the ads on television.

Next time you log on to your favorite health care website, look for the sponsor and the advertisers. Then consider whether the information is in your best interest, or whether it's designed to sell you something. If you'd like, I can point you to sites where all of the health care information is reviewed by competent medical professionals.

I suggest you use the following five criteria to evaluate the sites you visit. They were developed by George D. Lundberg, M.D., former editor of the Journal of the American Medical Association, *and health journalist William M. Silberg. Consider any online information unreliable unless you can answer these questions:*

1. *Who wrote what you're reading? The site should contain the name of a real person.*
2. *Where does that person work? A university? A web business? A product manufacturer? Can you easily find that information on the site?*
3. *Was the information created for the site? If not, is there clear attribution showing where the information originated?*
4. *Who owns the site, and who pays for it? The source of money and ownership should be clearly identified.*
5. *Can you tell when the article itself was posted, whether it has been updated, and when?*

If you can't answer these questions, you may want to look elsewhere for health information. Even if you can answer the questions easily, there's no guarantee that the information is accurate and unbiased. If you have any questions about anything you find on the Net, I'd be happy to discuss them with you.

Since so much information is available today, I may not know any more than you on any given medical subject the first time you raise it. However, I make a commitment to you to use my resources to get you responsible answers, in a timely fashion.

Happy and (responsible) surfing!

Sincerely,

Resources for the Nurse Practitioner

Cardiovascular

- American College of Cardiology: *www.aac.org*
- National Heart Lung Blood Institute: *www.nhlbi.nih.gov/*
- Society for Cardiovascular & Interventional Radiology: *www.scvir.org*

Case Studies

- Association of Cancer On-line Resources: *www.acor.org*
- Case Study RX: *www.casestudyrx.com/heart/index/php*
- John Hopkins Allergy & Asthma: *www.hopkins-allergy.org*
- Karolinska Institute Medical University: Clinical Case Studies, Grand Rounds: *www.mic.ki.se/Medcases.html*
- Medical Simulations: *www.medicalsimulations.com/*
- Medscape: *www.medscape.com/px/mscpsearch?QueryText=case+studies&searchfor=Clinical*
- Pediatric Virtual Hospital: *www.vh.org/pediatric/provider/pediatrics/ virtualpedspatients/pedsvphome.html*
- University of Pittsburgh School of Medicine: Pathology: *http://path.umpc.edu/ cases/dxindex.html*
- University of Virginia Health System: *www.healthsystem.virginia.edu/ internet/pediatrics* (search words: case studies)

Clinical Resources

- Agency for Healthcare Research and Quality: *www.ahcpr.gov*
- Doctor's Guide: *www.docguide.com*
- eMedicine: *www.emedicine.com*
- FDA Health Professional Site, online reporting of health issues: *www.fda. gov/oc/*
- HealthWeb: *http://healthweb.org/*
- Mayo Clinic: *www.mayoclinic.org*
- MedlinePlus: *www.nlm.nih.gov/medlineplus*
- National Heart Lung Blood Institute Clinical Guidelines: *www.nhlbi.nih.gov/ guidelines/*
- National Library of Medicine: *www.nlm.nih.gov*
- Reuters Health: *www.reutershealth.com/en/index.html*

- The Stanford Health Library: Diseases and Disorders: *http://healthlibrary.stanford.edu/resources/internet/bodysys.html*
- Virtual Hospital: *www.vh.org*
- Web MD Health: *www.webmd.com*

Dermatology

- American Academy of Dermatology: *www.aad.org*
- Electronic Textbook of Dermatology: *www.telemedicine.org/stamford.htm*
- Johns Hopkins University: *www.dermatlas.com/derm/*
- National Psoriasis Foundation: *www.psoriasis.org/*
- University of Iowa: *http://tray.dermatology.uiowa.edu:80/Home.html*

Drug Information and Therapies

- Medscape: *www.medscape.com*
- The Stanford Health Library: *http://healthlibrary.stanford.edu*
- U.S. Food and Drug Administration: *www.fda.gov/default.htm*

E-Journals and *Continuing Education

- AANP SmartBrief: *www.aanp.org*
- *Advance for Nurse Practitioners: *www.advancefornp.com*
- *EMedicine: *www.emedicine.com*
- Family Practice News: *www.efamilypracticenews.com*
- Hardin MD: *www.lib.uiowa.edu/hardin/md*
- *MedStudent MedPulse: *www.medscape.com/medstudentshome*

Elderly

- Alzheimer's Disease Education: *www.alzheimers.org*
- American Geriatrics Society: *www.americangeriatrics.org*
- National Conference of Gerontological Nurse Practitioners: *www.ncgnp.org*
- National Institute on Aging: *www.nih.gov/nia*
- The Stanford Health Library: *http://healthlibrary.stanford.edu/resources/ internet/bodysystems/seniors.html*

Emergency/ Emergency Preparedness

- American College of Emergency Physicians: *www.acep.org*
- American Red Cross, Disaster Services: *www.redcross.org*
- CDC, Agency for Toxic Substances/Disease Registry: *www.atsdr.cdc.gov*
- CDC, Bioterrorism Preparedness & Response: *www.bt.cdc.gov*
- Department of Health & Human Services (DHHS), Office of Emergency Preparedness (OEP): *www.oep-ndms.dhhs.gov*
- DHHS-OEP, National Disaster Medical System: *www.ndms.dhhs.gov*

- Environmental Protection Agency (EPA), Chemical Emergency Preparedness & Prevention Office: *www.epa.gov/ceppo*
- Federal Emergency Management Agency (FEMA), includes a family emergency plan: *www.fema.gov*
- National Institutes of Health (NIH): *www.nih.gov*
- Occupational Safety & Health Administration (OSHA): *www.osha.gov*

Endocrinology

- American Association of Clinical Endocrinologists: *www.aace.com*
- American Diabetes Association: *www.diabetes.org*
- The Endocrine Society: *www.endo-society.org/*
- The Stanford Health Library: *http://healthlibrary.stanford.edu/resources/ internet/bodysystems/endocrine5.html*

Gastroenterology

- American College of Gastroenterology: *www.acg.gi.org*
- American Gastroenterological Association: *www.gastro.org*
- American Liver Foundation: *www.liverfoundation.org*
- HCV Advocate: *www.hcvadvocate.org*
- Hepatitis C Association: *www.hepcassoc.org*
- Hepatitis Foundation International: *www.hepfi.org*

Hospice and Palliative

- American Academy of Hospice and Palliative Medicine: *www.aahpm.org*
- American Pain Society: *http://ampainsoc.org*
- Education for Physicians on End-of-Life Care (EPEC): *www.epec.net*
- Harvard Medical School Center for Palliative Care: *www.hms.harvard.edu/cdi/pallcare/*
- Hospice and Palliative Nurses Association: *www.hpna.org*
- National Hospice and Palliative Care Organization: *www.nhpco.org*

Immunology

- AIDS info: *www.aidsinfo.nih.gov/*
- American Academy of Allergy, Asthma, and Immunology: *www.aaaai.org/*

Infectious Disease and Epidemiology

- Association for Professionals in Infection Control and Epidemiology: *www.apic.org*
- Center for Disease Control and Prevention: *www.cdc.gov/*
- HIV Clinical Resource: *www.hivguidelines.org/index.html*
- HIV Insight: *http://hivinsite.ucsf.edu/*

Medical Equipment

- Allheart: *www.Allheart.com*
- TheMalls: *www.TheMalls.com*

Men's Health

- The Stanford Health Library:
  http://healthlibrary.stanford.edu/resources/internet/bodysystems/genital.html

Mental Health

- American Psychiatric Association: *www.psych.org*
- National Alliance for the Mentally Ill: *www.nami.org*

Miscellaneous

- Almanac, encyclopedia, dictionary, and atlas: *www.infoplease.com/*
- American Medical Association: HIPAA updates: *www.ama-assn.org/go/hippa*
- CNN Health News: *www.cnn.com/HEALTH/*
- Dictionary Search: *www.onelook.com/*
- Health on the Net Foundation (HON): *www.hon.ch*
- Map Quest: *www.mapquest.com/*
- McGraw Hill Healthcare and Medicine: Lists and rates health sites:
  http://web10.eppg.com/medical/lange/cmdt/index.html
- Medem Inc.: Provides secure e-mail connectivity: *www.medem.com*
- Mid-Level Practitioners: Job search:
  www.midlevelpractitioners.com/advertising.php
- The ePolicy Institute: *www.epolicyinstitute.com*
- VOLC-R Primary Care Resources: *www.intmed.vcu.edu/inm/general.shtml*
- Yellow Pages: *www.infospace.com/*

Neurology

- American Council for the Blind: *www.acb.org/index.html*
- The National Eye Institute: *www.nei.gov*

Nurse Practitioner Sites

- ADVANCE for Nurse Practitioners: *www.advanceweb.com*
- American Academy of Nurse Practitioners: *www.aanp.org*
- American College of Nurse Midwives: *www.acnm.org*
- American College of Nurse Practitioners: *www.acnpweb.org*
- American Nurses' Association: *www.nursingworld.org*
- American Nurses Credentialing Center: *www.nursingworld.org/ancc*
- Fitzgerald Health Education: *www.fhea.com*
- HealthyInfo: *www.healthyinfo.com*

- National Association of Nurse Practitioners in Women's Health: *www.npwh.org*
- National Conference of Gerontological Nurse Practitioners: *www.ncgnp.org*
- National Organization of Nurse Practitioner Faculties (NONPF): *www.nonpf.com*
- NP Central: *www.npcentral.net*
- Nurse Practitioner Association for Continuing Education: *www.npace.org*
- Uniformed Nurse Practitioner Association: *www.unpa.org*

Occupational Health

- Occupational Safety and Health Administration (OSHA): *www.osha.gov*
- The National Institute for Occupational Safety and Health: *www.cdc.gov/niosh/homepage.html*

Oncology

- American Society of Clinical Oncology (ASCO): *www.asco.org*
- National Cancer Institute: *www.cancer.gov*
- OncoLink: *www.oncolink.com*

Orthopedic

- American Academy or Orthopedic Surgeons: *www.aaos.org*
- American Academy of Physical Medicine and Rehabilitation: *www.aapmr.org*
- American College of Rheumatology: *www.rheumatology.org*
- American College of Sports Medicine: *www.acsm.org*

Pathology

- College of American Pathologist: *www.cap.org/*

Patient Support Links and Educational Resources for the Practitioner

- Adam.com: *www.adam.com*
- Drkoop: *www.drkoop.com*
- Healthfinder: *www.healthfinder.gov*
- InteliHealth: *www.intelihealth.com*
- Mayo Clinic Health Oasis: *www.mayohealth.org*
- National Campaign to Prevent Teen Pregnancy: *www.teenpregnancy.org*
- OncoLink: *www.oncolink.com*
- Oregon Health Sciences University: Multilingual educational material: *www.ohsu.edu/library/patiented/links.shtml*
- Polycystic Ovarian Syndrome: Soul Cysters support site: *www.soulcysters.com*

PDA Resources

- American Association of Critical Care Nurses: *http://aacn.pdaorder.com/welcome.xml*
- CollectiveMed: *www.collectivemed.com*
- Dr. Gadget: *www.doctorsgadgets.com*
- Ectopic Brain: *http://pbrain.hypermart.net*
- Epocrates: *www.epocrates.com*
- Franklin: Book reader software: *www.franklin.com*
- Freeware Home: *www.freewarehome.com*
- Handango: *www.handango.com/home.jsp?siteId=1*
- Handheldmed: *www.handheldmed.com*
- Healthy Palmpilot: *www.healthypalmpilot.com*
- Iscribe: Electronic prescription writing: *www.iscribe.com*
- Medical Pocket PC: *www.medicalpocketpc.com*
- PalmGear: *www.PalmGear.com*
- Palmzone: *www.palmzone.com/software.html*
- Patientkeeper: *www.patientkeeper.com*
- PDA Buyers Guide: *www.pdabuyersguide.com/tips/palm_vs_pocketpc.htm*
- PDA MD: *www.pdamd.com* or *http://acp.pdaorder.com/welcome.xml*
- PDx Handheld: *www.firstconsult.com/home/framework/fs_main.htm*
- Pocketgear: *www.pocketgear.com*
- Pocket PC Magazine: *www.pocketpcmag.com/*
- Statcoder: *www.statcoder.com*
- Skyscape: *www.skyscape.com*
- Zapmed: Program for point of service billing: *www.zapmed.com*

Pediatric

- American Academy of Pediatrics: *www.aap.org*
- HealthWeb: *http://healthweb.org/*
- Keep Kids Healthy: *www.keepkidshealthy.com/*
- National Association of Pediatric Nurse Practitioners: *www.napnap.org*
- National Center for Missing and Exploited Children: *www.missingkids.org/ missingkids/servlet/PublicHomeServlet?Language Country=en_US*
- National Clearinghouse on Child Abuse and Neglect: *http://nccanch.acf.hhs.gov/*
- The Stanford Health Library: *http://healthlibrary.stanford.edu/resources/ internet/bodysystems/ childrenshealth.html*
- UCFF University of California School of Nursing: *http://nurseweb.ucsf.edu/www/appnres.htm*
- Virtual Pediatric Hospital: *www.vh.org/pediatric/*

Podiatry

- American Podiatric Medical Association: *www.apma.org*

Political Resources

- FirstGov: *www.firstgov.gov/Agencies/Federal/Legislative.shtml*
- Michigan Legislature: *www.michiganlegislature.org*
- Thomas Legislative Information on the Internet: *http://thomas.loc.gov*

Primary Care

- Advance NP Complimentary Care Forum: *www.advancefornp.com/Common/CompCareForum/Welcome.aspx*
- American Academy of Family Physicians: *www.aafp.org*
- American Academy of Physician Assistants: *www.aapa.org*
- Antibiotic Consult: *www.antibiotic-consult.com*
- Department of Transportation: Safety hotline/teaching tools: *www.nhtsa.dot.gov/hotline*
- Doctor's Guide: *www.docguide.com*
- Journal of the American Academy of Physician Assistants: *www.jaapa.com/be_core/j/index.jsp*
- MD Consult: *www.mdconsult.com*
- Patient Care Best Clinical Practices for Today's Physician: *www.patientcareonline.com/patcare/article/articleDetail.jsp?id=119753*
- Patient Care for the NP: *www.patientcarenp.com/be_core/n/index.jsp*
- Primary Care Internet Guide: *www.uib.no/isf/guide/family.htm*

Pulmonary

- American Association of Respiratory Therapist: *www.aarc.org*
- American College of Chest Physicians: *www.chestnet.org*
- National Heart Lung Blood Institute: *www.nhlbi.nih.gov/*

Radiology

- American College of Radiology: *www.acr.org/flash.html*
- Society for Cardiovascular & Interventional Radiology: *www.scvir.org*

Research Sites

- Agency for Health Care Policy and Research Quality (AHRQ): *www.ahcpr.gov/*
- Centers for Disease Control and Prevention (CDC): *www.cdc.gov*
- Healthy People 2010: *www.healthypeople.gov/*
- Medscape: *www.medscape.com/px/urlinfo*
- National Institute of Health: *http://grants.nih.gov/grants*
- National Institute of Nursing Research: *http://ninr.nih.gov/ninr*
- National Library of Medicine's PUBMED: *www.nlm.nih.gov*
- National Occupational Research Agenda (NORA): *www.cdc.gov/niosh/nora/*
- Sigma Theta Tau International: *www.nursingsociety.org*
- Survey Monkey: Survey tool: *www.surveymonkey.com/home.asp*

Search Engines and Search Information

- Alltheweb.com: *www.alltheweb.com*
- AOL Search internal: *http://search.aol.com/aolcom/index.jsp*
- Ask Jeeves: *www.askjeeves.com*
- Boston University Medical Center: Search engine guide and tutorial: *http://med-libwww.bu.edu/library/engines.html*
- Dogpile: *www.dogpile.com/*
- Google: *www.google.com*
- HotBot: *www.hotbot.com/*
- Medical Dictionary Meta-Search Engine (CDC, Joslin, NFB, NIDDK, & UL): *http://medical-dictionary-search-engines.com/diabetes/*
- MSN Search: *www.search.msn.com*
- Yahoo: *www.yahoo.com*

Underserved

- Association for Clinicians for Underserved: *www.clinicians.org*
- National Commission of Correctional Health Care: *www.ncchc.org*

Urology

- Urology Associations/Societies/Foundations: *www.edae.gr/uro-ass.html*

Women's Health

- Association of Reproductive Health Professionals: *www.arhp.org*
- Breast Feeding Basics: *www.breastfeedingbasics.org*
- Center for Applied Reproductive Science: *www.ivf-et.com*
- Contemporary OB/GYN: *www.contemporaryobgyn.net*
- Contraception Online: *www.contraceptiononline.org/*
- La Leche League: *www.lalecheleague.org/home_intro.html*
- National Association of Nurse Practitioners in Women's Health: *www.npwh.org*
- National Campaign to Prevent Teen Pregnancy: *www.teenpregnancy.org*
- Obgyn: *www.obgyn.net/*
- Polycystic Ovarian Syndrome Association: *www.pcosupport.org*
- The Stanford Health Library: *http://healthlibrary.stanford.edu/resources/internet/bodysystems/womenshealth.html*
- Washington State Midwives Health Care Resources and Web Sites: *www.midwivesofwa.org/online.htm*

eRisk Working Group for Healthcare: Guidelines for Online Communication

November 2002

The eRisk guidelines have been developed by the eRisk Working Group for Healthcare, a consortium of professional liability carriers, medical societies, and state board representatives. These guidelines are meant to provide information to health care providers related to online communication. They are reviewed and updated regularly. These guidelines are not meant as legal advice, and providers are encouraged to bring any specific questions or issues related to online communication to their legal counsel.

Online Communications

The legal rules, ethical guidelines, and professional etiquette that govern and guide traditional communications between the health care provider and patient are equally applicable to e-mail, websites, listservs, and other electronic communications. However, the technology of online communications introduces special concerns and risks:

1. **Security.** Online communications between health care provider and patient should be conducted over a secure network, with provisions for authentication and encryption in accordance with eRisk, HIPAA, and other appropriate guidelines. Standard e-mail services do not meet these guidelines. Health care providers need to be aware of potential security risks, including unauthorized physical access and security of computer hardware, and guard against them with technologies such as automatic logout and password protection.
2. **Authentication.** The health care provider has a responsibility to take reasonable steps to authenticate the identity of correspondent(s) in an electronic communication and to ensure that recipients of information are authorized to receive it.

3. **Confidentiality.** The health care provider is responsible for taking reasonable steps to protect patient privacy and to guard against unauthorized use of patient information.

4. **Unauthorized Access.** The use of online communications may increase the risk of unauthorized distribution of patient information and create a clear record of this distribution. Health care providers should establish and follow procedures that help to mitigate this risk.

5. **Informed Consent.** Prior to the initiation of online communication between health care provider and patient, informed consent should be obtained from the patient regarding the appropriate use and limitations of this form of communication. Providers should consider developing and publishing specific guidelines for online communications with patients, such as avoiding emergency use, heightened consideration of use for highly sensitive medical topics, appropriate expectations for response times, etc. These guidelines should become part of the legal documentation and medical record when appropriate. Providers should consider developing patient selection criteria to identify those patients suitable for e-mail correspondence, thus eliminating persons who would not be compliant.

6. **Highly Sensitive Subject Matter.** The health care provider should advise patients of potential privacy risks associated with online communication related to highly sensitive medical subjects. This warning should be repeated if a provider solicits information of a highly sensitive nature, such as issues of mental health, substance abuse, etc. Providers should avoid active initial solicitation of highly sensitive topic matters.

7. **Emergency Subject Matter.** The health care provider should advise patients of the risks associated with online communication related to emergency medical subjects such as chest pain, shortness of breath, bleeding during pregnancy, etc. Providers should avoid active promotion of the use of online communication to address topics of medical emergencies.

8. **Doctor-Patient Relationship.** The health care provider may increase liability exposure by initiating a doctor-patient relationship solely through online interaction. Payment for online services may further increase that exposure.

9. **Medical Records.** Whenever possible and appropriate, a record of online communications, pertinent to the ongoing medical care of the patient, must be maintained as part of, and integrated into, the patient's medical record, whether that record is paper or electronic.

10. **Licensing Jurisdiction.** Online interactions between a health care provider and a patient are subject to requirements of state licensure. Communications online with a patient outside of the state in which the provider holds a license may subject the provider to increased risk.

11. **Authoritative Information.** Health care providers are responsible for the information that they provide or make available to their patients online. Information that is provided on a medical practice website should come either directly from the health care provider or from a recognized and credible source. Information provided to specific patients via secure e-mail from a health care provider should come either directly from the health care provider or from a recognized and credible source after review by the provider.

12. **Commercial Information.** Websites and online communications of an advertising, promotional, or marketing nature may subject providers to increased liability, including implicit guarantees or implied warranty. Misleading or deceptive claims increase this liability.

Fee-Based Online Consultations

A fee-based online consultation is a clinical consultation provided by a medical provider to a patient using the Internet or other similar electronic communications network in which the provider expects payment for the service.

An online consultation that is given in exchange for payment introduces risks. In a fee-based online consultation, the health care provider has the same obligations for patient care and follow-up as in face-to-face, written, and telephone consultations. For example, an online consultation should include an explicit follow-up plan that is clearly communicated to the patient.

In addition to the 12 guidelines stated earlier, the following are additional considerations for fee-based online consultations:

1. **Preexisting Relationship.** Online consultations should occur only within the context of a previously established doctor-patient relationship that includes a face-to-face encounter when clinically appropriate. State medical boards have begun enforcement actions.
2. **Informed Consent.** Prior to the online consultation, the health care provider must obtain the patient's informed consent to participate in the consultation for a fee. The consent should include explicitly stated disclaimers and service terms pertaining to online consultations. The consent should establish appropriate expectations between provider and patient.
3. **Medical Records.** Records pertinent to the online consultation must be maintained as part of, and integrated into, the patient's medical record.
4. **Fee Disclosure.** From the outset of the online consultation, the patient must be clearly informed about charges that will be incurred, and that the charges may not be reimbursed by the patient's health insurance. If the patient chooses not to participate in the fee-based consultation, the patient should be encouraged to contact the provider's office by phone or other means.
5. **Appropriate Charges.** An online consultation should be substantive and clinical in nature and be specific to the patient's personal health status. There should be no charge for online administrative or routine communications such as appointment scheduling and prescription refill requests. Health care providers should consider not charging for follow-up questions on the same subject as the original online consultation.
6. **Identity Disclosure.** Clinical information that is provided to the patient during the course of an online consultation should come from, or be reviewed in detail by, the consulting provider whose identity should be made clear to the patient.
7. **Available Information.** Health care providers should state, within the context of the consultation, that it is based only on information made available by the patient to the provider during, or prior to, the online consultation, including

referral to the patient's chart when appropriate, and therefore may not be an adequate substitute for an office visit.

8. **Online Consultation vs. Online Diagnosis and Treatment.** Health care providers should attempt to distinguish between online consultation related to preexisting conditions, ongoing treatment, follow-on question related to previously discussed conditions, etc., and new diagnosis and treatment addressed solely online. New diagnosis and treatment of conditions, solely online, may increase liability exposure.

_____

Source: Copyright © 2002 Medem, Inc.

Community Coalition Worksheets

HEALTH ISSUE/PROBLEM:

POPULATION AFFECTED:

DOCUMENTATION/DATA SUBSTANTIATING THE ISSUE

Data: Source:

COALITION COMPOSITION:

Type of Individual	Number	Organization/Group Represented:

PLANS FOR COALITION FORMATION:

Plans for bringing individuals together to form a coalition (when, where, how):
Evaluation of coalition formation:

Activities to Lay the Foundation	Steering Committee (Potential key leaders)	Key Research on the Issue (Facts, allies, opponents, uncontrollable factors, and ability to mobilize support)	Organization Timetables	Action Plan (Key actions based on the outcome of the problem solving worksheet analysis)

PROBLEM SOLVING WORKSHEET (Kaye, 1995, p. 161)

ACTORS (People or institutions who can help solve the problem)	IDEAL ROLES (One or two activities each actor could undertake to help with the problem)	BARRIERS (What "walls" might we run up against/why aren't these activities taking place?)	STRATEGIES/ PROGRAMS/ ACTIVITIES (Creative, collaborative ways to address problems, overcome barriers)	RESOURCES (Needed to effectively; implement strategies; H=have N=need)

Source: From Kaye, G. (1995). Developing action plans for your community coalition. In G. Kaye & T. Wolff (Eds.), *From the ground up: A workbook on coalition building and community development* (pp. 143-162). Amherst, MA: AHEC/Community Partners.

Example of Letter to a Legislator

Date

The Honorable Fred Upton
House of Representatives
2183 Rayburn House Office Building
Washington, DC 20515

Dear Representative Upton,

As a nurse educator and a member of your congressional district, I am writing to ask you to support H.R. 5324 the Nurse Education, Expansion, and Development Act of 2004. This bill will provide resources that are critical to expanding the number of nursing faculty that are needed to address the nursing shortage. I appreciate your support of the Nurse Reinvestment Act (Public Law 107-205), which increased the applications to schools of nursing by 60%. Unfortunately, without an increase in the number of nurse educators, many of these well-qualified applicants have had to be turned away. This year at _____ University where I teach, we turned away 300 qualified applicants. We cannot afford to do that if we are to reach the goal of 1,000,000 new and replacement nurses that are needed by 2012 (*Monthly Labor Review of the Bureau of Labor Statistics*, February 2004).

I have been a nurse educator for more than 30 years and am concerned about the following facts:

1. During the last few years more than 12% of nurses with doctoral degrees have chosen careers that do not include nursing education.
2. The number of master's level students who are preparing for roles as nurse educators has decreased during the last few years.
3. The average age of nursing faculty is 55 years and faculty usually retire at age 62.

We have to take immediate action to reverse this trend. In the current economic climate, neither state-supported nor private universities are able to expand their preparation of nurse faculty without help. H.R. 5324 will provide capitation grants to creatively expand the preparation of nurse faculty. Please feel free to contact me at [contact information] and I will be happy to provide you further data and illustrations, if that would be helpful.

Thank you for your continued efforts to support nursing and, thus increase the quality of health care.

Example of Testimony

Testimony for the Subcommittee on Appropriate Supply and Utilization of Michigan's Health Care Workforce of the Standing Committee on Health Policy

Testimony on Nursing Shortage August 27, 2001

Patricia W. Underwood, PhD, RN
Michigan Nurses Association, Past President
Professor
Kirkhof School of Nursing
Grand Valley State University
Grand Rapids, MI

As a past president of the Michigan Nurses Association, I am here to testify on behalf of the MNA and the more than 80,000 registered nurses actively practicing in Michigan. We commend the members of the Subcommittee on Appropriate Supply and Utilization of Michigan's Workforce for your initiative in seeking to understand how we can maintain, increase, and appropriately utilize our nursing workforce. As you are aware, nursing is a profession that demands a high level of skill and education to fulfill a critical role in meeting the health care needs of a diverse population. Before we consider strategies to achieve a sufficient supply of well-prepared nurses, it is critical that we understand the nature and dimensions of Michigan's nursing workforce supply problem. Therefore, I will do three things today:

1. Present some facts that suggest that we are facing a nursing workforce problem in Michigan.
2. Clarify what we mean when we talk about a shortage of nurses.
3. Identify areas in which to focus our efforts to address the supply of nurses in Michigan.

Michigan Nursing Workforce

Unfortunately, in Michigan, we do not have an adequate system of ongoing data collection sufficient to yield reliable projections of our future supply of nurses. This was one of the reasons that Public Act 256 was passed last year to mandate a study of the nursing workforce supply. It is anticipated that the Legislature will soon be receiving copies of the final report from the Department of Consumer and Industry Services. Formal and informal discussions have yielded the following data:

- As of 1998-1999 there were an estimated 106,195 nurses including 83,800 RNs and 22,395 LPNs actively practicing in Michigan
- In informal discussions, many hospitals report significant vacancies in nursing particularly in critical care, emergency rooms, and other specialty areas. One hospital administrator told me that she could hire 200 registered nurses tomorrow if they were available.

It does not bode well for the future that:

- While the Michigan population has increased by 0.8%, the number of working RNs and LPNs has increased only by 0.4%.
- The number of graduates from LPN, ADN, and BSN programs has generally declined throughout the state.
- National data indicates that the average age of the working RN is 43.4 years.
- Additionally, the average age of faculty is 55 years, so any attempts to increase the number of graduates from nursing programs must begin with efforts to recruit and develop more faculty.

The need and demand for nurses has increased in all settings and is expected to continue. Although patients are experiencing shorter stays in the hospital, the only reason they are there to begin with is because they need nursing care. The fact that they are sicker means that more registered nurses are needed to make the frequent checks and critical judgments that will prevent complications. When Jim Brady lay in the Intensive Care Unit after being shot in the attack on President Reagan, he was lucky to have the care of an experienced ICU nurse. Her experience made her concerned about her patient's condition one night. She reported her concerns to the physician who did not share them because the patient's vital signs were not unexpected. Nevertheless, the nurse remained vigilant. When a change in Brady's condition became more evident, she knew immediately and took the emergency steps that in fact saved his life. He had experienced a blood clot in the lungs that might have been fatal if it had not been treated quickly.

It is not just a case of needing more registered nurses. We need nurses with the experience, education, and expertise to anticipate and respond to patients' needs in the most complex and novel situations. Studies have shown that an inadequate supply of registered nurses in the acute care setting is associated with increased rates of hospital-acquired infections, falls, and decubitus ulcer formation. Lengths of stay increase, while patient satisfaction decreases. These occurrences also increase health care costs.

Inadequate staffing takes its toll on the nurses as well. I have talked with staff nurses around the state. They are frustrated by the significantly increased demands that are placed on them in the workplace. Their comments support the findings of national and international studies that report increased rates of burnout (as high as 36%) among nurses (Aiken et al., 2001). As many as 40% of the nurses reported that they leave aspects of care such as oral hygiene, skin care, patient teaching, comfort, and updating plans of care undone when they leave, because they simply do not have time. Nurses are sad that they cannot give the quality of care they believe patients need and are worried that fatigue and stress will lead to mistakes in care. In another study of 7,300 nurses, 75% stated that they believed the quality of care in their hospitals had decreased in the past year (ANA, 2001). The Michigan Nurses Association conducted a survey of nurses in the Grand Rapids area last year and found similar results.

Increasing numbers of nurses face patient and family complaints and verbal abuse (Aiken et al., 2001). In view of the increase in work stress, decrease in job satisfaction, and increase in verbal abuse, it is not surprising that 29% of nurses under the age of 30 report plans to leave their present job within the next year (Aiken et al., 2001). Thus, it is obvious that a problem exists, that the need for registered nurses will continue to increase, and that Michigan is likely following a path similar to the rest of the country.

Definition of Nursing Shortage

The supply of nurses in Michigan does not meet current needs and, unless things change, will not meet future needs. To find appropriate solutions to workforce needs, it is important to understand that we are experiencing two different shortages. The present shortage is typical of the cyclical shortages that occur as a result of reorganization in health care. Cutbacks, in the use of nurses, support the perception that job openings are limited. The effect of this perception is a decrease in the number of individuals who seek preparation for licensure as a nurse. This cycle is enhanced by the plethora of educational and professional opportunities open to young people today. It is also enhanced when stressed nurses do not encourage others to join their profession. In the past, we have tried to address this shortage but have failed to break the cycle.

Along with our present shortage, we are facing a future shortage that is unique, because it is a significant projected deficit of more experienced and educated nurses. It is a shortage that will not be amenable to the simple infusion of new graduates into the professional workforce. It is expected to arrive around 2010 as substantial numbers of faculty and nurses in direct care retire.

Focal Areas for Addressing the Shortage

Plans to address the nursing workforce in Michigan must focus on both types of shortages. Thus, it becomes evident that retaining nurses is as critical an issue as the recruitment into the profession. So where should we focus our efforts at solution? Quick-fix strategies such as mandated overtime or the infusion of undereducated and quickly trained assistive personnel are not the answers. None of us would choose to fly in a plane where the pilot was unduly fatigued. Nurses make equally critical life and death decisions and, therefore, should be equally rested. Likewise, none of us would willingly put the care of our family members in the hands of an individual who 3 weeks ago was flipping burgers. We want well-educated professionals available to make the critical checks and judgments needed to prevent complications and facilitate optimal health and well-being. If we are going to find a lasting, comprehensive solution to both nursing shortages, all of us—nurses, legislators, administrators, educators, physicians, other health care providers, payers, corporations, the media, and the public—are all going to have to work together. There are several places we can start:

1. Develop a center for the routine collection of Michigan nursing workforce data to more adequately describe the current reality and project future nursing workforce needs, availability of clinical resources, graduation rates, etc.
2. Support studies of new models of nursing care delivery in areas where our need is most critical. We need to see what levels of staffing and staff mix are necessary to achieve desired patient outcomes in a cost-effective way. Such studies should include the collection of nursing sensitive quality care data.
3. Encourage the implementation of best practices to more effectively retain nurses, even as they age with the rest of the population, and to support them in providing quality, nursing care. We know through a study of magnet hospitals, for example, that good communication between doctors and nurses and giving nurses more decision-making authority at the bedside and throughout the organization greatly enhance retention (Sochalski & Aiken, 1999). Decreasing stress in the workplace is an essential first step, but other strategies such as improved pay and providing retirement benefits are important in keeping nurses at the bedside.
4. Encourage and support a state-wide collaborative initiative aimed at further clarifying those aspects of the shortage of nurses in Michigan that are most amenable to lasting solutions. Through this collaboration we can develop creative strategies to address these areas and support their implementation. It will do absolutely no good if comprehensive reports and recommendations are developed only to languish on someone's shelf.

Conclusion

In conclusion, we should all recognize and help others to understand that when we talk about a shortage of nurses in Michigan, it is very real and we are talking about two shortages: a typical shortage that we are currently experiencing and a potentially devastating shortage that is barreling down on us. The second will occur as the result of the loss of our most experienced and educated nurses. Since the average age of nurse educators is 55, schools of nursing will potentially feel the shortage of faculty first. This may further constrain our ability to increase the numbers of qualified graduates needed in nursing service. While Michigan data are limited, they support a clear need for more registered nurses. Lasting solutions to the nursing shortage will only be developed through our collaborative efforts focused on:

1. Enhancing the image of nursing as a valued, rewarding, and appropriately compensated career.
2. Recruitment of a more diverse population of academically talented individuals.
3. Support for students' success in completing programs of initial professional education, obtaining licensure, and going on for advanced education.
4. Maximization of the capacity of existing educational programs in producing well-prepared graduates.
5. Encouraging nurses to obtain further education and prepare for roles as faculty.
6. Increasing the ability of employers to attract nurses to settings (geographic and clinical) where the needs are most critical.
7. Retention of a qualified and satisfied workforce.

In Michigan, the nursing shortage is here, and nurses welcome the partnership of legislators in addressing this issue so that the people of Michigan will continue to receive quality nursing care.

References

Aiken, L. et al. (2001, May-June). Nurses' reports of hospital quality of care and working conditions in five countries. *Health Affairs, 20.*

American Nurses Association. (2001). *Analysis of American Nurses Association staffing survey.* Warick, RI: Cornerstone Communications Group.

Sochalski, J., & Aiken, L. (1999). Accounting for variation in hospital outcomes: A cross-national study. *Health Affairs, 18,* 256-259.

APPENDIX 15-2

Exemplar: Oncology Specialty Practice Role Development

Sharon VanLeeuwen, MSN, AOCN, APRN-BC
Oncology Nurse Practitioner

Focusing Educational Experiences

For fifteen years I worked on a critical care unit before returning to school to obtain a graduate degree. I wanted to combine the expertise that I had gained in practice with my passion for end-of-life care. In my graduate program, I focused projects and papers, thesis work, and clinic experiences on quality, end-of-life issues. In the NP program, I worked on critical thinking skills and in diagnosing and establishing a treatment plan for acute and chronic problems. Through this process, I discovered that it was important to understand the clinical rotations and preceptors that are available to students. I had frequent contacts with the coordinator of our clinical rotations who assigns medical students, physician assistants (PA), and nurse practitioners to clinical sites and expressed my personal goals and clinical preferences. She understood the requirements of the program and was able to provide experiences that were essential in establishing my career in palliative care.

Over the next two years as a student in clinical rotations, I worked in a primary care and internal medicine office as well as an oncology practice. I consistently shared my passion and what I hoped to accomplish as an NP in an acute care setting working with families and patients in crisis as well as growing in patient-centered end-of-life care. I kept redefining and exploring what indeed was my passion in health care and specifically in nursing. I had always felt that advanced education was the key for opportunities in practice. In graduate school, I didn't want to miss the chance to gain confidence and expertise in what I knew to be true regarding care of a most unique patient population.

Applying and Securing an NP Position

Approximately two months from graduation, I was offered an interview in an oncology practice. The office had one acute care oncology NP working exclusively with a physician's patient population in the hospital. She had been my clinical preceptor and we had spent our days meeting patients' physical (both immediate and chronic), psychological, and spiritual needs. She was also involved in doctoral work and is a palliative care expert. It seemed like the perfect job.

Two physicians in the practice had initiated the job search and requested a second NP to provide similar types of services to their patients. The interview was challenging because neither physician clearly understood a NP role and scope of practice. Each had different expectations and needs even though they had closely watched the collaborative practice between their physician peer and the NP. They didn't know the specifics, but somehow having a NP created better care for both the patients and families. They noted that the patients seemed more confident in themselves, their treatment plan, and their health care providers with the NP-physician model of care.

Whatever one learns about job interviews, it never seems enough to sustain confidence about the experience. My interview was no exception. When asked my knowledge base in oncology and what led me to seek employment in this specialty in the midst of my career, I responded with a description of passion for improving care at the end of life. What I didn't realize is that end-of-life issues are not the favorite subject of oncologists! As clinicians, they are more interested in responses of the chemotherapy agents in slowing down or eradicating malignancies. The quality-of-life issues and patient-family response are to be considered, but are not on the top of their priority list.

I was able to articulate a 20-year history of strong clinical experience and patient management skills during the interview. I highlighted my leadership in managing family conferences and strategies for working with "challenging" family cases. Following the interview, I was certain that the experience gained through the interview was all that I could expect. I later learned that the lack of oncology experience was a weakness identified in the job interview, but that my strong clinical experience, positive references, and professional relationships as well as my ability to communicate with patients and families would land me the job. I felt especially proud about securing the oncology NP position because there are few NPs and PAs in specialty practice in our community.

Defining and Negotiating the Specialty Role

I learned early on that a NP must be able to articulate his or her unique role in the practice, provide a written job description, and describe the orientation and evaluation process. It became clear at the interview that neither physician had identified job expectations, communication strategies, orientation or mentoring, or standards for best practices for the NP role. These job components are important in the transition from being a novice to an expert. I was able to share my thoughts and plans for the new position. This is not ideal, because as a novice, I had limited understanding of the patient population I was to serve, and an incomplete depth of understanding concerning my scope of practice in this specialty area. However, my limited plan was better than no direction, and I had daily availability of my more experienced NP colleague.

In a collaborative practice, it remains a challenge to perceive the uniqueness of roles, and to allow the patient to benefit from various healthcare disciplines. The medical model requires diagnosis and treatment on a regular basis. As a NP in a busy oncology practice, I am expected to recognize and manage acute and chronic conditions as well as assessing and managing family issues, strengthening patient coping mechanisms, and teaching about the specific physiological needs of the patient in order to ensure a better patient outcome. The physicians in our practice realize the value-added component of these additional interventions as they experience the demands of a challenging medical practice.

Challenges in Practice

The challenge for me was to preserve the unique role as an advanced practice nurse in an oncology practice. This has been the most pressing issue over the past five months as our practice has merged with a larger one that employs PAs to provide care for the inpatient population. The new oncology practice looked at the amount of "work to be done," and ways to divide up the inpatients that needed to be covered between us. It soon became apparent that this would not be an easy task, since there were two different styles of practice.

As a NP, having partial ownership of the responsibility of patient treatment, I needed to assess and strengthen coping patterns of both the patient and family and then integrate these mechanisms into the treatment plan. The PAs were more task oriented, allowing for a greater number of patients to be seen, but narrowing the care to daily rounds, admissions, and discharges. Building relationships and following a patient over a length of time, both in the office and with readmissions, was very important to me. Although the PAs may have appreciated more continuity, they felt that working a specific schedule and focusing on the "work of the day" superseded any in-depth type of follow-up. I spend many hours in family conferences, follow up with patients after discharge, enroll patients in research studies, and work to broaden my knowledge base about the physiology of cancer as well as treatment strategies. What I learn helps me to be able to educate the patient and family about the specifics of their disease.

As the practice reviewed the PA and NP roles and scope of practice, the physicians were not unified in the support that they desired in the hospital. Some were comfortable with having admissions, discharges, and daily rounds managed on a fairly superficial level. The physicians who hired me wanted more of a partnership in patient care with a PA or NP. I soon realized that the collaborative practice we had developed over the past eighteen months was threatened. It took a number of discussions since both physicians I worked with had a strong desire to "blend into" the new practice. However, when it became apparent that the style being suggested by the medical director of the new practice was not based on a team approach but rather a "work list" model, I knew that I could not continue working under these circumstances.

I met again with the physicians who had hired me. After eighteen months, we could both articulate the components of a collaborative practice and a simple definition of the supporting pieces of our role. They were not willing to sacrifice our practice model to blend into a more homogeneous model with their new partners. The decision was to maintain our collaborative relationship in caring for our patients with the rest of the physicians using the PAs as they had before the merger.

Lifelong Learning

As an NP, it is important to become certified in your area of specialty. This is done through a national certification examination offered by the specialty professional organization. I was certified within the first year by the oncology nursing society as an advanced oncology nurse. This establishes a baseline of expertise, and it illustrates a desire to meet a specific standard of practice. I also attend a yearly national oncology nursing conference. Weekly, I attend either the tumor board that is specific to oncology patients or general grand rounds that review a variety of internal medicine topics. It is important to attend these activities because it is opportunity to build relationships with physicians, NPs and other health care providers such as clinical pharmacists, and PAs. Exposure to journals and making the effort to do literature searches on a variety of topics also aid in daily survival. After two years, I still have moments when I open a chart and feel very uncertain as to the direction of care. It is those times that one needs to take a deep breath and plunge in with resources and confidence. The critical thinking skills are cultivated over years of education, and they are developed to allow for success.

Defining a Unique Role

Entering a specialty practice is only one opportunity that a NP may seek upon completing his or her graduate education. It is important that one first has a clear understanding of his or her knowledge and skills gained through experience. It is also important to examine clinical opportunities provided by a graduate program, and attempt to engage in those that most closely align with your interests. It is essential that you articulate that what you can offer a practice. During precepted clinical experiences, ask to see coding and billing information so that you can understand what type of monetary benefit your services will be able to generate. Understanding the coding and billing criteria for both inpatient and outpatient is important.

The last two years have been a wonderful time of professional growth. Being a NP is a very satisfying and unique role. There are specific steps to be taken when entering practice, and being able to articulate one's scope of practice as well as specifics of role are important for success. The health care crisis continues to demand creative solutions in managing complex patient populations. Utilizing NPs in specialty practices is a viable and helpful option in promoting better care for distinct patient populations.

Sample Collaborative Contract between a University and a Private Practice

STATE UNIVERSITY AND _____

THIS AGREEMENT made and entered into this 11th day of August, 2005, by and between State University, a constitutionally created public corporation (hereinafter referred to as "University"), and the (hereinafter referred to as "Professional Corporation") for the nursing services of Assistant Professor, _____ a certified Nurse Practitioner ("Nurse Practitioner").

Statement of Facts

State University College of Nursing has nursing faculty members who are qualified and duly certified to practice nursing in the State of Michigan. State University's mission includes nursing education and research and through the performance of clinical services and clinical education at community hospitals, health care agencies, and professional corporations the University is able to promote its mission. State University desires _____, a certified nurse practitioner, to provide services at Professional Corporation in furtherance of the mutual goals and aims of the Professional Corporation and State University.

Agreement

In consideration of the mutual representations and agreements contained in this Agreement, the parties agree as follows:

I. Engagement of University

Scope of Engagement. Professional Corporation engages University through its College of Nursing to provide the nurse practitioner services of Assistant Professor _____.

II. Relationship with State University

A. In the performance of the services to be rendered pursuant to this Agreement, University and Nurse Practitioner shall be and at all times is acting and performing as an independent contractor. Except as provided in this Agreement, University reserves to itself the exclusive right to designate the hours, duties, and work assignments of Nurse Practitioner, and the Professional Corporation shall neither have nor exercise control or direction over Nurse Practitioner performing services on behalf of University except as provided in this Agreement.

B. Taxes. The University shall pay all federal, state and local income taxes, FICA, FUTA, and other required taxes for amounts paid to University by the Professional Corporation as compensation for professional services rendered by Nurse Practitioner.

III. Professional Services

A. Duties of Nurse Practitioner. Nurse Practitioner shall provide any service assigned by Professional Corporation and permitted under the Nurse Practice Act of the Public Health Code of Michigan.

B. Schedule. Nurse Practitioner's faculty responsibilities will be reduced to (__%) for Nurse Practitioner's normal teaching schedule during the University's academic year. Consequently, Nurse Practitioner shall be available to provide services to the Professional Corporation approximately (__) hours for each workweek for the term of this Agreement. For purposes of this provision, "workweek" shall be defined as any week during the academic year, excluding Saturday, Sunday, and holidays designated by the University, in which faculty must perform their assigned responsibilities. Further, the work schedule of Nurse Practitioner at the Professional Corporation shall not conflict with any of her University responsibilities as determined at least 90 days in advance of her scheduled work at the Professional Corporation by the Dean of the College of Nursing.

The Professional Corporation acknowledges that Nurse Practitioner will be allowed to bring University students, during those hours when providing services to the Professional Corporation, to provide students with clinical experiences in conjunction with the Nurse Practitioner's clinical practice. The number and extent of the student visits shall depend upon the number of students involved in the relevant nursing curriculum and the number of appropriate learning experiences available to Nurse Practitioner.

IV. Professional Corporation Services

Professional Corporation shall perform the following duties during the term of this Agreement:

A. *Facilities, equipment and services.* The Professional Corporation shall provide and maintain at the Professional Corporation's expense, such facilities, furnishings, equipment, medicine, and medical supplies consistent with accepted standards of health care.

B. *Personnel.* The Professional Corporation shall provide physician and support personnel required for proper functioning of the Professional Corporation.

C. *Evaluation.* The Professional Corporation shall be responsible for conducting an annual evaluation (calendar year) of the nurse practitioner's performance relative to clinic practice and related issues. The annual evaluation shall include, but not be limited to, standards of care, patient satisfaction, and inner office work relationships. A copy of the annual performance appraisal will be made available to the Dean of the College of Nursing no later than January 31 of each year.

V. Insurance

A. *Professional Corporation Liability Coverage.* The Professional Corporation shall provide professional liability, insurance coverage for Nurse Practitioner, for services provided pursuant to this Agreement. The Professional Corporation shall maintain a minimum professional liability coverage of $100,000 per incident, $300,000 aggregate. When coverage is on a claim made basis, however, tail insurance shall be provided by the Professional Corporation. Upon request, the Professional Corporation shall provide to University copies of appropriate certificate evidencing such insurance coverage.

The University shall receive at least 30 days written prior notice of the termination of any coverage covering Nurse Practitioner. Failure to provide notice is an automatic breach of this agreement and will subject Professional Corporation to 100% indemnity of University for any loss that would have been covered under liability coverage for Professional Corporation and its employees.

B. *Risk Management.* Each party agrees to cooperate with the other party in the operation of their respective Risk Management/Quality Assurance

Systems. Further, each party agrees to discuss facts related to any incident report so as to allow each party's Risk Management System/Quality Assurance System to operate effectively. It is understood between the parties that the information so exchanged shall be held strictly confidential to the extent permitted by law.

VI. Records and Reports

A. *Medical Records and Reports.* In performing her or his duties under this Agreement, Nurse Practitioner shall generate medical records pertaining to patients treated, which records shall be kept in the format determined by Professional Corporation. All such records shall be and remain the property of Professional Corporation. The parties recognize that Nurse Practitioner shall have a continuing right of access to the medical records of patients for which Nurse Practitioner participated in care, but only during such time as Nurse Practitioner is engaged at the Professional Corporation as a contracted nurse practitioner through the University.

B. *Access to Books and Records.* If it is determined, pursuant to Federal Regulations which may be issued pursuant to Section 952 of the Federal Omnibus Reconciliation Act of 1980, that University is a "subcontractor" of the Professional Corporation, that this agreement is a "contract for services," and that Section 952 applies to this agreement, University and Professional Corporation agree that the Secretary of the Department of Health and Human Services, the Comptroller General of the United States and their duly appointed representatives shall be entitled to access to this Agreement, books, documents, and records of University and Professional Corporation as necessary to verify the "cost" of this Agreement.

VII. Compensation and Billing and Financial Arrangements

A. *Billing.* The Professional Corporation shall have the right to bill patients and third parties for all services provided by the Nurse Practitioner and to collect from such persons all amounts owed for such services.

B. *Compensation.* Professional Corporation shall provide University $_____ for services for the period of this agreement. Compensation for services provided shall be renegotiated on an annual basis.

C. *Payment schedule.* Payment shall be made in monthly payments of $_____ beginning the 1st day of September 2006.

VIII. Term and Termination

This Agreement shall become effective as of August 11, 2006, and shall continue until April 23, 2007, unless earlier terminated pursuant to the provisions of this Agreement. The term of the agreement may be renewed by the mutual written agreement of the parties.

A. *Termination by mutual written agreement of the parties.*

This Agreement may be terminated at any time upon the mutual written agreement of the parties.

B. *Other Termination.*

1. Professional Corporation can terminate this Agreement, upon ninety (90) days prior written notice to University, with or without cause.
2. University may terminate this Agreement, upon ninety (90) days prior written notice to Professional Corporation, with or without cause.

IX. General

A. *Notice.* Any notice, offer, demand or communication required or permitted to be given under any provision of this Agreement shall be deemed to have seen sufficiently given or served for all purposes if delivered by registered or certified mail, postage and charges prepaid, addressed to the address of the parties set forth below. Either party may change its address for purposes of this agreement by giving the other notice thereof in the manner hereinbefore provided for the giving of notice. Unless otherwise required by the agreement, notices under this agreement shall be directed to the following persons:

To Professional Corporation:
To State University:

B. *Severability.* In the event any provision of this Agreement is held to be illegal or unenforceable, such provision of this agreement shall be deemed severed from this Agreement and shall not affect the legality or enforceability of the remaining provisions of this Agreement unless unable to perform without such provision or unless such omission would be destructive of the intent of the parties.

C. *Governing Law.* This Agreement shall be construed and enforced in accordance with, and governed by, the law of the State of Michigan.

D. *Entire Agreement.* This Agreement and the exhibits thereto constitute the entire agreement of the parties. There are no promises, terms, conditions, or obligations, other than those contained herein and this Agreement shall supersede all previous communications, representations, or agreements, either verbal or written, between the parties.

E. *Amendments.* No amendment or modification to this Agreement shall be effective unless the same is in writing and signed by both parties. Amendments to this Agreement shall be effective as of the date stipulated.

F. *Assignability.* Neither party may assign its rights or obligations under this Agreement except with the written consent of the other party. Any attempted assignment in violation of this provision shall be null and void.

G. *Reference Headings.* Headings used in this agreement are for convenience of reference only and shall not be used to interpret this Agreement.

H. *No Third Party Rights.* This Agreement is intended solely for the benefit of University and Professional Corporation, and it shall not be construed to create any benefits for or rights in any other person or entity, including patients, employees and their representatives.

I. *Non Discrimination.* In connection with the performance of services under this Agreement, the parties agree to comply with the provisions of the Elliott-Larsen Civil Rights Act, PA 453 of 1976, as amended, and specifically agree not to discriminate against an employee or applicant for employment with respect to hire, tenure, terms, conditions, or privileges of employment because of a handicap that is unrelated to the individual's ability to perform the duties of a particular job or position, or because of race, color, religion, national origin, age, sex, height, weight, or marital status. Breach of this covenant may be regarded as a material breach of this Agreement.

STATE UNIVERSITY   PROFESSIONAL CORPORATION
BY:_____   BY:_____

Notification of Practice Announcement

Grand Valley Family Practice

is pleased to welcome

their new associate

Mary Jane Smith, MSN, APRN-BC

Geriatric Nurse Practitioner

Now accepting new patients

510 Court Street, NE
Anytown, USA

Phone: 1-000-000-0000
Fax: 1-000-000-0000

Diabetes Flow Sheet

Diabetes Flow Sheet

Name: _____ Date of birth: _____ Date of diagnosis: _____ Chart # _____
Hospital of choice: _____ Medical power of attorney: _____
Allergies: _____ Medication: _____

PROPHYLACTIC: ASA: >40yr _____ **ACE-I/ARB** = 55 yr or risk factors CAD _____
STATIN >40 yr: _____ **Not part of the plan? Rationale:**
Pneumonia vaccine: _____

R O U T I N E	Date								
	A1C <7%								
	Bp = 130/80								
	Weight								
	BMI								
	Visual foot								
A N N U A L	Sensory, 5 pt microfilament								
	FLU vaccination								
	FBS								
	CHOL <200								
	LDL <100 mg/dl								
	HDL >40 mg/dl								
	TGL <150 mg/dl								
	BUN/CR / UA or								
	Microalbuminuria								
	*Serum K+ with (ACE, ARB, diuretic)								
	*TSH								
	*AST/ALT								
	*EKG								
REFERRALS									
	Ophthalmology								
	Dental								
	Podiatry								
	Diab. Educator								
	*Cardiology								

* Obtain these laboratory values if clinically indicated.

SELF-MANAGEMENT AND EDUCATION								
Tobacco/alcohol use								
Medication side effects								
Hypo/hyperglycemia								
Home BG								
Foot care								
Diet								
Exercise								
Sick day plan								
Support group								
Patient goals								
Barriers								
Strategies								
Advanced directives								

Specialist Name(s): _____ Cardiologist: _____
Ophthalmologist: _____ Diabetes educator: _____
Dentist: _____ Podiatrist: _____

These are general guidelines and do not take the place of the clinical judgment of the health care practitioner. Reference: American Diabetes Association. (2004). Standards of Medical Care in Diabetes. *Diabetes Care,* 27, s15-s35.

Developed by Leona Meengs: All rights reserved.

American Diabetes Association (ADA) Criteria for the Diagnosis of Diabetes

1. Symptoms of diabetes and casual plasma glucose 200 mg/dl (11.1 mmol/l). Casual is defined as any time of day without regard to time since last meal. The classic symptoms of diabetes include polyuria, polydipsia, and unexplained weight loss.

OR

2. FPG 126 mg/dl (7.0 mmol/l). Fasting is defined as no caloric intake for at least 8 h.

OR

3. 2-h PG 200 mg/dl (11.i mmol/l) during OGTT. The test should be performed as described by the World Health Organization using a glucose load containing the equivalent of 75-g anhydrous glucose dissolved in water.

In the absence of unequivocal hyperglycemia, these criteria should be confirmed by repeat testing on a different day. The OGTT is not recommended for routine clinical use, but may be required in the evaluation of patients with impaired fasting glucose (IFG) or when diabetes is still suspected despite a normal FPG.

Reference: American Diabetes Association. (2004). Standards of Medical Care in Diabetes. *Diabetes Care,* 27, s15-s35, p. s16.

American Diabetes Association Glycemic Control Recommendations for Adults with Diabetes

A1C	<7%
Preprandial plasma glucose	90-130 mg/dl (5.0-7.2 mmol/l)
Postprandial plasma glucose	<180 mg/dl (<10.0 mmol/l)
Norma A1C	4-6%

AANP Standards of Practice and a Proposal for a Code of Ethics for NPs

AANP Standards of Practice	Proposal for a Code of Ethics for NPs
Professional education	The NP should provide competent medical and nursing care with compassion, confidentiality, and respect for the individual, regardless of social, economic, or health status. The NP's primary commitment and responsibility is to the patient, whether that patient is an individual, family, group, or community
Patient education, consultation, and equal access	The NP shall support access to care for all patients and should strive to effect public policies that will result in equal access. The NP shall support the patient's efforts toward an optimal level of health through education, self-care promotion consultation, and collaboration with other health care team members.
Consultation and collaboration	The NP shall support the patient's efforts toward an optimal level of health through education, self-care promotion consultation, and collaboration with other health care team members.
Legal standards	The NP shall maintain and be accountable for accurate medical records for each patient. The NP shall not engage in fraud or deception and shall report any other health care provider who engages in such activities.
Advocacy and public health	The NP shall advocate for and strive to protect the rights, health, safety, and privacy of all patients. The NP should collaborate with other health professionals and the public on local, national, and international levels to promote this effort.

AANP Standards of Practice	Proposal for a Code of Ethics for NPs
Professional development Role interpretation for the public Research and advancement	The NP shall continue to advance personal and professional development through practice, education of the public, and lifelong continuous study, research, and activity in professional organizations The NP shall, in the provision of patient care, responsibly choose whom to serve, with whom to associate, and the environment in which to provide that care

Source: From Peterson, M., & Potter, R.L. (2004). A proposal for a code of ethics for nurse practitioners. *Journal of the American Academy of Nurse Practitioners, 16*(3), 123.

17-3

Patient Satisfaction Survey

Patient Satisfaction Survey

We want to be sure we are doing everything we can to serve you. Please take a minute to fill out this survey. All responses are confidential, and we don't want you to sign it or otherwise indicate your name. Just let us know what to do better!

Thank you.

On a scale from 1 to 5, with 5 being excellent and 1 being poor, how would you rate:

The time between your call to schedule an appointment and your appointment date? Did we fit you in fast enough? ☐1 ☐2 ☐3 ☐4 ☐5
Comments:

The time it took us to answer your call? ☐1 ☐2 ☐3 ☐4 ☐5
Comments:

The manners of the person(s) who scheduled your appointment? ☐1 ☐2 ☐3 ☐4 ☐5
Comments:

The convenience of our location? ☐1 ☐2 ☐3 ☐4 ☐5
Comments:

Parking convenience? ☐1 ☐2 ☐3 ☐4 ☐5
Comments:

The convenience of our office location? ☐1 ☐2 ☐3 ☐4 ☐5
Comments:

The professionalism and helpfulness of your reception. Was the receptionist polite? Were your questions answered? ☐1 ☐2 ☐3 ☐4 5
Comments:

Your wait time in the office? ☐1 ☐2 ☐3 ☐4 ☐5
Comments:

The comfort, cleanliness and amenities of the reception? ☐1 ☐2 ☐3 ☐4 ☐5
Comments:

Your health care provider:

I saw   X   Y   Z   A (circle one) [enter your health care providers names here]

The amount of time spent with your physician?	☐1 ☐2 ☐3 ☐4 ☐5
Comments:	

His or her listening?	☐1 ☐2 ☐3 ☐4 ☐5
Comments:	

His or her explanation of procedures, diagnoses, or treatment regimen?	☐1 ☐2 ☐3 ☐4 ☐5
Comments:	

His or her "bedside manner"?	☐1 ☐2 ☐3 ☐4 ☐5
Comments:	

If you have visited our practice before, how convenient did you find: Prescription refills (if appropriate)?	☐1 ☐2 ☐3 ☐4 ☐5
Comments:	

Getting lab results (if appropriate)?	☐1 ☐2 ☐3 ☐4 ☐5
Comments:	

Overall, how would you rate our practice?	☐1 ☐2 ☐3 ☐4 ☐5
Comments:	

Source: Adapted from Burnie, Glen, M.D. (2005). *Physicians Practice, The Business Journal for Physicians.* Accessed February 3, 2005, at *www.physicianspractice.com/tools/satisfaction.doc*

Nurse Practitioner Peer Review Record

SECTION I: ONGOING CARE FOR PREVENTION, MINOR ILLNESSES, AND CHRONIC ILLNESS

In this section, answer the questions as they relate to:
- Prevention
- Minor illnesses
- Chronic illness
  ⇒ include exacerbations of those illnesses unless they are severe enough to meet criteria for acute illness, as described below.

Exclude care for acute illness: Acute illness is further defined under Section II. Acute illnesses are those that may result in relatively immediate severe morbidity or death *and* require timely action by the provider.

PREVENTIVE CARE

Instructions for the next question:
Consider preventive care in relation to the table below and rate the amount and appropriateness of preventive care for this patient. The table lists some screening recommendations. Although they are not universally accepted as necessary (e.g., yearly depression screening), providers who follow them should receive a high rating. This question is meant to identify care that meets or exceeds standards for preventive care, rather than to penalize providers for not providing all potentially indicated care.

Definitions:
- *Not done* = A period of care greater than 1 year was reviewed and no evidence of preventive care was recorded.
- *Unable to assess* = The care being reviewed encompasses less than 1 year and no preventive care is recorded. If a period less than 1 year is reviewed and evidence of preventive care is present, rate that care as adequate or excellent.
- *Adequate* = At least one appropriate preventive measure was taken and documented.
- *Excellent* = Most, if not all, appropriate prevention measures were taken and documented.

TYPE OF PATIENT/CONDITION	SCREENING RECOMMENDATION	
Everyone	• Yearly depression screening • Smoking screening and cessation counseling for smokers every visit • Yearly alcohol screening and counseling • Yearly exercise counseling • Yearly blood pressure evaluation	• Yearly nutrition counseling • Cholesterol screening every 5 years • Tetanus (every 10 years) • Advance directive (once)
Women	• Yearly pap • Yearly breast exam (age 50 and over)	• Yearly mammogram (age 40 and over)
Age 50 and above	• Yearly stool guaiac or flex sig/colonoscopy every 10 years	• Yearly rectal exam
Age 65 and above or relevant chronic illness	• Pneumovax (once)	• Yearly influenza vaccine
Overweight (BMI>25)	• Yearly weight control counseling	
Diabetes	• Yearly pedal pulses/foot exam • Yearly proteinuria screen	• Yearly eye exam • Hemoglobin A1c: At goal every 6 mo. not at goal every 3 mo.
Hypertension	• Yearly counseling on fluid/sodium restriction	
Congestive Heart Failure	• Yearly counseling on fluid/sodium restriction	• Echocardiogram/ejection fraction (1)

1. **According to the above definitions, how would you rate the *preventive care* this patient received during the interval of time reviewed?**

Not done (>1 yr reviewed)	Unable to assess (<1 yr reviewed)	Adequate	Excellent
Continue with Q1A	**GO TO Q2**	**GO TO Q2**	**GO TO Q2**

> **Instructions for the next question:**
> If there is an explanation, other than poor care, for the lack of preventive care recorded, choose the appropriate answer.

1A **If you answered "Not done" in question 1, which, if any of the following, explain or mitigate the failure to screen?** *Mark all that apply.*

Patient had a terminal illness.

Physician acting in a consultative role only (primary physician care not reviewed).

Patient refused to undergo screening.

Other, please specify. _____

OR

None of the above.

PROBLEM LIST

> **Definitions for the next question:**
> - *Not done* = A period of care greater than 1 year was reviewed and no problem list is found.
> - *Unable to assess* = The care being reviewed encompasses less than 1 year and no problem list found. If a period less than 1 year is reviewed and a problem list *is* found, rate that care as adequate or excellent.
> - *Adequate* = A problem list is present, although it may not be complete.
> - *Excellent* = The problem list contains all relevant problems and is up-to-date.

2. **According to the above definitions, how would you rate the problem list for this patient's record?**

NOTE: A problem list may be a separate document, or it may be part of the notes for a given visit. Consider a scenario where you are covering for this patient's primary care provider, and base your rating on the extent to which you would have to search through the records to identify important problems if the record was your only information source.

Not done (>1 yr reviewed)	Unable to assess (<1 yr reviewed)	Adequate	Excellent

USE OF SERVICES FOR MINOR AND CHRONIC ILLNESSES

3. **Did the patient receive care for a chronic medical or psychologic illness (e.g., diabetes, congestive heart failure, osteoarthritis, depression) or a minor short-term illness, such as an upper respiratory infection, during the period reviewed?**

> NOTE: Mark *"minor only"* if the patient has no chronic illnesses. *Mark one box only.*

Yes; chronic   ⟶ **Continue with Q4**

Yes; minor only ⟶ **Continue with Q4**

No   ⟶ **GO TO Q6**

Instructions for the next question (on the following page):
This question asks about the use of particular types of services related to care for minor and chronic illnesses. Answer about both quantity (overuse and underuse) and quality (timeliness and appropriateness) of these services. Only consider visits at which providers delivered care for **minor** or **chronic** problems. Care that relates to visits for **prevention** should be considered under the subsection "Preventive Care." Care that relates to visits for severe **acute** problems should be considered under Section II, "Acute Illness Episodes."

- **Definitions for quantity:**
  - ⟹ *Too little* = Most patients would have better outcomes if more of this service were used.
  - ⟹ *About right* = Appropriate amount of that service given the patient's status at the time of use (even if the treatment was done to treat a complication of prior mismanagement). **INCLUDE** circumstances in which the service was **not** needed **AND** not used.
  - ⟹ *Too much* = The equivalent health benefits for the patient could have been achieved without using as much of the indicated service.

- **Definitions for quality:**
  - ⟹ *Poor* = Unacceptable quality.
  - ⟹ *Adequate* = Acceptable, although minimally so.
  - ⟹ *Good/excellent* = Care significantly increases the chance of a good outcome.
  - ⟹ *N/A* = The service was not provided, or its quality could not be assessed.

4. According to the previous definitions, what is your assessment of the quantity and quality of the following tests or treatments?

NOTE: Integrate your findings across the entire period covered by the records you reviewed. Judge the importance of any particular episode of better or worse care in terms of its potential impact on the patient's health status, and weigh that episode accordingly in your judgments.

	QUANTITY:			QUALITY:			
	Too little	About right	Too much	Poor	Adequate	Good/ excellent	N/A
TESTS AND PROCEDURES	Mark one box on each line.			Mark one box on each line.			
a. Blood, urine, and stool tests; other noninvasive tests and imaging (including CT imaging without IV contrast)							
b. Invasive procedures and tests (including imaging with IV contrast and procedures requiring conscious sedation)							
CLINICAL CARE							
c. Primary care provider(s) visits				PRIMARY PHYSICIAN CARE IS RATED IN QUESTION 5.			
d. Primary care provider referrals or consultations (e.g., neurology, psychiatry, surgery, internal medicine subspecialties or any MD with a special area of expertise)							
e. Non–primary care provider consultations (e.g., respiratory therapist, dietitian, social worker, physical therapist, psychologist)							
f. Long-term care (e.g., home care, skilled nursing facility, rehabilitation facility, hospice)							
g. Surgery (inpatient and outpatient)							
MEDICATIONS							
h. Prophylactic medications (not including treatment for pain)							
i. Therapeutic medications (not including treatment for pain)							
j. Prophylactic and therapeutic treatment of pain							
OTHER							
k. Use of durable medical goods (e.g., walkers, canes)							

CLINICAL MANAGEMENT FOR MINOR AND CHRONIC ILLNESS

Instructions for the next question:
The previous question addresses the use of specific services. This question examines the **quality** of the primary care provider's problem detection and management in relation to the patient's minor and chronic conditions. Only consider visits at which providers delivered care for **minor** or **chronic** problems. Care that relates to **prevention** should be considered under the subsection "Preventive Care." Care that relates to **acute** problems should be considered under Section II, "Acute Illness Episodes." Integrate your findings across the entire period of time covered by the records you reviewed. Judge the importance of any particular episode of better or worse care in terms of its potential impact on the patient's health status, and weigh that episode accordingly in your judgments.

Definitions:
- **Items a-d:** Imagine you are suddenly asked to take over care for this patient. Consider each one of the patient's complaints or problems, and evaluate the extent to which pertinent assessments have been performed and documented.
  - ⇒ **Excellent** = All the data you need for diagnosis and therapy have been gathered.
  - ⇒ **Adequate** = Evaluation is minimally acceptable and would allow you to make the most important decisions.
  - ⇒ **Very poor** = You would need to start over evaluating this patient.

- **Item e:**
  - ⇒ **Excellent** = All important diagnoses are mentioned.
  - ⇒ **Adequate** = Minimally acceptable, because although some significant diagnoses are missing, the most important are mentioned.
  - ⇒ **Very poor** = Important errors in diagnosis that decrease the likelihood of a good outcome.

- **Item f:** Consider only problems or diagnoses that were identified by the provider. Poor problem identification should be rated under the subsection "Preventive Care" or in Items 5 a-d (assessment). For example, if you think the provider should have identified a problem of liver disease, based on abnormal test results, but the provider did not, **do not** rate management of liver disease.
  - ⇒ **Excellent** = Ideal treatment.
  - ⇒ **Adequate** = Minimally acceptable because important treatments are given, although some significant treatments are omitted.
  - ⇒ **Very poor** = Wrong treatments are given or important correct treatments are omitted, such that the probability of a good outcome is substantially reduced.

5. **According to the previous definitions, how would you rate the quality of each of the following components of care as they relate to minor or chronic illnesses?**

NOTE: Exclude severe acute illness episodes likely to have major health impacts within 1 month and requiring timely provider action (these are rated in Section II).

REMINDER:
Consider all patient complaints and identified active problems and then judge assessment, diagnosis, and management of them.

Mark one box on each line.

	Very poor	Poor	Adequate	Good	Excellent	Not needed/ not done
a. Assessment by primary care providers of patient's medical and surgical history, allergies, and current medications						
b. Assessment by primary care providers of functional status and psychosocial situation						
c. Physical examination						
d. Laboratory testing: Selection and timing of tests						
e. Primary care providers' integration of clinical information and development of appropriate diagnoses and problem list						
f. Development and execution of treatment plans						

SECTION II: **ACUTE ILLNESS EPISODES**

In this section, answer the questions as they relate to illnesses that meet both of the following criteria:
1. The illness might result in hospitalization, death, or severe morbidity within 1 month without treatment.
2. The illness requires timely action on the part of the provider to maximize the chance of a good outcome.

Consider illnesses meeting this definition to be acute, even if they represent exacerbations of preexisting chronic illnesses.

6. **Was there an acute illness episode during the period of care reviewed?** *Mark one box.*

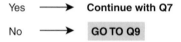

    Yes   ⟶   **Continue with Q7**

    No   ⟶   **GO TO Q9**

USE OF SERVICES FOR ACUTE ILLNESS EPISODES

Instructions for the next question (on the following page):
This question asks about the use of particular types of services related to **acute illness** care. Answer about both quantity (overuse or underuse) and quality (timeliness and appropriateness) of these services.

- **Definitions for quantity:**
    ⇒ *Too little* = Most patients would have better outcomes if more of this service were used.
    ⇒ *About right* = Appropriate amount of that service, given the patient's status at the time of use (even if the treatment was done to treat a complication of prior mismanagement). **INCLUDE** circumstances in which the service was **not** needed **AND** not used.
    ⇒ *Too much* = The equivalent health benefits for the patient could have been achieved without using as much of the indicated service.

- **Definitions for quality:**
    ⇒ *Poor* = Unacceptable quality.
    ⇒ *Adequate* = Acceptable, although minimally so.
    ⇒ *Good/excellent* = Care significantly increases the chance of a good outcome.
    ⇒ *N/A* = The service was not provided, or its quality could not be assessed.

7. **According to the previous definitions, what is your assessment of the quantity and quality of the following tests or treatments?**

NOTE: Integrate your findings across the entire period covered by the records you reviewed. Judge the importance of any particular episode of better or worse care in terms of its potential impact on the patient's health status, and weigh that episode accordingly in your judgments.

	QUANTITY:			QUALITY:			
	Too little	About right	Too much	Poor	Adequate	Good/ excellent	N/A
TESTS AND PROCEDURES	*Mark one box on each line.*			*Mark one box on each line.*			
a. Blood, urine, and stool tests; other noninvasive tests and imaging (including CT imaging without IV contrast)							
b. Invasive procedures and tests (including imaging with IV contrast and procedures requiring conscious sedation)							
CLINICAL CARE							
c. Primary care provider(s) visits				PRIMARY CARE PROVIDER IS RATED IN QUESTION 8.			
d. Primary care provider referrals or consultations (e.g., neurology, psychiatry, surgery, internal medicine subspecialties or any MD with a special area of expertise)							
e. Non–primary care provider consultations (e.g., respiratory therapist, dietitian, social worker, physical therapist, psychologist)							
f. Long-term care (e.g., home care, skilled nursing facility, rehabilitation facility, hospice)							
g. Surgery (inpatient and outpatient)							
h. Inpatient acute hospital admissions							
i. Emergency department services							
MEDICATIONS							
j. Prophylactic medications (not including treatment for pain)							
k. Therapeutic medications (not including treatment for pain)							
l. Prophylactic and therapeutic treatment of pain							
OTHER							
m. Use of durable medical goods (e.g., walkers, canes)							

CLINICAL MANAGEMENT FOR ACUTE ILLNESS

Instructions for the next question:
The previous question addresses the use of specific services. This question examines the quality of the primary care provider's problem detection and management in relation to the patient's acute illnesses, over the 2 to 4 weeks after the beginning of the episode. Only consider visits at which providers delivered care for **acute illness**, as defined at the beginning of Section II. Care that relates to ongoing issues, including prevention, minor illness, and chronic illness, should have been considered under Section I. Integrate your findings across the entire period covered by the records you reviewed. Judge the importance of any particular episode of better or worse acute care in terms of its potential impact on the patient's health status, and weigh that episode accordingly in your judgments.

Definitions:
- **Items a-d:** Imagine you are suddenly asked to take over care for any one of the acute illness episodes included in your review. You arrive just in time to make diagnoses and initiate treatment based on the assessment data already collected. Evaluate the extent to which pertinent assessments have been performed and documented.
  ⇒ **Excellent** = All the data you need for diagnosis and therapy have been gathered.
  ⇒ **Adequate** = Evaluation is minimally acceptable and would allow you to make the most important decisions.
  ⇒ **Very poor** = You would need to start over evaluating this patient.

- **Item e:**
  ⇒ **Excellent** = All important diagnoses are mentioned.
  ⇒ **Adequate** = Minimally acceptable, because although some significant diagnoses are missing, the most important are mentioned.
  ⇒ **Very poor** = Important errors in diagnosis that decrease the likelihood of a good outcome.

- **Item f:** Consider only problems or diagnoses that were identified by the provider. Poor problem identification should be rated under Items 5 a-d (assessment). For example, if you think the provider should have identified a problem of liver disease, based on abnormal test results, but the provider did not, **do not** rate management of liver disease. If, on the other hand, a needed treatment is given, you can infer that an associated problem has implicitly been identified, and then judge the quality of the treatment. For example, if insulin is given, you can infer that the physician detected diabetes, and rate the quality of the management, even if no note states the diagnosis in the record.
  ⇒ **Excellent** = Ideal treatment.
  ⇒ **Adequate** = Minimally acceptable because important treatments given, although some significant treatments are omitted.
  ⇒ **Very poor** = Wrong treatments are given or important correct treatments are omitted, such that the probability of a good outcome is substantially reduced.

8. **According to the previous definitions, how would you rate the quality of each of the following components of care as they relate to acute illnesses?**

REMINDER:
Consider all patient complaints and identified active problems and then judge assessment, diagnosis, and management of them.

Mark one box on each line.

	Very poor	Poor	Adequate	Good	Excellent	Not needed/ not done
a. Assessment by primary care providers of patient's medical and surgical history, allergies, and current medications						
b. Assessment by primary care providers of functional status and psychosocial situation						
c. Physical examination						
d. Laboratory testing: selection and timing of tests						
e. Primary care provider's integration of clinical information and development of appropriate diagnoses and problem list						
f. Development and execution of treatment plans						

SECTION III: **COMMUNICATION, EDUCATION, AND ACCESS TO CARE**

Instructions for Questions 9, 10, and 11:
To answer these questions, think about all of the care delivered, regardless of who delivered it. Weigh each piece of information you are trying to integrate based on how important it was to the patient's care, then provide a single answer that sums up the overall care the patient received.

Definitions:
- ***Excellent*** = Both the patient and his/her family had all their questions answered, and they were educated about the important issues with their care.
- ***Adequate*** = The most important questions were answered, though some may have been neglected, and relevant complications (e.g., bleeding on coumadin) were discussed, albeit perhaps not in great detail.
- ***Very poor*** = There is evidence that such communication was inadequate, misleading, or relayed incorrect information.
- ***Unable to judge*** = There is inadequate information to assess communication or education in this case.

In your assessment of communication and education, include:
- Quality of assessment and management of patient preferences (e.g. for particular treatments)
- Education of patient and family

9. **According to the previous definitions, how would you rate the quality of communication?**

	Unable to judge or N/A	Very poor	Poor	Adequate	Good	Excellent
			Mark one box on each line.			
a. Between primary care provider(s) and this patient?						
b. Between other providers (e.g., consultants) and this patient?						

10. **According to the definitions above, how would you rate the overall quality of the education provided to the patient and family by primary care provider(s) and by consultants (physician and non–physician)?**

Unable to judge	Very poor	Poor	Adequate	Good	Excellent

Instructions for the next question:
Rate the quality of communication and coordination between providers. Base your rating on the extent to which each provider knows and understands the actions of other providers and the extent to which there is a clear overall plan guiding clinical care.

Definitions:
- ***Very poor*** = There is evidence that important information about the patient was not communicated among providers.
- ***Adequate*** = Communication was acceptable, although minimally so.
- ***Excellent*** = Each provider knew relevant details of care provided by the patient's other providers and took these into account.
- ***Unable to judge*** = There is inadequate information to assess communication/coordination in this case.

---

11. **According to the definitions above, how would you rate coordination and continuity of care throughout the period of care you received?**

Unable to judge	Very poor	Poor	Adequate	Good	Excellent

12. **How would you rate patient access to his/her primary care provider?**

   NOTE: In your assessment of access to care, consider such things as telephone contacts, prompt office visits as needed, and proactive office staff case management.

Unable to judge	Very poor	Poor	Adequate	Good	Excellent

SECTION IV: **OVERALL QUALITY OF CARE**

---

13. **Considering everything you know about this patient, how would you rate the overall quality of care delivered to this individual during the period of care you reviewed?**

   NOTE: When rating overall care, consider that standard care refers to the minimal care primary care providers agree **should** be given, regardless of whether the general practice is to administer this care.

Extreme, below standard	Below standard	Standard	Above standard	Extreme above standard

Instructions for the next question:
For this next question, consider a scenario in which your mother is ill and in need of medical care.

Definitions:
- *Definitely not* = You would do almost anything possible to make sure she was **not** cared for by this patient's primary care providers, even to the extent of delaying her treatment.
- *Probably not* = You would try to transfer her if transfer were easy, but you would not do anything extreme to have her treated by other primary care providers.
- *Probably yes* = You would not try to transfer her care to other primary care providers.
- *Definitely yes* = You would actively seek out these primary care providers to care for your mother.

14. **Would you send your mother to be cared for by these primary care providers?**

    Definitely not   Probably not   Not sure   Probably yes   Definitely yes

SECTION V: COMMENTS ON YOUR REVIEW

15. **If there were any question(s) on this form you did not feel qualified to answer regarding this patient (given your own background and knowledge), please indicate which ones.** *Mark all that apply.*

    1. **1A**
    2.
    3.
    4. a. b. c. d. e. f. g. h. i. j. k.
    5. a. b. c. d. e. f. g.
    6.
    7. a. b. c. d. e. f. g. h. i. j. k. l. m.
    8. a. b. c. d. e. f. g.
    9. a. b.
    10.
    11.
    12.
    13.
    14.

16. **If you did not feel qualified to rate all aspects of this patient's care, which other kind(s) of primary care provider(s) should also review the diagnostic and treatment issues in this record?** *Mark all that apply.*

    General Internist
    Internal Medicine Subspecialist   (Specify) _____
    General Surgeon
    Surgical Subspecialist   (Specify) _____
    Obstetrician/Gynecologist
    Other kind of physician   (Specify) _____
    Nurse Practitioner   _____

Source: Adapted from RAND Corporation, Santa Monica, CA. © 2005.

Nurse Practitioner Job Performance Evaluation Tool

ST. JOSEPH HOSPITAL
NASHUA, NEW HAMPSHIRE

JOB PERFORMANCE STANDARDS

Position: Palliative Nurse Practitioner
Responsible to: Palliative Care Director
Department Service: Palliative Care

Job Grade:
Location: Nashua
Date: 05/20/05

METHODS OF MEASUREMENT:

Exemplary Performance = 4 points
This employee provides a "model" for this standard for other employees. Requires little or no oversight or supervision concerning this standard.

Exceeds Performance = 3 points
This employee regularly performs above the level required to meet performance expectations. Requires occasional oversight and supervision regarding this standard.

Meets performance = 2 points
This employee is viewed as competent on this standard. Requires moderate supervision regarding this standard. "Doing a good job."

Marginal Performance = 1 point
This employee's performance is not meeting expectation in this area and requires improvement. Requires close oversight and supervision regarding this standard.

Unsatisfactory performance = 0 points
This employee is substantially below competency in this area and requires marked improvement. Specific action is required to improve performance with supervisor observation and documentation.

Job Duty Number	Relative Weight	Performance is adequate on this job when:
1.	20	**Assessment and Planning** 1. Elicits and records physical and mental status, psychosocial history, including review of bodily systems. 2. Performs focused bedside physical examinations. 3. Initiates appropriate diagnostic tests to screen or evaluate the care-recipient's current health status. 4. Assesses finding of history, review of systems, physical examinations and diagnostic tests, and formulates a diagnosis prior to implementing a treatment regime. 5 Identifies health problems and learning needs of the care recipient. 6. Works in collaboration with members of the interdisciplinary team to support the highest quality of patient care delivered. 7. Assists with diagnosis, treatment, and management of acute and chronic health conditions. 8. Orders, performs, and interprets laboratory and radiology tests. 9. Prescribes medications including controlled substances to the extent delegated and licensed. 10. Orders treatments and durable medical equipment as indicated. 11. Performs other therapeutic or corrective measures as indicated, including urgent care. 12. Has a sophisticated knowledge of pharmacologic and nonpharmacologic approaches to the management of symptom distress in seriously ill and dying patients. Source of Measurement: Supervisor observation or complaint, patient satisfaction, M.D. satisfaction, patient outcome measurements, program evaluations.
2.	20	**Education** 1. Plans, teaches, promotes, and manages palliative care in a continuous program improvement model. 2. Plans, teaches, and facilitates educational programs for Palliative Care Team and allied health professions on care for patient and family at the end of life. 3. Plans, teaches, and facilitates community educational programs on advanced illness and palliative care. 4. Has excellent communication skills.

Continued

Job Duty Number	Relative Weight	Performance is adequate on this job when:
		Source of Measurement: Supervisor observation or complaint, patient satisfaction, M.D. satisfaction, patient outcome measurements, program evaluations.
3.	20	**Intervention and Evaluation** 1. Implements and manages treatment regimens and prescribes pharmacological agents for identified health problems. 2. Arranges appropriate referrals. 3. Ensures that there is continuous improvement of services through assessment, planning, intervention, and evaluation. 4. Utilizes approved reference and procedure manuals when providing care. 5. Performs focused bedside evaluation of patients. 6. Has board clinical knowledge and demonstrated experience and expertise in palliative care. Source of Measurement: Supervisor observation or complaint, patient satisfaction, M.D. satisfaction, patient outcome measurements, program evaluations.
4.	10	**Palliative Care** 1. Provides services related to promoting excellence in palliative and end-of-life care. 2. Consults with PC M.D. or designees as needed, informs attending physician of services provided and collaboration with another physician if ordered, provides written reports to attending physician on request. 3. Demonstrates commitment to improving care for the seriously ill and those nearing the end of life.
5.	20	**Professional Development** 1. Supports and participates in appropriate clinical professional organization(s). 2. Attends and participates in development and implementation of palliative care educational programs. 3. Establishes environment within the hospital to promote ongoing clinical research, inquiry, and expansion of palliative care services. 4. Exhibits a strong theory-based practice. 5. Is a skilled teacher with nurses at all levels of training and in diverse educational settings (bedside, classroom, professional meetings). 6. Is a confident mentor and coach for colleagues and staff.

Job Duty Number	Relative Weight	Performance is adequate on this job when:
		7. Is an integral member of a team composed of physicians, trainees, and other professional staff. Has credibility, confidence, knowledge, and high level of clinical competency. 8. Is an effective problem solver. 9. Has strong interpersonal communication skills. 10. Is self-directed and a self-starter; able to take initiative, but equally comfortable in seeking guidance and assistance when needed. 11. Is committed to ongoing professional development. Source of Measurement: Supervisor observation or complaint, patient satisfaction, M.D. satisfaction, patient outcome measurements, program evaluations.
6.	10	**Mission Integration** 1. Is responsible for promoting the Standards of Excellence for St. Joseph Healthcare (Policy HR-48). Demonstrates the philosophy, mission, and core values of St. Joseph Healthcare in performance of job responsibilities. Demonstration includes courteous and cooperative behavior toward patients, visitors, volunteers, and peers; initiative/decision-making abilities; and work flexibility. Source of Measurement: Supervisor observation or complaint, patient satisfaction, M.D. satisfaction, patient outcome measurements, program evaluations.

Job Summary

Primary Responsibilities: Member of interdisciplinary professional team providing teaching and hospital-based palliative care consultation for seriously ill patients and their family caregivers. All work done in close collaboration with primary physicians, attending physician, nursing staff, and social services.

Clinical Activities: Medical and psychosocial evaluation of patient and family; skilled and meticulous symptom management; extensive involvement in discharge planning and continuity of care efforts; and support and collaboration with primary medical and nursing staff responsible for the patient.

Educational Responsibilities: In-service teaching of medical, nursing, and other professional colleagues and students; role modeling for physicians and nurses at all levels of training; attendance at weekly administrative and team meetings. Case finding initiatives will require strong interpersonal and collegial skills with colleagues from a broad range of professional disciplines throughout the hospital.

The standards in this job description, which is used in the annual performance appraisal process, are reflective of the expectation that patient care is delivered in a manner that is appropriate to patient age, physical ability, and intellectual development. It is expected that patient care will be adapted to meet one or more of the following populations: (a) *infancy* – birth to 11 months; (b) *toddlers* – 1 to 3 years of age; (c) *preschool children* – 4 to 5 years of age; (d) *school-age children* – 6 to 12 years of age; (e) *adolescents* – 13 to 18 years of age; (f) *adults* – 19 to 65 years of age; and (g) *geriatrics* – more than 65 years of age.

Qualifications

1. Education: Master's degree in nursing
2. Experience: 3-5 years NP experience
3. Skills required:

   - BCLS
   - NH RN licensure
   - NP certification
   - Registered DEA number

Reference – New Hampshire Code of Administrative Rules Nur 304.05

Department Director: _____ Date: _____

Human Resources: _____ Date: _____

Vice-President: _____ Date: _____

Rev: 4/2000, 5/2002; 05/2005

Source: Adapted from material available from the Center to Advance Palliative Care (CAPC) and reprinted with permission from St. Joseph Hospital, Nashua, New Hampshire.

Preceptor Letter

Date

Dear Preceptor,

Thank you for your willingness to participate as a preceptor in our nurse practitioner program. We recognize the additional responsibility that is inherent in providing optimal patient care while preceptoring the novice practitioner.

In addition, we are attentive to the reality that both preceptors and students have individual teaching and learning preferences and that a good *fit* between preceptors and students enhances the clinical rotation experience. Our goal is to facilitate positive experiences for both the student and preceptor. Please help us to achieve our goal by completing the enclosed preceptor matching form and survey.

Thank you for your participation as a preceptor as well as your assistance in the preceptor/student matching process. We hope that this clinical rotation is an enjoyable experience for you. If you have any questions or concerns please contact our nursing faculty liaison at _____ at any time during the rotation.

Sincerely,

Preceptor Matching Survey and Key

Even though you may use all of the following teaching techniques and apply each according to individual student learning needs, please indicate which techniques you tend to enjoy or use most often by numbering the list below from 1 through 8 with 1 being the most used and/or enjoyed technique.

a _____Prepare and guide students as they perform new skills and procedures.

b _____Stand behind appropriate student decisions even though their decision may not be your first choice.

c _____Ensure optimal patient care while promoting student learning by providing straightforward guidance.

d _____Guide and supplement student learning with mini lectures, case studies, references, and computer access.

e _____Expect the student to shadow for the first few days to assimilate them into the practice philosophy and setting.

f _____Focus on incorporating basic information that the student will need as a novice practitioner.

g _____Expect students to complete assignments and to consult with you regarding their impressions.

h _____Provide immediate feedback and correction with positive reinforcement.

Key:

Direct: c, e
Coach: a, d
Support: f, h
Delegate: b, g

Preceptor and Clinical Site Survey

1. How many clients or patients do you usually see per day? _____
2. Is your client population diverse? If so, how? _____
3. If you had to choose one practice area of expertise, what would it be?
_____
4. Are you certified in any other practice areas? _____
5. What procedures do you perform in the office and which ones can the student observe or perform? _____
6. Are you routinely available for student discussions? _____
7. Do you review and evaluate with students their progress toward their goals on a daily, weekly, or midterm basis? _____
8. What are your expectations of the beginning, intermediate, or advanced nurse practitioner student? _____
9. What do you consider the most important factor in developing an optimal student preceptor relationship? _____
10. Do you participate with an on-site interdisciplinary team? _____
11. Which methods do you use most often in patient care and/or interactions with staff: directing, coaching, supporting, or delegating? _____

Student Matching Survey and Key

Learning Style Assessment: Please number the statements below from 1 through 12 with 1 being your most preferred learning style.

a_____ I am familiar with the tasks and skills, but lack confidence in performing them.

b_____ I prefer straightforward guidance.

c_____ I appreciate immediate feedback or correction with positive reinforcement.

d_____ I am eager to try to perform skills and procedures, but feel unprepared or unskilled.

e_____ I tend to be hesitant in performing new skills and prefer assistance.

f_____ I prefer to consult with team members.

g_____ I usually ask for clarification of preceptor expectations and review of the patient's plan of care.

h_____ I enjoy case studies, multiple references, and mini lectures.

i_____ I prefer general rules and clinical pearls over interactive mini lectures, puzzles, and strategic games.

j_____ I am usually able to take on new skills and complete them as requested with minimal direction.

k_____ I tend to be self-motivated and proactive.

l_____ I prefer to shadow a preceptor for the first couple of days.

Key to Assess Learning Needs

Direct: b, e, l
Coach: d, g, h
Support: a, c, i
Delegate: f, j, k

Nurse Practitioner Student Assessment

1. Please describe your graduate classroom work that has prepared you for this clinical rotation. _____
2. What classes are you taking now? _____
3. Do you have any nursing experience? Please list. _____
4. Do you have any specialty certifications? _____
5. What interdisciplinary team experiences have you had? _____
6. Have you had any previous NP clinical rotations? Please list. _____
7. What are your clinical objectives for this rotation? _____
8. What procedures have you observed? _____
9. Have you performed office laboratory and screening tests (urinalysis, strep screen, FBS, and EKG monitor)? _____
10. Are you familiar with the medication formulary of the large insurance companies in the area? _____

Please attach your Ambulatory Care Procedural and Experiential Log.

Ground Rules and Expectations

This sheet lists the issues to be clarified with students early in the rotation. You may find it helpful to place initials of the individual responsible for conveying the information in the space to the left of the item.

Student's Name _____

Staff	Information
Practice Site Details	
	Introduction to critical staff and their responsibilities
	Weekly office schedule routine
	Standard operating procedures (appointments, location and operation of dictation equipment, where to make chart entries)
	Paperwork and coding procedures
	Telephone and paging protocols/important numbers to know
	Introduction to in-house laboratory and procedures
	Characteristics of the types of patients the student is likely to see
	Location of reference materials or teaching file
	Computer station for student reference work
	Student work space
Clarification of the Student's Role	
	What goals/objectives should the student be aware of?
	How many patients is the student likely to see in clinic? In hospital?
	How much involvement in patient care/decision making will the student have?
	What is meant by "focused history and physical"?
	What format should be used for case presentations?
	How should notes be taken or dictated?
	What are the student's work hours? On-call hours?

Staff	Information
	What procedure should the student take when making rounds on hospital patients?
	Who supervises the student when the physician has time off?
Preceptoring and Teaching Issues	
	Will teaching occur in front of the patient?
	Will the student be observed during the course of the rotation?
	How often will the student observe other members of the practice?
	What does the teaching schedule/pattern look like? (e.g., lecture en route to hospital or nursing home, teaching in hallway after each patient, reserved time at the end of the day)
	What procedures should take place when a situation becomes too complex or time consuming for the student to handle?
	What are the expectations regarding reading assignments? How often are they given?
	What forms and frequency of feedback should the student expect?
	When will you meet to evaluate progress and performance?

Source: Adapted from the work of Lesky, L.G., & Hershman, W.Y. (1995). Practical approaches to major educational challenge. *Archives of Internal Medicine, 155 (9)*, 897-904, and the Society of Teachers of Family Medicine, Preceptor Education Project Instructors' Manual, Kansas City, MO.

Ambulatory Care Procedural and Experiential Log

Student's Name _____

Procedure	Diagnosis	Date Procedure Performed	Certification Expiration Date	Preceptor or Supervisor Signature
ACLS or BLS				
Allergy Testing				
Anoscopy				
Auricular Hematoma Removal				
Bartholin's Abscess I & D				
Biopsy: Curettage				
Biopsy: FNA				
Biopsy: Incisional				
Biopsy: Punch				
Biopsy: Shave				
Urethral Bladder M Catheterization F P	_____	_____	_____	_____
Burn: Debridement				
Burn: DSG Change, ABX				
Cast Removal				
Casting Type				

Procedure	Diagnosis	Date Procedure Performed	Certification Expiration Date	Preceptor or Supervisor Signature
Cerumen Impaction Removal: Cur/Irr/ Suct				
Cervical Conization				
Cervical Polyps Removal				
Colposcopic Examination				
Comedone Removal				
Conscious Sed w/Analg				
Contraceptives: Cervical Caps				
Diaphragm				
IUD Insert/Remove Implants: Norplant Insertion/Removal				
Cryosurgery				
Electrocardiogram				
Endometrial Biopsy				
Epidural Anesth/Analg				
Epistaxis: Nasal Packing/Topical				
Fecal Impaction Management				
Fishhook Removal				
Flexible Sigmoidoscopy				
Foreign Body Removal: Ear/Nose				

Continued

Procedure	Diagnosis	Date Procedure Performed	Certification Expiration Date	Preceptor or Supervisor Signature
Incision & Drainage				
Injection				
Keloid: Corticosteroid				
Laceration Repair				
Laser Ablation				
Local Anesthesia				
Lumbar Puncture				
Microdermabrasion				
Nail Plate Removal				
Orthostatic BP				
Pap Smear/Thin Prep				
Perianal Abscess I & D				
Pediatric Sedation				
Peripheral Nerve Block				
Peritonsillar Abscess Drainage				
Reimplantation of Avulsed Tooth				
Ring Removal				
Skin Stapling				
Slit-Lamp Examination				
Spirometry				
Staple Removal				
Steroid Inj: Knee				
Synvisc Inj: Knee				
Suture/hand				
Suture Lab				
TCA 85% Application				

Procedure	Diagnosis	Date Procedure Performed	Certification Expiration Date	Preceptor or Supervisor Signature
Tissue Glues				
Tonometry				
Topical Anesthesia				
Trigger Point Inject				
Tympanometry				
Unna Paste Boot				
Venipuncture				
Verruca: Candida Antigen				
Visual: Snellen				
Wet Smear & KOH				
Woods Light Exam				
Other:				
Other:				
Other:				
Other:				
Other:				
Other:				
Other:				

Procedure Skills
1. Verbalizes indications and contraindications.
2. Assembles supplies and equipment.
3. Explains procedure to patient and potential complications.
4. Obtains informed patient consent with patient signature.
5. Performs appropriate patient preparation, sterile or clean technique as appropriate.
6. Performs procedure with pain management as needed.
7. Postprocedure patient management and teaching.

Index

Note: Page numbers followed by the letter *f* refers to figures and those followed by *t* and *b* refers to tables and boxes respectively.

A

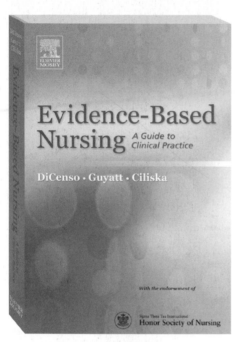